Kristen M Swanson
543-8228

P9-DWJ-304

HEALTH PROMOTION IN NURSING PRACTICE

Second Edition

HEALTH PROMOTION IN NURSING PRACTICE

Second Edition

Nola J. Pender, R.N., Ph.D., F.A.A.N.
Professor
School of Nursing
Northern Illinois University
DeKalb, Illinois

With a contribution by:

Albert R. Pender, Ph.D.
Associate Professor
Department of Business Education and
  Administrative Services
College of Business
Northern Illinois University
DeKalb, Illinois

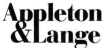

Appleton & Lange

Norwalk, Connecticut/Los Altos, California

0-8385-3674-3

Notice: The author(s) and publisher of this volume have taken care that the information and recommendations contained herein are accurate and compatible with
the standards generally accepted at the time of publication.

Copyright © 1987 by Appleton & Lange
A Publishing Division of Prentice-Hall

All rights reserved. This book, or any parts thereof, may not be used or reproduced
in any manner without written permission. For information, address Appleton &
Lange, 25 Van Zant Street, East Norwalk, Connecticut 06855.

90 91 / 10 9 8 7 6 5

Prentice-Hall of Australia, Pty. Ltd., Sydney
Prentice-Hall Canada, Inc.
Prentice-Hall Hispanoamericana, S.A., Mexico
Prentice-Hall of India Private Limited, New Delhi
Prentice-Hall International (UK) Limited, London
Prentice-Hall of Japan, Inc., Tokyo
Prentice-Hall of Southeast Asia (Pte.) Ltd., Singapore
Whitehall Books Ltd., Wellington, New Zealand
Editoria Prentice-Hall do Brasil Ltda., Rio de Janeiro

Library of Congress Cataloging-in-Publication Data

Pender, Nola J., 1941-
  Health promotion in nursing practice.

  Includes index.
  1. Health promotion. 2. Preventive health services.
3. Nursing. I. Pender, Albert R. II. Title. [DNLM:
1. Health Promotion—nurses' instruction. 2. Nursing
Care. WY 100 397h]
  RT67.P56 1987 613 86-25872
  ISBN 0-8385-3674-3

Design: M. Chandler Martylewski
Cover: Kathleen Peters

PRINTED IN THE UNITED STATES OF AMERICA

To Al, my husband and companion in the quest for health
To Andrea, my daughter and exercise partner
To Brent, my son and athlete
To Eileen and Frank, my parents and cheering section

Contents

Preface

Since the first edition of this book was published, interest in health promotion has burgeoned among policy makers, health professionals, and the general public. Many individuals and families have made significant positive changes in their life styles in an effort to optimize the quality of life as well as to extend longevity. No longer satisfied with defining health as merely the absence of disease or illness, many Americans have redefined health as exuberant physical, mental, social, and spiritual well-being. The essence of humanness is not only to exist but to experience growth toward increasing richness and complexity throughout the life span. Such growth presupposes a life style that is health producing and energy generating.

A "National Survey of Personal Health Practices and Consequences" conducted by the federal government in 1979–1980 revealed that 92 percent of the people surveyed agreed that eating more nutritious food, smoking less, maintaining proper weight, and exercising regularly would do more to improve the health of Americans than anything the organized health care system could do. Such agreement on the importance of healthful patterns of living is truly encouraging.

The ground swell of interest in disease prevention and health promotion has occurred, in John Naisbitt's words in *Megatrends*, "from the bottom up." The public began to look critically at its pressured, sedentary life styles in the 1970s. Health food stores started to flourish, jogging and running paths were developed in communities, health spas proliferated with rapidly expanding enrollments, and stress management became a popular topic at executive seminars. While some people predicted that health promotion was a fad that would not last, others ridiculed the notion that individuals and families would take responsibility for their own health. More than a decade later, such negative predictions have been proved wrong. Today, the American public exhibits more interest in health information, health magazines, and a variety of health-protecting and health-promoting practices than ever before. The potential of disease prevention and health promotion for improving the health status of people throughout the world has captured the imagination of the public, and health professionals alike.

National health policy has responded to public pressure and changed dramatically, with disease prevention and health promotion emerging as major goals. The next wave in health care evolution will involve changes in health care reimbursement plans, services provided by health professionals, and expenditures for research to reflect more accurately the *health rather than illness* emphasis in national health policy. Currently, it is estimated that only 2.5 percent of the total national health budget is spent on disease prevention and a miniscule 0.5 percent on health promotion. This means that 97 cents of every health-care dollar is still spent on the treatment and care of illness. Such a trend cannot continue. Lack of funding for health promotion initiatives is fiscally irresponsible and humanistically untenable. Health expenditures should reflect national commitments in health care policy. A major challenge to the federal government and the private sector during the next decade and into the twenty-first century will be to eliminate the chasm that currently exists between health policy and health programs.

The changing health care scene offers all health professionals, including nurses, an unprecedented opportunity to re-examine their contributions to health care. Settings for the delivery of health services are changing from hospitals to schools, corporations, shopping malls, ambulatory clinics, emergicenters, and surgicenters. It is predicted that many hospitals, the traditional employment setting for nurses, will close in the coming decade. The work settings for new graduates will shift, with fewer jobs available in hospitals and more jobs available in other types of agencies and nontraditional settings. Nursing as the largest health profession needs to evaluate carefully its education programs for current and future societal relevancy. Education for professional nurses should be based on a health–wellness model rather than an illness–disease model.

Nursing research, the basis for scientific practice, is already undergoing change. The 1985 publication of the American Nurses' Association Commission on Research, *Directions for Nursing Research: Toward the Twenty-first Century,* outlines a blueprint for knowledge generation that gives major emphasis to health promotion for individuals, families, and communities. Emphasis on research that addresses human health processes has promise for generating scientific knowledge that will undergird the practice of nurses in a variety of settings in the coming years.

Clearly, this is an exciting time to be in or entering the nursing profession. Career options have never been more challenging and the opportunities for creativity more plentiful.

In light of accelerating changes in health care, my purpose for preparing the second edition of this book is twofold: (1) to stimulate thinking among nurses concerning the conceptual frameworks and theories needed for understanding human health and health behaviors, and (2) to provide an overview of "state-of-the-art" nursing strategies for health promotion among individuals, families, and communities. A deliberate attempt has been made to write this book to reflect the way that professional nurses "ought to think" about practice—that is, with thoughtful consideration of research findings and integration of relevant findings into the clinical decision-making process. While an increasing number of books are being written on health promotion, few integrate empirical data with discussion of health care issues and strategies. Other books offer few specific tools for use by the practitioner or, conversely, present health promotion stagies in isolation from relevant theoretical frameworks. In this book, I offer the reader an approach to health promotion that integrates theory, research, and practice. Research findings are cited in support of many of the concepts and ideas offered. I trust that readers will find this approach both informative and stimulating.

I am convinced that the public is ready and waiting for more professional nurses who are knowledgeable and skilled in strategies for disease prevention and health promotion. For nursing students and nurses in practice who are interested in careers in health promotion, this book will provide an orientation to frameworks and strategies for the provision of preventive and promotive care. For all nurses, this book will enhance appreciation of the diversity of health care services that professional nurses can provide to clients. In addition, students and practitioners alike will gain an understanding of the need for interdisciplinary efforts in health promotion programs. The best programs combine the knowledge, skills, and talents of multiple health professionals into an integrated team that offers quality services to individuals and families.

The content of the book is organized into five sections. In Part I, various approaches to defining health are examined, and models with potential for explaining or predicting health-protecting (preventive) behavior and health-promoting behavior are presented.

Establishing professional relationships with clients is examined in Part II, with a discussion of the diverse settings for providing illness prevention and health promotion services and the nature of the nurse–client relationship for health promotion. Part III presents strategies for health promotion during the decision-making phase. These strategies include health assessment, values clarification, developing clients' competencies for self-care, and structuring a health protection–promotion plan. Part IV focuses on health promotion during the action phase. Strategies useful during this phase include: modification of life style, exercise and physical fitness, nutrition and weight control, stress management, and building social support. Aggregate strategies for health promotion, such as social and environmental change and the development of economic incentives, are the focus of Part V. Suggestions for future initiatives in health promotion are also presented.

The term *client* rather than *patient* will be used throughout the book to denote individuals, families, groups, and communities who are guided by nurses toward the realization of their self-care competencies and health potential. *Health* and *wellness* will be used as interchangeable terms.

I am deeply indebted to the many individuals who used the first edition of this book and provided positive reinforcement as well as constructive suggestions. I have made every attempt in the second edition to incorporate suggested changes in order to enhance the usefulness of the book to students, teachers, and nurses in practice.

Appreciation is extended to Marion Kalstein-Welch, Executive Editor, Nursing, Appleton & Lange, for her encouragement and assistance throughout preparation of the manuscript. I want particularly to acknowledge the chapter, "Economic Incentives for Prevention and Health Promotion," contributed by my husband, Al, and express appreciation for his unwavering support of my revision efforts that culminated in the second edition. The superb work of Karen Hancock, graduate assistant, in searching the literature and abstracting articles greatly expedited preparation of this edition. Her warm support and extremely efficient working style were invaluable. The assistance of Cindy Dugan in putting portions of the manuscript on the word processor is acknowledged. Special thanks are also expressed to Andrea and Brent, who tolerated their mother's many hours at the computer and who, I trust, will be a living expression of the ideas presented in this book.

Nola J. Pender

HEALTH PROMOTION IN NURSING PRACTICE

Second Edition

Health Promotion and Prevention Throughout the Life Span

This chapter traces the restructuring of health policy in the United States from a reactive stance focused on treatment of disease to a proactive stance emphasizing prevention of disease and promotion of health. The importance of health promotion and prevention throughout the life span is emphasized. In addition, the sources of motivation for health behavior are discussed, as well as the individual–family–community–environment–society interactional patterns that must be considered in understanding the fundamental dynamics of human health.

TOWARD A PROACTIVE HEALTH POLICY

In 1979, *Healthy People*, a landmark document, was published by the Surgeon General of the United States. Based on the realization that major health gains throughout the rest of the century would result more from advances in nutrition, physical fitness, personal life styles, immunization, and environmental modification than from traditional medical care, the report introduced a set of broad national goals for improving the health of Americans by 1990. The goals, one for each stage of the life span, are as follows:

1. To continue to improve infant health, and, by 1990, to reduce infant mortality by at least 35 percent, to fewer than 9 deaths per 1000 live births

1

2. To improve child health, foster optimal childhood development, and, by 1990, reduce deaths among children ages 1 to 14 years by at least 20 percent, to fewer than 34 per 100,000
3. To improve the health and habits of adolescents and young adults, and, by 1990, to reduce deaths among people ages 15 to 24 by at least 20 percent, to fewer than 93 per 100,000
4. To improve the health of adults, and, by 1990, to reduce deaths among people ages 25 to 64 by at least 25 percent, to fewer than 400 per 100,000
5. To improve the health and quality of life for older adults and, by 1990, to reduce the average annual number of days of restricted activity due to acute and chronic conditions by 20 percent, to fewer than 30 days per year for people aged 65 and older[1]

In 1980, a companion document, *Health Promotion–Disease Prevention: Objectives for the Nation,* was published. The objectives focused on three major areas: health promotion, health protection, and preventive health services, and on five specific strategy targets within each area:

Health promotion—any combination of health education and related organizational, environmental, and economic interventions designed to support behavior conducive to health.

1. smoking and health
2. misuse of alcohol and drugs
3. nutrition
4. physical fitness and exercise
5. control of stress and violent behavior

Health protection—protective measures in the environment that can be used by governmental and other agencies, as well as by industries and communities, to protect people from harm.

1. toxic agent control
2. occupational safety and health
3. accident prevention and injury control
4. fluoridation and dental health
5. surveillance and control of infectious diseases[2]

Preventive health services—key preventive services that can be delivered to individuals by health providers.

1. high blood pressure control
2. family planning
3. pregnancy and infant health
4. immunization
5. sexually transmitted diseases

A year later, a document entitled *Strategies for Promoting Health for Specific Populations* was issued; it focused on the priorities and strategies for health promotion efforts among Asian–Pacific, black, Hispanic, and elderly Americans and American Indians.[3]

The action steps that the federal government plans to take in order to achieve the objectives set forth for the nation were published in a Supplement to the September–October 1983 issue of *Public Health Reports*.[4] The implementation plans embody the directions of the Public Health Service in health promotion, health protection, and disease prevention for the remainder of the 1980s. Public Health Service agencies hold monthly review sessions to discuss the status of national progress toward the objectives.

The Centers for Disease Control are working with state and local governments to stimulate use of the national objectives as their framework for prevention and health promotion activities. Special attention is also being devoted to working with private-sector and voluntary organizations to enlist their assistance in realization of the objectives by 1990. A comprehensive information tracking system is being developed by the federal government in order to use public and private data sources to track progress toward each objective. Other federal initiatives in health promotion focus on nutrition, school health, wellness at the worksite, risk assessment, and health promotion among the elderly.[5]

An effort has been spearheaded by the Bureau of Health Professions, National Advisory Council for Health Professions Education, and National Advisory Council for Nurse Training to study the implications of national health promotion objectives for the education of health professionals. Five workshops on this topic were conducted between January and July 1984. The Bureau of Health Professions has initiated strategies to disseminate the results of the workshops to professional associations; academic institutions; accreditation, certification and licensure groups; voluntary health groups; private industry; and the public. Such efforts are directed toward maintaining the relevancy of health professions education to the current and future needs of the population.

The private sector is also attempting to collect data and develop policy–program initiatives reflective of the increasing emphasis on health promotion. As an example, Louis Harris and Associates, Inc., conducted a national survey of a random sample of 1254 adults within the United States in 1983 for the Prevention Research Center. The Prevention Index Project was designed to answer the following questions: Who are the prevention-oriented people, and exactly what are they doing? What aspects of their life style can be emulated by other Americans to promote their own health? The health behaviors that interviewees reported engaging in most frequently were: avoiding smoking in bed, moderate use of alcohol, socializing regularly, and having their blood pressure checked. Approximately half of the persons studied indicated that they consumed adequate fiber, and restricted fat, sodium, and sugar in their diet. The health behaviors performed least frequently were: exercising strenuously, maintaining weight within recommended limits, and wearing seat belts.[6] In 1985, a second survey was conducted. This survey showed that Americans had improved in five areas of health behavior since 1983. They reported taking more steps to control stress and to avoid accidents at home. They were also more likely to own a smoke detector, wear a seat belt, and cut back on their fat intake. On the downside, the survey indicated that fewer people obeyed the speed limit when driving and fewer made an effort to include adequate sources of vitamins and minerals in their daily diet. About 28 percent of those surveyed still smoke cigarettes. Unfortunately, the current national emphasis on prevention and health promotion has had less impact on persons of lower socioeconomic status than on persons who are highly educated, have high incomes, and are in managerial or professional positions. According to the Louis Harris survey, the latter are more likely to follow a health-promoting life style.[7] The results of these periodic surveys are used to construct a Prevention Index, the "Dow Jones average" of the nation's health. In addition, study results will be used to direct initiatives in the private sector to improve the health of the public.

Examples of other private sector efforts include the "Know Your Body Program" of the American Health Foundation, which is a prevention education program for grades K–12; YMCA/YWCA Fitness and Health Promotion Programs; corporate programs such as the Live for Life Program of Johnson & Johnson and the Stay Well Program of Control Data Corporation; and organizations and centers such as the National Center for Health Education and the National Foundation for Prevention of Disease.

National, state, and local initiatives in prevention and health promotion within both the public and private sectors will escalate in the years ahead. An informed public, activated communities, and concerned health professionals can encourage and energize such efforts.

HEALTH PROMOTION AND ILLNESS PREVENTION: IS THERE A DIFFERENCE?

Before proceeding any further in this book, it is important for the reader to differentiate between the concepts of health promotion and illness prevention. While the terms are often used interchangeably, there are distinguishable differences in underlying motivational mechanisms and in goal orientations. Definitions for health promotion and three levels of prevention are presented in the following excerpt.

> Health promotion consists of activities directed toward increasing the level of well being and actualizing the health potential of individuals, families, communities, and society.

> Primary prevention consists of activities directed toward decreasing the probability of specific illnesses or dysfunctions in individuals, families, and communities, including active protection against unnecessary stressors.

Secondary prevention emphasizes early diagnosis and prompt intervention to halt the pathological process, thereby shortening its duration and severity and enabling the individual to regain normal function at the earliest possible point.

Tertiary prevention comes into play when a defect or disability is fixed, stabilized, or irreversible. Rehabilitation, the goal of tertiary prevention, is more than halting the disease process itself; it is restoring the individual to an optimum level of functioning within the constraints of the disability.[8]

First, the reader should note that health promotion is not disease- or health–problem-specific; prevention is. Second, health promotion is "approach" behavior, while primary prevention is "avoidance" behavior. Third, health promotion seeks to expand positive potential for health, while prevention or health protection seeks to thwart the occurrence of pathogenic insults to health and well-being. Brubaker[9] has argued that even the dictionary definitions support the differentiation between health promotion and prevention. To "prevent" is to keep from occurring, while to "promote" is to help or encourage to exist or flourish. In this book, a distinction will be made between health promotion and prevention. Health promotion will be presented as a positive, dynamic process in its own right rather than merely an extension of illness–avoidance behavior. *Prevention* and *health protection* will be used interchangeably. Health promotion and prevention while distinguishable are complementary processes. Their integrated manifestation in person–environment interactions is critical to health enhancement throughout the life span.

HEALTH PROMOTION AND PREVENTION: A LIFE LONG QUEST

Experts have estimated that at least half the deaths in the United States each year result from health-damaging life styles. Habits detrimental to health that are established in early childhood and carried into adolescent and adult years not only decrease the potential for healthful and productive living but increase morbidity and mortality. The five health goals set forth in *Healthy People* address the developmental span for health promotion–prevention activities from infancy and childhood through the older adult years.

Promotion of health and prevention of illness among children have received much less attention than they deserve. Pediatric medical clinics, often the only settings in which preschool and school-age children interact with health personnel, focus on the treatment of illness almost to the exclusion of the promotion of health. In addition, schools with financial constraints have cut back on staff, including school health personnel. Thus, school nurses may not be available to segments of the student population just at the time when health personnel are critically needed to accomplish national health goals. The early development of regular exercise patterns, nutritious eating habits, strategies for managing stress, and productive interpersonal relationship styles is paramount for a healthy and vigorous childhood as well as for quality of life in later adult years.

Adolescence as a period in the life span is of major developmental significance and has special relevance for health.[10] This is the stage of life during which individuals may experiment with behaviors such as smoking, use of alcohol and drugs, fad diets, reckless driving, sexual promiscuity, and aggressive–violent behavior that can be health-damaging or life-threatening. Adolescents try out adult roles, begin to stabilize their social identity, develop interpersonal skills, and lay down patterns of values and behaviors from which their adult life style will evolve. The rapidity of change during adolescent years makes anticipatory guidance and peer support for healthy life styles especially critical during this period of development. It is interesting to note that positive health behaviors developed during adolescent years are resistant to change and can persist over time. It is much easier to develop the habit of regular exercise or good nutritional practices as an adolescent than as an adult. Thus, adolescents are an important target group for well-planned health promotion programs.

Life styles during the young and middle adult years can either augment or drain vital energy needed to meet personal needs and the needs of dependent others as well as job demands. High-level wellness is essential if adults are to deal constructively with the multiple and sometimes conflicting roles that they adopt. The workplace is an ideal setting for reaching many young and middle-aged adults, since a significant portion of their day is spent in occupational activities.

Many changes occur with aging that can be delayed or minimized through a healthful life style. For instance, lean body mass tends to decrease as part of the aging process, yet this can be slowed by regular exercise. Fatty tissue also tends to increase but can be controlled through proper diet and activity. Social support is threatened by loss of spouse, loss of close friends, and geographic relocation. However, social support systems can be augmented and reinforced to "cushion" such losses and promote well being. Proper nutrition can minimize disconcerting and uncomfortable body symptoms as well as increase resistance to infectious and chronic diseases. With the dramatic increase in the number of individuals over 65 years of age expected during the next decade, prevention and health promotion planning for this age group is a major challenge to health professionals.

Throughout this book, the frame of reference for prevention and health promotion activities will be the total life span from infancy–childhood to the older adult years. Every developmental stage must be considered in formulating national health policy and programs if the quality of life for people of all ages is to be significantly enhanced through health promotion efforts.

THE MULTIDIMENSIONAL NATURE OF HEALTH PROMOTION

The health of individuals and families is affected markedly by the community, environment, and society in which they live. The nature of individual–family–community–environment–society interaction patterns can either sustain and expand health potential at each system level or inhibit the emergence of health and well-being. It is important that nurses appreciate and consider the complexity of health promotion endeavors. Dunn has provided the following schema for health promotion efforts:

- Individual wellness
- Family wellness
- Community wellness
- Environmental wellness
- Societal wellness[11]

Individuals play a critical role in the determination of their own health status, since self-care represents the dominant mode of health care in our society. Many decisions are made by individuals daily that shape their life style and social and physical environment. Individuals can be viewed as subsystems within families.

The family, the smallest aggregate, plays a particularly critical role in the development of health beliefs and health behaviors. Almost all individuals can identify with a traditional or nontraditional family group in which members influence one another's ideas and actions. Each family has a characteristic value, role, and power structure as well as unique communication patterns. In addition, families fulfill affective, socialization, health care, and coping functions.[12] Families are subsystems within communities.

According to Dunn, community wellness is achieved by a multiplicity of actions that improve the conditions of family and community life.[13] A number of benefits of community-based health promotion programs can be identified:

1. They enhance opportunities for information exchange and social support among members of the target population
2. They reduce the unit cost of programming because large groups, rather than individuals, receive health promotion services[14]
3. They allow for use of interorganizational networks that can facilitate and coordinate health promotion efforts
4. They promote change in social norms regarding health and health behavior
5. They provide a coordinated rather than piecemeal approach to the promotion of health in large populations
6. They can access a broad array of media for dissemination of health information
7. They allow aggregate indices to be used for tracking the health status of the population

8. They utilize the talents and resources of community residents resulting in a sense of commitment to health promotion programming

Community programming for prevention and health promotion can result
in rapid dissemination of health information and in marked changes in cultural norms relevant to health and health behavior.

The level of environmental wellness affects the extent to which individuals, families, and communities can achieve their optimum potential. *Environment* is a comprehensive term meaning the physical, interpersonal, and
economic circumstances in which we live. The quality of the environment is
dependent on the absence of toxic substances, the availability of aesthetic
experiences, and the accessibility of human and economic resources needed
for healthful and productive living. Environmental wellness is manifest in
harmony and balance between human beings and their surroundings.

Societal wellness depends largely on the passage of laws and the establishment of policies that protect the health and welfare of all age groups.
Recent policy initiatives in health promotion by the federal government
represent attempts to deal at the societal level with health issues. A well
society is one in which all members have a standard of living and way of life
that allows them to meet basic human needs and engage in activities that
express their human potential. A well society recognizes the dignity of all
human beings, adopts policies to maintain that dignity, and avoids policies
and programs that are demeaning or belittling to its members. A well society
allows its members to utilize their talents throughout the life span without
premature retirement or relegation to a status of lesser value with age. Pre-
requisites for a well society include:

1. A belief that disease and illness are not inevitable consequences of
human existence
2. A vision for the population beyond that of immediate survival
3. Awareness of the close relationship between individual, family, and
community health assets and the well-being and productivity of the
society
4. Acceptance of high-level wellness as the goal of the society

Such a society recognizes the rights of all human beings:

1. The right to personal fulfillment
2. The right to make decisions about health as long as the health of
others is not endangered
3. The right to accurate information about personal health status as a
basis for informed decision making
4. The right to accurate information regarding the action alternatives
with the highest probability of enhancing health and minimizing health
threats
5. The right of access to comprehensive health care
6. The right to nursing care for health promotion and illness prevention

Societal wellness provides the framework in which individual, family, community, and environmental wellness can exist. Decisions made at all levels of bureaucracy in the public and private sectors affect the range of health-promoting options that are available to individuals and families and the ease with which individuals or groups can select health-promoting options as opposed to health-damaging ones. Humans are social beings who develop their values, beliefs, attitudes, and behaviors through interaction within groups. Thus, intervention at the aggregate level (family, community, and society) may be the most cost efficient and effective approach for many health promotion efforts.

THE MOTIVATIONAL BASE FOR HEALTH BEHAVIOR

Motivation plays a critical role in the initiation and maintenance of health-protecting (preventive) and health-promoting behavior. Two sources of motivation seem to characterize individuals and groups: the actualizing tendency and the stabilizing tendency. The *actualizing tendency* is directed toward increasing states of positive tension in order to promote change, growth, and maturation. The *stabilizing tendency* is evident in the functioning of homeokinetic mechanisms and is directed toward maintaining balance and equilibrium. The figure on page 10 depicts the stabilizing and actualizing tendencies as the two major sources of motivation for human behavior.

The Actualizing Tendency
Human beings are unique in exhibiting a distinct psychological form of the actualizing tendency, which is expressed as the need to experience all facets of self and the world about them. The actualizing tendency is not directed at tension reduction but at positive experiences of tension increase. A state of increased positive tension is often experienced as challenge. Increased tension when serving the actualizing tendency does not result in anxiety or distress but is perceived as a positive state that facilitates performance and growth.

The actualizing tendency is proposed as the driving force toward increased levels of well-being. Individuals and families are motivated to engage in health-promoting behaviors when they are aware of their own capacity for growth and their inherent and learned potentialities.

The Stabilizing Tendency
The stabilizing tendency is responsible for protective maneuvers, primarily maintaining the internal and external environments within a range compatible with continuing existence. This range is known as the *steady state*. Although the internal and external environments are constantly fluctuating, an input of energy or information that is less than or in excess of parameters of the steady state constitutes distress or a negative form of tension increase.

Major Sources of Motivation for Human Behavior

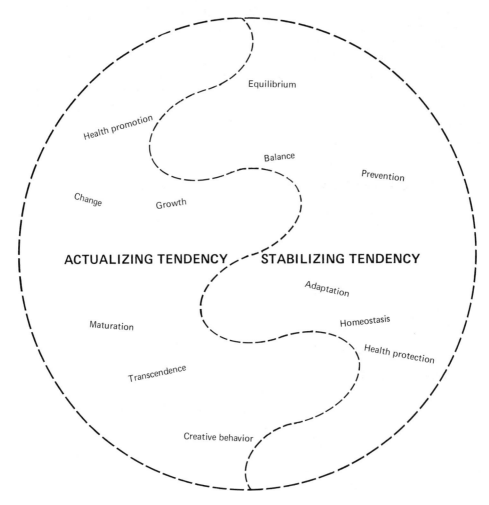

Two types of stressors may occur: a *lack stress* and an *excess stress*. In a lack stress, the input or output rate falls below the range characteristic of the steady state. In extreme cases of lack stress, hallucinations and other forms of abnormal behavior may occur. In an excess stress, the input or output rate goes above the range of the steady state. Examples of excess stress include high noise levels and continuous job strain. *Adaptation* refers to behaviors used by individuals and families to maintain the steady state when faced with disruptive internal or external stimuli. Preventive or health-protecting behaviors are manifestations of the stabilizing tendency, since they occur in response to potential or actual threats to health.

At any point in time, the actualizing or stabilizing tendency may be dominant, depending on the perceived needs of the individual or family. Expression of both tendencies is critical to integrated and healthy human functioning. Since the two tendencies are complementary, specific health behaviors may represent the integrated expression of both actualizing and stabilizing tendencies.

THE CONTRIBUTION OF NURSES TO PREVENTION AND HEALTH PROMOTION

Nurses, because of their recognized expertise and frequent, continuing contact with clients, have the unique opportunity of providing leadership in the promotion of better health among individuals, families, and communities. Nurses should also serve as role models of health-promoting life styles. The expected outcomes of nursing care directed toward prevention and the promotion of health include:

1. Increased levels of health and well-being among individuals, families, and communities
2. Decreased incidence of illness and disability for individuals and families
3. Improved ability on the part of individuals, families, and communities to make decisions related to health and well-being
4. Competence on the part of individuals and families in self-care
5. Increased ability of individuals and families to assess their needs for professional health care
6. Increased convenience of health promoting as opposed to health-damaging behavioral options within the community
7. Greater prevalence of health-promoting life styles within the society as a whole

Providing health care in a societal context that places primary emphasis on health promotion rather than treatment of illness is an exciting challenge to the nursing profession.

REFERENCES

1. *Healthy People: The Surgeon General's Report on Health Promotion and Disease Prevention.* U.S. Department of Health, Education, and Welfare Publication No. (PHS) 79–55071, U.S. Public Health Service, 1979.
2. *Promoting Health/Preventing Disease: Objectives for the Nation.* U.S. Department of Health and Human Services, U.S. Public Health Service, 1980.
3. *Strategies for Promoting Health for Specific Populations.* U.S. Department of Health and Human Services Publication No. (PHS) 81–50169, U.S. Public Health Service, 1981.

4. *Promoting Health/Preventing Disease: Public Health Service Implementation Plans for Attaining the Objectives for the Nation. Public Health Reports* (Supplement), September–October 1983.

5. McGinnis, J. M. Recent history of federal initiatives in prevention policy. *American Psychologist,* 1985, *40,* 205–212.

6. The Prevention Index: A report card on the nation's health (Summary Report), Conducted for *Prevention* Magazine by Louis Harris and Associates, Inc., October–November, 1983.

7. '85 Prevention Index (Summary Report). Conducted for *Prevention* Magazine by Louis Harris and Associates, Inc., Emmaus, PA, Rodale Press, 1985.

8. Shamansky, S. L., & Clausen, C. L. Levels of prevention: Examination of the concept. *Nursing Outlook,* 1980, *28,* 104–108.

9. Brubaker, B. H. Health promotion: A linguistic analysis. *Advances in Nursing Science,* 1983, *5* (3), 1–14.

10. Jessor, R. Adolescent development and behavioral health. In J. D. Matarazzo, S. M. Weiss, J. A. Herd, et al. (Eds.), *Behavioral health: A handbook of health enhancement and disease prevention.* New York: Wiley, 1984, pp. 69–90.

11. Dunn, H. L. *High-level wellness.* Arlington, Va.: Beatty, 1973.

12. Friedman, M. M. *Family nursing: Theory and assessment.* New York: Appleton-Century-Crofts, 1981.

13. Dunn, op. cit.

14. Weiss, S. M. Community health promotion demonstration programs: Introduction. In J. D. Matarazzo, S. M. Weiss, J. A. Herd, et al. (Eds.), *Behavioral health: A handbook of health enhancement and disease prevention.* New York: Wiley, 1984, pp. 1137–1139.

PART I

The Human Quest for Health

In this section, various definitions of health will be contrasted, compared, and analyzed. Conceptual models for health-protecting behavior (prevention) and health-promoting behavior will be described as a basis for structuring nursing interventions. The reader will be assisted in understanding the differences between health-protecting and health-promoting behaviors and the sources of motivation for each.

CHAPTER 1

Toward a Definition of Health

Most nurses would agree with the statement that the goal of nursing is the promotion of health among individuals, families, and communities. In fact, health is a focal concept in almost all conceptual and theoretical frameworks in nursing. During recent years, health, health behaviors, and the fundamental mechanisms underlying human health processes have received increasing attention from nurse-theorists and nurse-researchers. Such attention is indeed needed, given the limited information currently available about healthy functioning of individuals throughout the life span.

Mortality and morbidity have been the traditional methods used by public health and medicine for defining and measuring the level of health within a given population. Mortality and morbidity data provide information about the prevalence of illness; they do not provide information about the level of health within a given population. Thus, what are erroneously called "health status indexes" are really illness indexes. Attempts to measure health in terms of mortality and morbidity are based on the assumption that only deviations from health, not health itself, can be measured adequately. The following "levels of health" frequently used by the medical profession to describe client states illustrate the inappropriate use of disease-oriented criteria for determining health status:

- Level I —no clinical evidence of disease and low-risk profile for disease
- Level II —no clinical evidence of disease, but a risk profile that indicates an incubation period for disease that may emerge in the future

- Level III—subclinical evidence of disease detected in the early stages and amenable to treatment, and prevention of the occurrence of illness

Recent scientific and sociocultural developments, such as stabilization of the death rate, improved methods for prevention and early detection of illness, a renewed interest in the human sciences as well as the natural sciences, and increased leisure time with emphasis on aesthetic dimensions of existence, mandate reexamination of the concept of health as defined by medicine.

The following questions illustrate some of the dilemmas that must be addressed in explicating health:

1. Is health a separate and distinct concept from illness or is illness subsumed within the broad concept of health?
2. Does health represent a state to be attained or an ongoing dynamic process throughout the life cycle?
3. Are health and wellness the same or different constructs?
4. Is the definition of health universal or culturally specific?
5. Is health a multilevel concept applicable to individuals, families, communities, and societies?

Descriptions of health as a human phenomenon are needed to provide direction for health research, health policy, and health-care delivery. The development of health rather than illness indexes is critical to the effective assessment of the health status of individuals, families, and communities.

HEALTH AS AN EVOLVING CONCEPT

A brief review of the historical development of the concept of health will provide the context for examining recent definitions of health found in professional literature. The word *health* as it is commonly used did not appear in writing until approximately 1000 A.D. It is derived from the Old English word *hoelth*, meaning being safe or sound and whole of body.[1] Historically, physical wholeness was of major importance for acceptance in social groups. Persons suffering from disfiguring diseases like leprosy or from congenital malformations were ostracized from society and left to exist on whatever subsistence nature provided them. Not only was there fear of contagion of physically obvious disease, there was also repulsion at the grotesque appearance. Being healthy was construed as natural or in harmony with nature, while being unhealthy was thought of as unnatural or contrary to nature. The presence of disease marked the person as "unclean"; consequently, no attempt was made to effect cure or to maintain or enhance the integrity of bio–psycho–socio–spiritual functions not affected by disease.[2]

The concept of mental health as we know it did not exist until the latter part of the nineteenth century. Individuals who exhibited unpredictable or hostile behavior were labeled "lunatics" and ostracized in much the same way as were those with disfiguring physical ailments. Being put away with little if any human care was considered their "just due," since mental illness was often ascribed to evil spirits or satanic powers. Ostracizing the sick was a way for society to block out the painful aspects of human existence that they wished to ignore. The visibility of the ill only served to remind them of their own vulnerability and mortality.

With the advent of the scientific era and the resultant increase in the rate of medical discoveries, illness came to be regarded with less disgust, and society became concerned about assisting individuals to escape its catastrophic effects. *Health* in this context was defined as "freedom from disease." Since disease could be traced to a specific cause, often microbial, it could be diagnosed as a particular pathology. The notion that health was a disease-free state was extremely popular into the first half of the twentieth century and was recognized by many as *the* definition of health.[3] Health and illness were viewed as extremes on a continuum; the absence of one indicated the presence of the other. This definition is still in use today. The assumption is made frequently that a disease-free population is a healthy population.

For several decades, the importance of mental health became obscured in the rapid barrage of medical discoveries for treatment of physical disorders. However, the psychological trauma resulting from the high-stress situations of combat during World War II enlarged the scope of health as a concept to include consideration of the mental status of the individual. Health began to be defined as a biopsychological phenomenon. Mental health was manifest in the ability of an individual to withstand the stresses imposed by the environment. When individuals succumbed to the rigors of life around them and could no longer carry out the functions of daily living, they were declared to be mentally ill. Despite efforts to develop a more holistic definition of health, the dichotomy between individuals suffering from physical illness and those suffering from mental illness persisted.

In 1974, the World Health Organization (WHO) proposed a definition of health that emphasized the positive qualities of health: "Health is a state of complete physical, mental, and social well-being and not merely the absence of disease and infirmity."[4] While this definition enlarged the number of factors that needed to be taken into consideration in assessing health, it was difficult to deduce from it the criteria for recognizing health as a positive human experience. Many people believe that the WHO definition addresses the complexity of health but represents an ideal rather than a goal that can be achieved. The definition:

1. Reflects concern for the individual as a total person rather than the sum of parts
2. Places health in the context of the environment
3. Equates health with productive and creative living

With this brief historical perspective as background, more recent definitions of health will be examined. The definitions will be discussed in
three categories: (1) definitions emphasizing stability, (2) definitions emphasizing actualization, and (3) definitions emphasizing both stability and
actualization.

DEFINITIONS OF HEALTH FOCUSING ON STABILITY

The impetus for stability-based definitions derives from the physiologic concepts of homeostasis and adaptation. René Dubos, an early advocate of the
stability position, defined health as a state or condition that enables the
individual to adapt to the environment. The degree of health experienced is
dependent on one's ability to adjust to the various internal and external
tensions and stresses that one faces. Dubos considered optimum health to be
a mirage because man in the real world must face the physical and social
forces that are forever changing, frequently unpredictable, and often dan-
gerous for the individual and for the human species as a collective. According
to Dubos, the nearest approach to high-level health is a physical and mental
state free of discomfort and pain that permits one to function effectively as
long as possible within the environment.[5]

Aubrey conceptualized health as structural wholeness, in which sensory
processes are intact and function in such a way that balance and adaptability
characterize the individual. Health reflects the coordinated activity of
component parts, each functioning within its normal range. Aubrey defined
mental health as separate from physical health, perpetuating a mind–body
dualism. He characterized mental health as emotional stability, integration,
and adaptation of the individual to surroundings so that the person remains
viable and unharmed in spite of changing conditions. The healthy individual
should experience three conditions: subjective feelings of contentment and
balance, adequate performance of functions that societal living and human
existence require, and cognitive efficiency.[6]

Definitions of health based on normality can be described as stability
oriented. Statistical norms for a variety of human functions are already well
defined. Many physiological parameters are easily measured and ascertained.
In contrast, the normal range for holistic dimensions of man, such as rate of
energy exchange, boundary permeability, and structural complexity are not
presently known.

A major problem with normative definitions of health is that they predict
"what could be" based on "what is," leaving little room for incorporating
growth, maturation, and evolutionary emergence into a definition of health.
A norm represents average or middle-range effectiveness rather than excellence or exceptional effectiveness in human functioning.

Parsons defined health in terms of social norms rather than physiological
norms almost three decades ago. He described health as "the effective per-

formance of valued roles and tasks for which an individual has been social-ized."[7] According to Parsons, health status can be determined by application of normative standards of adequacy for present and future role and task performance.

Similar to Parsons' sociological model of health, Patrick, Bush, and Chen have defined health in terms of functional norms. They define health as:

> ... evidence of socially valued function levels in the performance of activities usual for a person's age and social roles with a minimum probability of change to less valued function levels.[8]

The desirability of the immediate function level, as well as the probability that the current condition or state will change to a higher or lower preference function level, must be considered in assessing present health status. The probability of change in function level can be thought of as prognosis. *Prognosis* is the probability that the human condition will deteriorate, remain constant, or improve with time.

A number of nurse–theorists have proposed definitions of health emphasizing stability. Levine defined health as a state in which there is balance between input and output of energy and in which structural, personal, and social integrity exist.[9]

Dorothy Johnson in her behavioral system model does not explicitly define health. However, a conception of health focusing on stability can be inferred from her writings. Health or wellness is balance and stability among the following behavioral systems: attachment or affiliative, dependency, ingestive, eliminative, sexual, aggressive, and achievement. Behavioral system balance and stability is demonstrated by efficient and effective behavior that is purposeful, goal-directed, orderly, and predictable.[10]

Betty Neuman has defined health or wellness as a condition in which all subsystems—physiological, psychological, and sociocultural—are in balance and in harmony with the whole of man. It is also a state of saturation, of inertness, free of disruptive needs. Disrupting forces or noxious stressors with which individuals cannot cope create disharmony, reducing the level of wellness. In a wellness state, total needs are met and more energy is built and stored than expended. A strong, flexible line of defense is maintained, providing the individual with considerable resistance to disequilibrium.[11]

Roy also ascribes to a stability definition of health. The central concept in Roy's model is adaptation. Health is a state and process of successful adaptation that promotes being and becoming an integrated whole person. The four adaptive modes through which coping energies are expressed are: physiological, self-concept, role performance, and interdependence modes. Adaptation promotes integrity. Integrity implies soundness or an unimpaired condition that can lead to completeness and unity. The person in an adapted state is freed from ineffective coping attempts that deplete energy. Available energy can be used to enhance health.[12]

Several additional homeostatic or stability definitions of health have been proposed recently by nurse-authors. Dixon and Dixon propose an evo lutionary model of health. They define health as:

> a condition in which positive viability emotions such as feelings of acceptance, usefulness, optimism and life clarity exist resulting in psychological comfort, productive behavior and normalcy of physiologic function. Viability emotions result in behaviors directed toward self-maintenance.[13]

This definition explicitly links health to the extent to which persons contribute to the stability and evolutionary survival of the group or groups in which they hold membership. The Alemeda County studies of longevity are sited as a rationale for incorporating social connectedness into a definition of health. Of the 7000 people in the Alemeda County study, those with the least extensive social and community ties had a higher death rate than those with the most extensive ties.[14]

Tripp-Reimer proposed a model for health that is stability oriented. The health state is conceptualized as two-dimensional: an *etic* dimension (disease–nondisease), which reflects the objective interpretation of health state by a scientifically trained practitioner; and the *emic* dimension (wellness–illness), which represents the subjective perception and experiences of an individual and social group as to health state. The various quadrants of the resultant grid—disease–wellness, disease–illness, nondisease–wellness, and nondisease–illness—indicate either congruence or incongruence between the perspectives of client and practitioner. This definition focuses on normality or homeostasis as medically defined. The model is proposed as particularly useful crossculturally when perceptions of scientifically trained personnel and clients of differing ethnic background may disagree regarding health status.[15]

The last definition of health to be presented in this section is that of Grossman, an economist. This definition, although emphasizing balance, stands out as markedly different from the others. Grossman defines health as:

> . . . a durable commodity to be purchased, an investment to be made. The end goal is an economic balance between the money and time spent in health behaviors, health services, health supporting products, health-related services and the level of health achieved by an individual, family or society.[16]

Grossman proposed that individuals inherit an initial "stock" of health that depreciates over time and can be increased by investment. Death occurs when the stock falls below a specified level. A novel feature of the economic model of health is that it proposes that an individual can choose to some degree the length of life or the amount of health desired during any given period of life by the extent and type of investments made. Examples of direct investments in the stock of health include time, medical care, diet, exercise, and housing. Grossman believes that health is being demanded increasingly by consumers for two major reasons: (1) as a commodity, health enters consumer preference profiles, and (2) sick days are a source of loss or disutility. Since depreciation of health occurs at an increasing rate after a certain point in the life span, more money must be spent to produce the same or a lesser degree of health. A stability definition of health such as that of Grossman provides an approach for quantification and cost–benefit analysis of health and investments in health at the societal level.

DEFINITIONS OF HEALTH FOCUSING ON ACTUALIZATION

Among health theorists, Halbert Dunn is the leading proponent of definitions of health emphasizing actualization. Dunn coined the term *high-level wellness*, which he defined in the following way:

> An integrated method of functioning which is oriented toward maximizing the potential of which the individual is capable. It requires that the individual maintain a continuum of balance and purposeful direction within the environment where he is functioning.[17]

While the definition advanced by Dunn identifies balance as a dimension of health, major emphasis is on the realization of human potential through purposeful activity.

Dunn stated that high-level wellness, or optimum health, involves three components: (1) progress in a forward and upward direction toward a higher potential of functioning, (2) an open-ended and ever-expanding challenge to live at a fuller potential, and (3) progressive integration or maturation of the individual at increasingly higher levels throughout the life cycle.[18] Dunn conceptualized wellness as being a direction of progress as well as levels to be reached. In optimum health, individuals function at a high level amid a dynamic and constantly changing environment.

According to Dunn, the essential need of an individual is freedom, if one is to realize personal uniqueness through creative expression and thereby achieve a high level of wellness. The importance of one's relationship with the environment is illustrated in Figure 1–1. In the health grid proposed by Dunn, high-level wellness can only emerge in a favorable environment. One is never isolated from the effects of surroundings.

Dunn identified nine points of attack for promoting high-level wellness:

1. Improvement of conditions of family living and community life
2. Education to assist individuals and families in application of knowledge to promote health
3. Education in principles of human relations
4. Development of high-level wellness among individuals in leadership positions

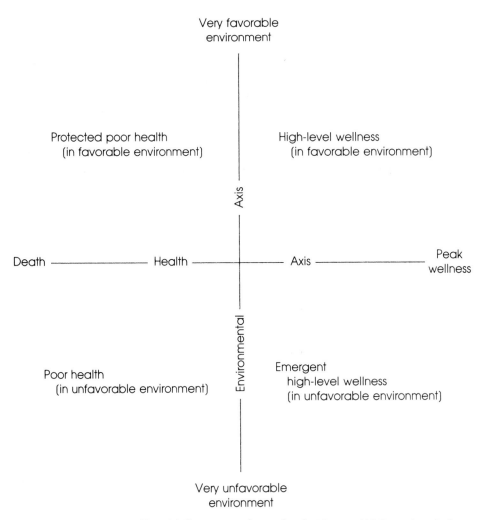

Figure 1–1. The health grid, its axes and quadrants. (*Source: U.S. Department of Health, Education and Welfare, Public Health Service, National Office of Vital Statistics.*)

5. Maintenance of open information channels and free access to knowledge available for intelligent decision making
6. Enhancement of opportunities for creative expression
7. Promotion of caring relationships and concern for the welfare of others
8. Understanding of the concept of maturity and methods of its promotion as a realistic goal
9. Extension of the human life span with the opportunity to utilize for the benefit of society those who have become fully mature and have reached the highest attainable level of wellness[19]

Health, according to Dunn, is not simply a "passive state of freedom from illness in which the individual is at peace with his environment";[20] it is an emergent process characteristic of the entire life span.

Another definition of health that focuses on actualization as opposed to stability is the description of health by Hoyman as "optimal personal fitness for full, fruitful, creative living."[21] Hoyman states that health is a dynamic process involving the total human being. Hoyman's model of health focuses on the interaction of heredity, environment, and behavior and the way in which the quality and quantity of interaction determines the level of health. The importance of vigor, vitality, and a zest for living are emphasized as factors profoundly affecting the search of the individual for health, meaning, and fulfillment.

Bermosk and Porter focus on holism and human evolution in their definition of health:

> Holistic health involves the ongoing integration of mind, body, and spirit. A person evolves from one level of wholeness to another level of wholeness.[22]

They view holistic health as integrated energies of mind, body, spirit, and environment. Integration within the human system is synonymous with healing. According to Bermosk and Porter, individuals are responsible for their own health and evolve toward greater levels of zest and well-being as they continually heal themselves and expand their consciousness.

Orem, in developing the self-care theory of nursing, used health and well-being to refer to two different but related human states. She defined health as a state characterized by soundness or wholeness of human structures and bodily and mental functions. Well-being was defined as a state characterized by experiences of contentment, pleasure, and happiness; by spiritual experiences; by movement toward fulfillment of one's self-ideal; and by continuing personalization. According to Orem, personalization is movement toward maturation and achievement of human potential. Engaging in responsible self-care and continuing development of self-care competency are facets of the process of personalization. Well-being is associated with success in personal endeavors and with sufficiency of resources. Individuals can experience well-being even under conditions of adversity, including disorders of human structure and functioning. The combined definitions of health and well-being express an actualizing state of existence.

Orem addressed the "state of the art" in defining health when she commented that health as a holistic phenomenon must still be understood in a compound sense. That is, there are as yet no valid and reliable measures for holistic health. Thus, man must be understood according to a composite of various dimensions of health, such as organic functioning, psychological functioning, and social functioning.[23]

Newman, building on the work of Martha Rogers, defined health as the totality of the life process, which is evolving toward expanded consciousness.[24] This definition emphasizes the actualizing properties of individuals throughout the life span. Four dimensions of health as a concept are identified:

1. Health is a fusion of disease and nondisease
2. Health is the manifestation of an individual's unique pattern
3. Health is expansion of consciousness. Time is a measure of consciousness and movement is a reflection of consciousness
4. Health encompasses the entire life process which evolves toward higher and greater frequency of energy exchange. Key life process phenomena include: consciousness, movement, space and time[25]

Newman's model of health addresses holistic characteristics of human beings. However, empirical referents for many of the terms used within the model need to be identified to facilitate the testing of hypotheses that can be derived from the model.

Parse, in describing her man–living–health theory of nursing, presents five assumptions about health that essentially define the term from her perspective:

1. Health is an open process of becoming, experienced by man
2. Health is a rhythmically coconstituting process of the man-environment relationship
3. Health is man's patterns of relating value priorities
4. Health is an intersubjective process of transcending with the possibles
5. Health is unitary man's negentropic (toward increasing order, complexity, and heterogeneity) unfolding[26]

Parse proposes that health is cocreated through relationships with others. Health reflects a synthesis of personal values, life style, and man–environment energy exchange. The theory proposed by Parse builds on Martha Rogers' theory of unitary man, as did Newman's model of health. Both represent early attempts to define health in terms of holistic man as opposed to defining health in terms of man's component parts. The emergent nature or actualization potential of the healthy individual and the capacity for open energy exchange with the environment are characteristics of both Newman's and Parse's definitions of health.

DEFINITIONS OF HEALTH FOCUSING ON BOTH ACTUALIZATION AND STABILITY

The definitions of health presented in this section represent mixed models. That is, the definitions incorporate the themes of stability and actualization. As early as 1974, Oelbaum identified 26 functions or behaviors of adults in optimum health.[27] The behaviors that she identified can be categorized under the two dimensions of actualization and stabilization, as illustrated in Table 1–1. Behaviors under the heading of actualization reflect self-direc-

TABLE 1–1. FUNCTIONS OF ADULTS IN OPTIMUM HEALTH

Actualization	Stability
1. Provides for own comfort and relaxation	1. Performs activities of daily living
2. Obtains and maintains an environment conducive to well-being	2. Has a stable body image perceived as being socially acceptable
3. Maintains optimum motor function	3. Efficiently disposes of metabolic wastes
4. Obtains, digests, and metabolizes appropriate amounts of food that promote optimal nutrition	4. Has an appropriate intake and healthy distribution of excretion of fluids and electrolytes
5. Builds and maintains meaningful interpersonal relationships, is comfortable with interdependence	5. Guards self against overwhelming changes; regulatory and defense systems intact and helpful
6. Accumulates knowledge and skills that bring one success in one's chosen life roles	6. Maintains good hygiene
7. Demonstrates personality growth and creative expression appropriate to one's developmental level and prized by one's culture	7. Juxtaposes the tasks of various life roles with minimal conflict while keeping in touch with own needs
8. Demonstrates high quality cerebral functioning	8. Holds expectations and makes decisions reflecting understanding of his own limitations and situational realities
9. Is a team member of own prevention/rehabilitation team; has sufficient understanding, initiative, self-control, and financial resources to maintain health	9. Efficiently uses oxygen
10. Recognizes and cherishes the uniqueness of own identity and the uniqueness of each other person	10. May have symptoms, but they are yielding to prescribed therapy; uses therapies to help carry out own wellness work
11. Humanistically expresses love and respect for all life and the quality of that life	11. Receives and recognizes sensory input
12. Mobilizes resources to meet own needs; begins by expressing needs freely to another person	12. Demonstrates functional verbal and nonverbal communication
13. Demonstrates a zeal for living	13. Attains healthful balance of productive work and rest

Copyright © 1974, American Journal of Nursing Company. Adapted from *American Journal of Nursing*, September 1974, *74*(9), p 1623.

tion and initiative, while behaviors under the heading of stabilization represent reactive adjustment and adaptation responses.

Oelbaum suggested a 4-point ordinal scale that could be used with the 26 descriptive statements to assess specific levels of health attained by individuals:

- 4 points—self-reliance and proficiency in carrying out the function or behavior
- 3 points—ordinarily performs the task on one's own fairly well
- 2 points—usually reliant on others or performs the task poorly
- 1 point —total dependence on others for performance of the task or complete avoidance of the task[27]

Wu has described health as:

. . . a feeling of well-being, a capacity to perform to the best of one's ability, and the flexibility to adapt and adjust to varying situations created by the subsystems of man or the suprasystems in which he exists.[28]

Wu proposed that wellness and illness represent distinct entities, with a repertory of behaviors for each. Within this frame of reference, both wellness and illness can exist simultaneously. Evaluation of both are critical to comprehensive health assessment.

King proposed a definition of health that emphasized both stabilizing and actualizing tendencies. She defined health as:

Dynamic life experiences of a human being which implies continuous adjustment to stressors in the internal and external environment through optimum use of one's resources to achieve maximum potential for daily living.[29]

Maintenance of health enables a person to perform activities of daily living in such a way that a useful, satisfying, productive, and happy life results. King indicates that polarity between health and illness are outmoded ideas. Instead, health should be viewed as a functional state in the life cycle, with illness defined as interference in the cycle.

Smith offered an exposition and analysis of four distinctive ideas of health, three focused on stability and one on actualization. Each of the models of health is defined by the extremes of the health-illness continuum that it identifies.

Clinical model—Health extreme: absence of signs or symptoms of disease or disability as identified by medical science; Illness extreme: conspicuous presence of these signs or symptoms

Role-performance model—Health extreme: performance of social roles with maximum expected output; Illness extreme: failure in performance of roles

Adaptive model—Health extreme: the organism maintains flexible adaptation to the environment, interacts with environment with maximum advantage; Illness extreme: alienation of the organism from environment, failure of self-corrective responses

Eudaimonistic model—Health extreme: exuberant well-being; Illness extreme: enervation, languishing debility[30]

Smith proposes that each model requires distinct approaches to the client. The nature of practice and the modes of intervention are different depending on which model is being used as the framework for care.

The following definition of health incorporating both actualizing and stabilizing tendencies has been proposed by the author of this book:

Health is the actualization of inherent and acquired human potential through goal directed behavior, competent self-care, and satisfying relationships with others while adjustments are made as needed to maintain structural integrity and harmony with the environment.

Criteria for evaluating health based on this definition appear in Table 1–2. According to this definition and related criteria, individuals in optimum health actively seek new information relevant to the attainment of life goals, derive pleasure from experiences of personal and environmental mastery, and exhibit a high tolerance for new and unusual internal and external stimuli. Health reflects a process of development characterized by frequent experiences of challenge, achievement, and satisfaction.

TABLE 1–2. PROPOSED CRITERIA FOR EVALUATING HEALTH

---

1. Exhibits personal growth and positive change over time
2. Identifies long-term and short-term goals that guide behavior
3. Prioritizes identified goals
4. Exhibits awareness of alternative behavioral options to accomplish goals
5. Perceives optimum health as a primary life purpose
6. Engages in interpersonal relationships that are satisfying and fulfilling
7. Actively seeks new experiences that expand knowledge or increase competencies for personal care
8. Displays a high tolerance for new and unusual situations or experiences
9. Derives satisfaction from the experience of daily living
10. Expends more energy in acting on the environment than in reacting to it
11. Recognizes barriers to growth and deals constructively in removing or ameliorating them
12. Uses self-monitoring and feedback from others to determine personal and social effectiveness
13. Maintains conditions of internal stability compatible with continuing existence
14. Anticipates internal and external threats to stability and takes preventive actions

---

NEED FOR AN INTEGRATED VIEW OF HEALTH

The importance of nursing's avoiding a fragmented view of health and espousing an integrated biopsychosocial view of human health phenomenon has been described by Shaver.[31] Rationale for an integrated view includes:

1. The scope of clinical indicators on which diagnostic decisions can be based will be greater. Indicators could include interpersonal behaviors, social support, socioeconomic status, mood state, cognitive efficiency, symptom complaints, hormone levels, neurotransmitter breakdown products, neurochemical substrates, immunoglobulin status or any combination of the above.
2. Study of human response patterns could determine what combination of indicators is predictive of healthy and unhealthy outcomes.
3. An integrated view enlarges the scope of therapeutic options for treating health problems or responses to health problems.
4. An integrated approach offers greater potential for targeting therapy and individualizing prescriptions for intervention.[31]

An integrated approach represents a step in the direction of a holistic approach to the definition of health. Until holistic phenomenon have been identified that can be measured with some degree of reliability, a composite biopsychosocial approach to defining and assessing health is needed. The approach to health assessment presented in Chapter 6 is an attempt to implement an integrated definition of human health processes.

HEALTH AND ILLNESS: DISTINCT OR OPPOSITE ENDS OF A CONTINUUM?

The issue of whether health and illness are separate entities or opposite ends of a continuum has fascinated scientists for some time. Are health and illness quantitatively or qualitatively different?

Theorists presenting health and illness as a continuum usually identify possible reference points such as (1) optimum health, (2) suboptimal health or incipient illness, (3) overt illness and disability, (4) very serious illness or approaching death.[32] This scale has only one point representing health, while three points on the scale represent varying states of illness. Dunn proposed a more balanced continuum, with death representing one end of the scale and peak wellness representing the opposite end.[33] The continuum described by Dunn allows the differentiation of varying levels of health as well as varying levels of illness.

When health and illness are assumed to represent a single continuum, it is difficult to discuss healthy aspects of the ill individual. The presence of illness ascribes the "sick role", and the individual is expected to direct all energies toward finding the cause of the illness and engaging in behaviors that will result in a return to health as soon as possible.

Manifestations of health in the presence of illness have lead some theorists to propose separate but parallel continuums for health and illness. Sorochan commented that everyone free from disease is not equally healthy. He proposed gradations of health separate from gradations of illness, which would allow individuals to be at any stage of health regardless of their position on the illness continuum.[34] Oelbaum stressed the interrelationship of health and illness, even though she considers the concepts to be separate entities rather than opposite ends of a continuum. She stated that apathy toward the work of wellness is the precursor of disease. The particular health behaviors or functions that are poorly performed will influence the type of disease, disorder, or damage that will follow.[35]

It is the belief of the present author that health and illness are qualitatively different but interrelated concepts. In Figure 1–2, differing levels of health are depicted in interaction with the experience of illness. Illness is diagrammed as representing discrete events throughout the life process of short or long duration. These illness experiences can thwart or facilitate one's continuing quest for health. Thus, optimum health or poor health can exist with or without overt illness.

DEFINITIONS OF HEALTH FOCUSING ON FAMILY

Much more attention has been given to defining health and wellness as a state or process characteristic of individual human beings than as a state or process descriptive of family systems. Health as a concept applicable to

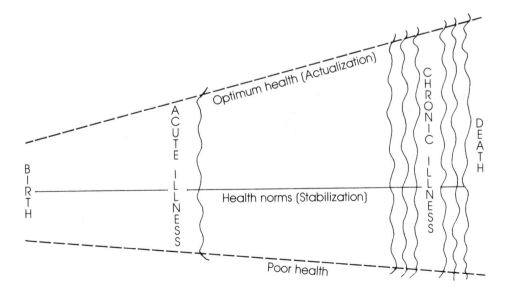

Figure 1–2. The health continuum throughout the life span.

families will be discussed here. Almost all family theorists would agree that health of families is more than a composite of the individual health assessments of family members. Feetham[36] has commented in her review of family research that by focusing on the individual family member, often a member with pathology, family researchers have generated little knowledge about the normal, well-functioning family. Few conceptual frameworks proposed for nursing have given attention to the family. The individual system rather than the family system has been the basic unit of analysis. O'Brien[37] has observed that conceptualization and measurement of family health and wellness has not been a priority in nursing research. Several definitions of family health will be presented here that are explicit or implicit in family literature.

A family can be defined as "a small social system made up of individuals related to each other by reason of strong reciprocal affections and loyalties and comprising a permanent household (or cluster of households) that persists over years or decades."[38] Families as systems are characterized by structure, function, and developmental stages. In discussing the assessment of families, Roberts and Feetham[39] identified three major areas that should be considered in defining family health:

- The relationship between the family and broader social units such as family and community, and family and economy

- The relationships between the family and subsystems such as parental dyad or sibling subsystem

- The relationships between the family and each individual focusing on reciprocity

While not specifically defining family health, Wright and Leahey imply that healthy families are characterized by stability and integrity of structure, adaptive rather than maladaptive functioning, and mastery of developmental tasks leading to progressive differentiation and transformation to meet the changing requisites for survival of the system.[40] This definition focuses on stability as the primary criterion for family health.

Petze, in discussing health promotion for the well family, does not provide an explicit definition of family health. However, the following definition of family health focusing on stability can be inferred from the discussion of competent and effectively functioning families:

> Family health is the continuing viability of the family unit as a functional and productive network. The healthy family has a sense of togetherness that promotes the capacity for change, a balance between mutual and independent action on the part of family members, and adaptation to life events.[41]

Smilkstein offered an actualizing definition of family health that can be paraphrased as follows:

> Family health is a state of cohesiveness in which nurturance and resources
> necessary for personal growth and sustenance in the face of life's challenges
> are available to family members.[42]

Another actualizing definition has been offered by Johnson, who defined
family health as a process that includes the promotion and maintenance of
physical, mental, spiritual, and social health for the family unit and for
individual family members. Johnson comments that to achieve wellness the
family must be an integrated unit striving to develop its fullest potential.
Family wellness contributes to both individual wellness of family members
and the level of wellness within the community.[43]

It is evident from a review of the literature that family health processes
must be given increased attention by nurse researchers along with scientists
in other disciplines. The development of models for describing family health
will assist health professionals in identifying predictors of family well-being
and in promoting the health of families.

DEFINITIONS OF HEALTH FOCUSING ON THE COMMUNITY

The community has been defined as a locality based entity, composed of
systems of formal organizations reflecting societal institutions, informal groups,
and aggregates that are interdependent, and whose function or expressed
intent is to meet a wide variety of collective needs.[44] This definition focuses
on the spatial, personal, and functional dimensions of a community.

Community health, a term used increasingly in current literature, is
complex and difficult to define. It is often defined implicitly through discussion of the community assessment process rather than explicitly through
identification of the dimensions or attributes of a healthy community. Dever,
in describing holistic models of health as a basis for community health analysis, identified the following attributes of the community to be assessed in
determining community health:

1. Environment—fetal, physical, sociocultural, education, and employment milieu
2. Population behavior or life style—self responsibility, self-care competency
3. Human biology—genetic characteristics of population
4. Systems of health care—prevention, cure, and rehabilitation[45]

Dever observed that holistic models of health have engendered new belief
systems about what constitutes both individual and aggregate health.

Goeppinger described community health as having three dimensions
which are assessed currently by multiple measures:

1. Status dimension—morbidity, mortality, life expectancy, risk factors,
   consumer satisfaction, mental health, crime rates, functional levels,
   worker absenteeism, infant mortality

2. Structural dimension—community health resources measured by utilization patterns, treatment data, and provider–population ratios; social indicators measured by dependency ratios, socioeconomic and racial distributions, and median education level
3. Process dimension—effective community functioning or problem-solving which results in community competence as evidenced by: Commitment, self-other awareness and clarity of situational definitions, articulateness, effective communication, conflict containment and accommodation, participation, and management of relations with larger society[46]

Incorporating all of these dimensions, community health is defined as "the meeting of collective needs through problem identifying and managing interactions within the community and between the community and the larger society."[47]

Tinkham, Voorheis, and McCarthy[48] define community health as a process. Community health is identified as "those activities and concerns which are designed to enhance the quality of life and promote the well being of the total population in the community." While Archer, Kelly, and Bisch[49] do not define community health per se, by describing a community as an open system, they imply that community health is characterized by openness to energy exchange, interdependence among community groups, hierarchical organization, self-regulation, dynamic activity, goal-directedness, and the synthesizing processes of wholeness. Community health is more than the sum of the health states of its individual members; it encompasses the characteristics of the community as a whole.

Building on the unitary man framework proposed by Kim and Moritz[50] and Maslow's hierarchy of needs, West identified three factors to be used in the assessment of community health:

- Factor One—interaction: exchanging, communicating, and relating patterns within the community
- Factor Two—action: valuing, choosing, and moving
- Factor Three—awareness: waking, feeling, and knowing[51]

West developed a community assessment tool to analyze these dimensions of man–environment interaction or patterns of energy within the community.

In describing a group or community intervention model for the promotion of health, Hogue suggests some group health indicators that might be selected as indices of the health of the community. The indices and examples of measures are presented here.

1. Level of social functioning—work attendance, school attendance, dependency ratio
2. Symptoms and complaints—reasons for absence from school or work, accident rates

    3. Disabilities and impairments—proportion of children with learning disabilities or physical, visual, or auditory impairment
    4. Biologic correlates of disease or risk factors—blood pressure, cholesterol, triglycerides
    5. Disease categories—cases of acute and chronic diseases
    6. Mortality—by specific causes
    7. Measurements of population growth and pressure—birth, fertility, death rates, divorce rate, proportion living at poverty level, rate of unemployment
    8. Measurements of growth and nutritional status—heights and weights of adults and children, iron-deficiency anemia
    9. Measures of health care utilization—prenatal care, immunization of infants and children, hospital admissions[52]

According to Hogue, any or all of these indicators could be used to describe the health of a community. However, in the view of the author of this book, most of the indexes suggested by Hogue represent only a clinical or disease-oriented definition of health with little attention given to role performance, adaptive or endaimonistic perspectives.

    It is evident from the various definitions and dimensions of community health described that there are a multiplicity of approaches proposed for evaluating the health of a community. Definitions of community health range

---

TABLE 1–3. TYPOLOGY OF HEALTH CRITERIA

  I. Health as a physiologic process or state (biological orientation)
    A. Medicine—absence of disease
    B. Physiology—predictability and integrity of cellular structures
    C. Anatomy—integrity of cellular structures
    D. Microbiology—absence of abnormal microbial activity
 II. Health as a feeling state (psychological orientation)
    A. Psychiatry—absence of cognitive, affective, and psychomotor disorders
    B. Psychology—continuing behavioral adjustment to changing environmental contingencies and the ongoing development of human personality
III. Health as a capacity to function (sociological orientation)
    A. Sociology—performance of roles and tasks within society appropriate for a given level of growth and development
    B. Social work—effective implementation of occupational and familial roles resulting in economic solvency and societal efficiency
IV. Health as a holistic process (biopsychosocial orientation)
    A. Nursing—actualization of human potential through integrated functioning of individuals and groups in interaction with their environment
    B. Public Health—the physical, social, economic and ecological well-being of world populations

---

from those that are highly disease oriented to those that focus on the actualizing potential of the community. With increasing emphasis on health as more than the absence of disease, community health personnel who rely heavily on disease-oriented indices of community health need to rethink their approach to community assessment. Population-based prevention and health-promotion interventions must be based on the assessment of community competence and actualizing potential as well as on morbidity and mortality indexes. During the next decade, systematic attempts to define community health more holistically and to measure community health as a positive state in all its richness and complexity will be critically needed.

SUMMARY

In this chapter, an attempt has been made to present varying definitions of individual, family, and community health. Such definitions provide the foundation on which health promotion efforts for persons and aggregates can be based. To address the promotion of health, one must know what the desired outcome—health—is and how its achievement will be measured at individual, family, and community levels. The survey of existing definitions of health presented in this chapter represents a beginning step toward the specification of health as a dynamic process inherent in the life experience of individuals and families and communities. In summary, a typology of major health criteria from various disciplines is presented in Table 1–3.

REFERENCES

1. Sorochan, W. Health concepts as a basis for orthobiosis. In E. Hart & W. Sechrist, (Eds.), *The dynamics of wellness.* Belmont, Calif.: Wadsworth, 1970, p. 3.
2. Dolfman, M. L. The concept of health: An historic and analytic examination. *Journal of School Health*, 1973, *43*, 493.
3. Wylie, C. M. The definition and measurement of health and disease. *Public Health Reports*, February 1970, *85*, 100–104.
4. Tempkin, O. What is health? Looking back and ahead. In I. Galdston (Ed.), *Epidemiology of health.* New York: Academy of Medicine, Health Education Council, 1953, 21.
5. Dubos, R. *Man adapting.* New Haven: Yale University Press, 1965, p. 349.
6. Aubrey, L. Health as a social concept. *British Journal of Sociology*, June 1953, *4*, 115.
7. Parsons, T. Definitions of health and illness in the light of American values and social structure. In E. G. Jaco, (Ed.), *Patients, physicians and illness.* New York: Free Press, 1958, 176.
8. Patrick, D. L., Bush, J. W., & Chen, M. M. Toward an operational definition of health. *Journal of Health and Social Behavior*, 1973, *14*, 6.

9. Levine, M. E. *Introduction to Clinical Nursing*, 2nd ed. Philadelphia: F. A. Davis, 1973.
10. Loveland-Cherry, C., & Wilkerson, S. A. Dorothy Johnson's behavioral system model. In J. Fitzpatrick, & A. Whall, (Eds.), *Conceptual models of nursing: Analysis and application*. Bowie, Md.: Robert J. Brady, 1983.
11. Neuman, B. *The Neuman system's model: Application to nursing education and practice*. Norwalk, Conn.: Appleton-Century-Crofts, 1982, 9, *10*, 138.
12. Roy, C. *Introduction to nursing: An adaptation model*, 2nd ed. Englewood Cliffs, N.J.: Prentice-Hall, 1984.
13. Dixon, J. K., & Dixon, J. P. An evolutionary based model of health and viability. *Advances in Nursing Science*, 1984, *6*(3), 1–18.
14. Berkman, L. F., & Syme, S. L. Social networks, host resistance and mortality: A nine-year follow-up study of Alemeda County residents. *American Journal of Epidemiology*, 1979, *109*, 186–204.
15. Tripp-Reimer, T. Reconceptualizing the concept of health: Integrating emic and etic perspectives. *Research in Nursing and Health*, 1984, 7, 101–109.
16. Grossman, M. *The demand for health: A theoretical and empirical investigation*. New York: Columbia University Press, 1972, pp. 1–8.
17. Dunn, H. L. What high-level wellness means. *Canadian Journal of Public Health*, November 1959, 447.
18. Dunn, H. L. High-level wellness for man and society. *American Journal of Public Health*, 1959, *49*, 789.
19. Dunn, H. L. Points of attack for raising the level of wellness. *Journal of the National Medical Association*, 1975, *49*, 223–235.
20. Dunn, H. L. *High level wellness*. Thorofare, N. J.: Charles B. Slack, 1980, p. 4.
21. Hoyman, H. S. Our modern concept of health. *Journal of School Health*, September 1962, 253.
22. Bermosk, L. S., & Porter, S. E. *Women's health and human wholeness*. New York: Appleton-Century-Crofts, 1979, p. 11.
23. Orem, D. E. *Nursing: Concepts of practice*, 3rd ed. New York: McGraw-Hill, 1985.
24. Newman, M. *Theory development in nursing*. Philadelphia: F. A. Davis, 1979, p. 58.
25. Engle, V. Newman's model of health. In J. Fitzpatrick, & A. Whall, (Eds.), *Conceptual models of nursing: Analysis and application*. Bowie, Md.: Robert J. Brady, 1983, pp. 263–273.
26. Parse, R. R. *Man-living-health: A theory of nursing*. New York: Wiley, 1981, pp. 25–36.
27. Oelbaum, C. H. Hallmarks of adult wellness. *American Journal of Nursing*, 1974, *74*, 1623.
28. Wu, R. *Behavior and illness*. Englewood Cliffs, N.J.: Prentice-Hall, 1973, p. 112.
29. King, I. M. *A theory for nursing: Systems, concepts, processes*. New York: Wiley, 1981, p. 5.
30. Smith, J. *The idea of health: Implications for the nursing profession*. New York: Teachers College Press, 1983, p. 31.
31. Shaver, J. F. A biopsychosocial view of human health. *Nursing Outlook*, 1985, *33* (4), 186–191.
32. Sorochan, op. cit., p. 5.
33. Dunn, 1980, op. cit., p. 5.

34. Sorochan, op. cit., p. 4.
35. Oelbaum, op cit., p. 1623.
36. Feetham, S. L. Family research: Issues and directions for nursing. In H. H. Werley, & J. J. Fitzpatrick (eds.), *Annual Review of Nursing Research*, 1984, *2*, 3–25.
37. O'Brien, R. A. A conceptualization of family health. In *ANA's clinical and scientific sessions.* New York: American Nurses' Association, 1979, 19–31.
38. Terkelson, K. Toward a theory of the family lifecycle. In E. Carter, & M. McGoldrick (eds.), *The family lifecycle: A framework for family therapy.* New York: Gardner Press, 1980, 21–52.
39. Roberts, C. S., & Feetham, S. L. Assessing family functioning across three areas of relationships. *Nursing Research*, 1982, *31*, (4), 231–235.
40. Wright, L. M., & Leahey, M. *Nurses and families: A guide to family assessment and intervention*, Philadelphia: F. A. Davis, 1984.
41. Petze, C. F. Health promotion for the well family. *Nursing Clinics of North America*, 1984, *19* (2), 229–237.
42. Smilkstein, G. The cycle of family function: A conceptual model for family medicine. *Family Practitioner*, 1980, *11*, 223.
43. Johnson, R. Promoting the health of families in the community. In M. Stanhope & J. Lancaster (Eds.), *Community health nursing: Process and practice for promoting health.* St. Louis: C. V. Mosby, 184, pp. 330–360.
44. Goeppinger, J. Community as client: using the nursing process to promote health. In M. Stanhope & J. Lancaster (Eds.), *Community health nursing: Process and practice for promoting health.* St. Louis: C. V. Mosby, 1984, p. 384.
45. Dever, G. E. A. *Community health analysis: A holistic approach.* Germantown, Md.: Aspen, 1980, 12–15.
46. Goeppinger, op. cit., pp. 384–385.
47. Goeppinger, ibid, p. 386.
48. Tinkham, C. W., Voorheis, E. F., & McCarthy, N. C. *Community health nursing: Evolution and process in the family and community*, 3rd ed. Norwalk, Conn.: Appleton-Century-Crofts, 1984, p. 180.
49. Archer, S. E., Kelly, C. D., & Bisch, S. A. *Implementing change in communities: A collaborative process.* St. Louis: C. V. Mosby, 1984, pp. 5–6.
50. Kim, M., & Moritz, D. (Eds.). *Classification of nursing diagnoses: Proceedings of the 3rd and 4th national conferences.* New York: McGraw-Hill, 1981.
51. West, M. Community health assessment: The man-environment interaction. *Journal of Community Health Nursing*, 1984, *1* (2), 89–97.
52. Hogue, C. C. An epidemiological approach to nursing practice. In J. E. Hall, & B. R. Weaver: *Distributive nursing practice: A systems approach to community health*, 2nd ed. Philadelphia: Lippincott, 1985, pp. 293–294.

CHAPTER 2

Health-Protecting (Preventive) Behavior

Prevention, or health-protecting behavior, has been the focus of increasing interest among the general public and health professionals within the past decade. The chronic nature of health problems that are the leading causes of morbidity and mortality, the lack of curative therapies for chronic diseases, and the expense of long-term control measures for chronic problems make prevention an attractive alternative to traditional medical approaches focused on relief of symptoms of chronic disease or minimization of resultant disability. The antecedents of chronic illness develop over a prolonged period of time, starting in early childhood. Chronic illnesses appear to reflect not only the impact of heredity but an unhealthy environment and health-damaging behaviors. Since the interaction of heredity, behavior, and environment is a dynamic process that can be altered to some degree, prevention offers a promising approach for decreasing the prevalence of chronic illness, particularly in the middle and older adult years.

Nurses and other health professionals can assist individuals, families, and communities in establishing effective plans for health protection that are flexible, tailored to specific needs, and periodically revised as needed to fit changing conditions and goals. Comprehensive plans for preventive care for individuals, families, and communities are as essential as plans for the management of illness.

The major focus of scientific inquiry in prevention since the 1950s has been on individual behavior. The model that has emerged as the dominant paradigm for describing determinants of preventive or health-protecting behavior, the Health Beliefs Model, will be described in this chapter.

Since illness frequently thwarts the attainment of high-level well-being, maintaining an illness-free state through preventive efforts is highly desirable. Freedom from illness and the resultant stresses and strains allows individuals and families to direct more energy toward the promotion of health. The primary goal of health protection is the removal or avoidance of encumbrances throughout the life cycle that may prevent the emergence of optimum health. Encumbrances go beyond illness and may include disturbed interpersonal relationships or social disruption. In current professional literature, prevention has a narrow "biologic-disease" orientation. Further progress in understanding prevention will require exploration of its multidimensional nature. The interpersonal, social, and environmental dimensions of prevention must be described and relevant theories developed and refined.

Prevention is best described as *health-protecting behavior* because major emphasis is placed on guarding or defending an individual or group against specific illness or injury.[1] Prevention is a defensive posture or set of actions that ward off specific illness conditions or their sequelae that threaten the quality of life or longevity.

In 1979, Harris and Guten introduced the term *health-protective behavior* into the literature, using it as a term inclusive of both prevention and health promotion activities. They defined health-protective behavior as "any behavior performed by a person, regardless of his or her perceived or actual health status, in order to protect, promote or maintain his or her health, whether or not such behavior is objectively effective toward that end."[2] This definition obscures rather than clarifies the differing motivational mechanisms that underlie health-protecting behavior as opposed to health-promoting behavior. While to some readers such a differentiation may seem insignificant, it is the view of this author that such a distinction may be critical to understanding differences in the fundamental dynamics underlying the respective behaviors.

In *Healthy People: The Surgeon General's Report on Health Promotion and Disease Prevention*, health protection is defined as "protective measures in the environment that can be used by governmental and other agencies, as well as by industries and communities, to protect people from harm." Preventive health services are described as "services that can be delivered to individuals by health providers."[3] These definitions separate protective acts on the part of agencies, industries, and communities from protective acts that require use of health care providers. Since the focus of both types of activity is the avoidance of disease, the two categories of activities simply represent two subcategories of protective phenomena.

LEVELS OF PREVENTION

While the levels of prevention have been defined in the introductory chapter, a more detailed discussion of what each level of prevention entails will be provided here.

Primary Prevention

Providing specific protection against disease to prevent its occurrence is the most desirable form of prevention. Primary preventive efforts spare the client the cost, discomfort, and threat to the quality of life that illness poses or, at the least, delay the onset of illness. Early breakthroughs in primary prevention centered on control of acute infectious disease and resulted in mass immunization efforts for childhood health problems such as diphtheria, pertussis, and smallpox. Effective measures for producing artificial active immunity to polio, measles, mumps, and influenza were developed later. Immunization clinics within health departments, mandatory immunization requirements for school admission, and mass media have been used to promote a high level of immunization against infectious diseases among children.

Primary prevention of chronic health problems presents a different kind of challenge for health care professionals. Preventive measures for such illnesses generally consist of counseling, education, and adoption of specific health practices or changes in life style by the client. Examples of counseling and educative efforts directed toward primary prevention include weight control to prevent the onset of diabetes, nutrition education (low-sodium diet) to maintain normal systolic and diastolic blood pressure, smoking cessation programs for prevention of cancer of the lung and cardiovascular disorders, and education concerning the danger of overexposure to direct sunlight as a risk factor for skin cancer. Primary prevention also encompasses counseling and education of women of childbearing age to prevent birth defects that may result from use of drugs, alcohol, or tobacco during pregnancy. Accident-prevention programs, use of protective equipment to prevent blindness or deafness, and self-care education to prevent frequent colds or respiratory disorders that may lead to chronic lung disease also represent forms of primary prevention for chronic health problems.

Primary prevention is also important in the area of mental health. Counseling individuals and families to help them recognize, avoid, or deal constructively with problems or situations that may pose a threat to mental health is an important preventive measure. Family and individual counseling by the nurse or use of peer support groups are two ways in which clients can learn to manage life stress or cope successfully with specific life crises.

Another approach to primary prevention that the nurse must be aware of is environmental control. While individual protective measures to avoid

illness are increasingly available for a number of health problems, control
of air, water, and noise pollution represent complementary approaches to
disease control. Minimizing contamination of the work or general environment by asbestos dust, silicone dust, smoke, chemical pollutants, and excessive noise represents a critical organizational–political approach to primary prevention of acute and chronic illness.

Secondary Prevention

Secondary prevention consists of organized, direct screening efforts or education of the public to promote early case finding of individuals with disease
so that prompt intervention can be instituted to halt pathologic processes
and limit disability. Early diagnosis of a health problem can decrease the
catastrophic effects that might otherwise result for the individual and family
from advanced illness and its many complications. Public education to promote breast self-examination, use of home kits for detection of occult blood
in stool specimens, and familiarity with the seven cancer danger signals are
all directed toward identification of signs of possible illness by individuals
in order to promote prompt use of health services for early detection. Screening programs for hypertension, diabetes, uterine cancer (Pap smear), breast
cancer (examination and mammography), glaucoma, and sexually transmitted diseases are continuing public health efforts for secondary prevention.
Vision and hearing screening, scoliosis screening, and assessment of children
for developmental delays or disabilities are preventive programs frequently
carried out within the school setting. Careful and systematic observation of
children and adolescents for malnutrition (undernutrition or overnutrition),
neurological disorders (seizures, tics, and other abnormal behaviors), drug
abuse, alcohol abuse, and other behavioral problems also constitute important secondary prevention efforts.

While individuals are often the initial focus of secondary prevention,
such efforts may also be extended to families or significant others. The early
identification of syphilis or gonorrhea should prompt the investigation of
contacts and their treatment, while detection of hypertension or diabetes
should result in further exploration of family history and screening of other
family members who could potentially have the same illness. Secondary
preventive efforts in the area of mental health may consist of assisting family
members to deal with the stress of mental illness or the anxiety and stigma
of hospitalization of a family member for a mental health problem. Such
efforts are directed toward enhancing the ability of families to cope with the
current crisis and decreasing the possible aftereffects of highly stressful
experiences.

Where primary prevention is not available, secondary prevention (early
diagnosis and treatment) represents the first line of defense against disease.
In other situations, primary preventive measures may be available but not
used, resulting in the need for secondary-level intervention. In either case,

organized screening programs and public education efforts will continue to be critical for the detection of health problems in their early stages.

Tertiary Prevention

Tertiary prevention begins early in the period of recovery from illness and consists of such activities as consistent and appropriate administration of medications to optimize therapeutic effects, moving and positioning to prevent complications of immobility, and passive and active exercises to prevent disability. Continuing health supervision during rehabilitation to restore an individual to an optimal level of functioning is an important role of the professional nurse. Minimizing residual disability and helping the client learn to live productively with limitations are the goals of tertiary prevention. Tertiary preventive measures are appropriate for clients of all ages: the child with cerebral palsy or cystic fibrosis and the adult following a stroke or other neurological insult are examples.

Rehabilitation programs are frequently offered during the posthospitalization phase of illness and provide an intensive period of restorative care. Often the nurse must assist the client and family in dealing with feelings of hopelessness about the illness, interpret the rationale for rehabilitation, and teach client and family self-care rehabilitation measures.[4] Cardiac rehabilitation programs following myocardial infarction or cardiovascular surgery are excellent examples of tertiary prevention services. Emphasis in such programs is on meeting the physical and emotional needs of clients and promoting life style changes, e.g., dietary and exercise habits, or environmental modifications, e.g., decreased stress, that minimize the probability of recurrence of the problem.

Follow-up of client and family after the intensive phase of rehabilitation is critical to maintain the health level or benefits achieved during the initial phase. The dynamic nature of chronic illness mandates continuity of care and support of the client over time to ensure stability and progress. When deterioration and increasing disability is inevitable over time, slowing the pace of progressive disability and maintaining the optimum level of health of the client is vital to continuing self-actualization and personal fulfillment. As negative forces (exacerbations and social visibility of illness) that disrupt health increase, positive actions to thwart movement to lower levels of health and functioning must increase through health-promotion efforts. The ultimate goal of tertiary prevention is to help clients live full and productive lives, managing the problems of chronicity successfully.[5]

In summary, prevention is an important responsibility of nurses in all care settings. Minimizing the occurrence of disease and its complications as well as promoting optimum restoration can greatly enhance the quality of life for individuals of all ages. Examples of primary, secondary, and tertiary preventive measures are presented in Table 2–1.

TABLE 2–1. EXAMPLES OF PREVENTIVE MEASURES

Disease or Condition	Before Disease or Condition Occurs: Measures of Primary Prevention	After Disease or Condition Occurs: Measures of Secondary and Tertiary Prevention
Pertussis Diphtheria Tetanus Smallpox Poliomyelitis Measles German measles Mumps	For each of these diseases there are safe, specific, effective measures to produce artificial active immunity.	Early diagnosis and prompt treatment, isolation of contacts where indicated, prevention and/or treatment of complications, restorative and rehabilitative measures.
Rheumatic fever	Maintenance of good general health and nutrition, treatment of predisposing streptococcal infections, prophylactic treatment of contacts.	Early diagnosis and prompt treatment to prevent cardiovascular-renal complications, nutrition counseling, health teaching regarding activities of daily living, postoperative rehabilitation (if heart surgery performed).
Diabetes	Genetic counseling, weight control, control of stressful situations.	Early diagnosis, prompt treatment, instructions for administering insulin, nutrition counseling, prevention of infections, care of skin and toenails, self-management in altered lifestyle, emotional support for good mental hygiene.
Hypertension	Nutrition education, control of stress, regular medical check-up, avoidance of smoking.	Early diagnosis and treatment, antihypertensive medication where indicated, self-management in altered lifestyle, adherence to prescribed dietary regimen, restorative and rehabilitative measures for late manifestations and complications.

TABLE 2–1. (continued)

Disease or Condition	Before Disease or Condition Occurs: Measures of Primary Prevention	After Disease or Condition Occurs: Measures of Secondary and Tertiary Prevention
Syphilis	Health education, family living and sex education, treatment of pregnant syphilitic women to prevent congenital syphilis, investigation of contacts with treatment where necessary.	Early diagnosis and prompt treatment, case finding and follow-up of patients and contacts, prevention and/or treatment of manifestations of late syphilis (e.g., blindness, heart disease, central nervous system involvement), rehabilitation of patient with late symptomatic syphilis.

From Benson, E.R., & McDevitt, J.C. *Community health and nursing practice.* Englewood Cliffs, N.J., Prentice-Hall, 1976, with permission.

MODELS OF HEALTH-PROTECTING BEHAVIOR

For several decades, investigative efforts of behaviorally oriented health scientists have focused on the development of theoretical models to explain why people engage in preventive behavior.[6] Understanding the determinants of preventive behavior is critical for the development of effective interventions that health professionals can use to assist clients in altering behaviors that increase risk for specific diseases.

The Health Belief Model

The Health Belief Model was developed in the early 1950s by Rosenstock,[7] Hochbaum,[8] and Kegeles[9] to provide a framework for exploring why some people who are illness free take actions to avoid illness, while others fail to take such protective actions. At the time the model was formulated, the major concern within the public and private health sectors was the widespread reluctance of individuals to accept screening for tuberculosis, Pap smear for detection of cervical cancer, immunizations, and other preventive measures that were often free or provided at nominal charge. The model was viewed as potentially useful to predict those individuals who would or would not use preventive measures and to suggest interventions that might increase predisposition of resistant individuals to engage in preventive or health-protecting behaviors.

The model is derived from social–psychological theory, primarily the work of Lewin. In his writings, Lewin conceptualized that the life space in which an individual exists is composed of regions, some having negative valence (negatively valued), some having positive valence (positively valued), and others being relatively neutral.[10] Diseases are conceived to be regions of negative valence that can be expected to exert a force moving the person away from the region.[11] Preventive behaviors are strategies for avoiding the negatively valued regions of illness and disease.

Results of early studies partially supported the predictive potential of the Health Belief Model and provided the impetus for continuing model refinement and testing. The model as modified by Becker is presented in Figure 2–1. Components of the model are divided into individual perceptions, modifying factors, and variables affecting the likelihood of initiating action. Individual perceptions directly affect predisposition to take action, while demographic, sociopsychological, and structural variables act as modifying factors that only indirectly affect action tendencies. It should be noted that the critical individual perceptions in the model are beliefs about the seriousness of a specific disease and personal susceptibility. These factors combine to provide a measure of the threat or negative valence of the life-space region designating a particular disease.

The Health Belief Model is appropriate as a paradigm for health-protecting or preventive behavior, but clearly inappropriate as a paradigm for health-promoting behavior. In addition, the model may only be able to explain medically based preventive actions, that is, use of preventive services in a provider–consumer context. Further research is needed to determine the sphere of preventive behavior that the model can explain or predict. Specific components of the model will be described.

Individual Perceptions

Perceived Susceptibility. Individuals' estimated probability that they will encounter a specific health problem constitutes perceived susceptibility.[12] Any individual falls somewhere on a continuum from high to low in estimating personal degree of risk for developing a specific illness. A person may deny any possibility of contracting a particular illness, accept a slight statistical possibility but consider the chances slight, or be strongly convinced that at some point in life the illness will occur. A number of studies have clearly supported the importance of perceived susceptibility as a predictor of preventive behavior.[13] Relatively high subjective estimates of susceptibility have been shown to be correlated with obtaining screening for cervical cancer, breast cancer, cardiovascular disorders, tuberculosis, Tay-Sachs disease, and dental problems. In addition, obtaining immunizations and acceptance

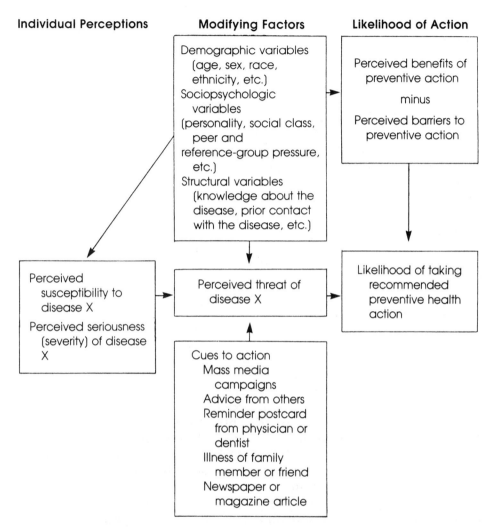

Individual Perceptions   **Modifying Factors**   **Likelihood of Action**

Demographic variables
(age, sex, race,
ethnicity, etc.)
Sociopsychologic
variables
(personality, social class,
peer and
reference-group pressure,
etc.)
Structural variables
(knowledge about the
disease, prior contact
with the disease, etc.)

Perceived benefits of
preventive action

minus

Perceived barriers to
preventive action

Perceived
susceptibility to
disease X

Perceived seriousness
(severity) of disease
X

Perceived threat of
disease X

Likelihood of taking
recommended
preventive health
action

Cues to action
Mass media
campaigns
Advice from others
Reminder postcard
from physician or
dentist
Illness of family
member or friend
Newspaper or
magazine article

Figure 2–1. The Health Belief Model. *(From Becker, M. H., Haefner, D. P., Kasl, S. V., et al. Selected psychosocial models and correlates of individual health-related behaviors. Medical Care, 1977, 15, 27–46, with permission.)*

of accident prevention measures have also been shown to be correlated with perceived susceptibility.[14]

Hochbaum[15] conducted one of the earliest studies on the role of perceived susceptibility in preventive behavior. He studied 1200 adults in an attempt to determine the key factors underlying the decision to obtain an x-ray for the detection of tuberculosis. In the group with high perceived susceptibility, 82 percent had obtained a chest x-ray during a specified period of time prior to the interviews, while only 21 percent of the individuals with low perceived susceptibility had obtained an x-ray.

Because of the limitations of retrospective studies, Kegeles[16] conducted a prospective study in which beliefs concerning susceptibility to dental disease were measured initially and use of preventive dental services was determined at a later time. He found that perception of susceptibility was correlated with subsequent number of dental visits. Fifty-eight percent of those believing themselves highly susceptible to dental disease made visits, while only 42 percent of those with low perceived susceptibility made such visits. Haefner and Kirscht[17] conducted an experimental study in which attempts were made to increase readiness to engage in preventive behaviors among the study population through communications about specific health problems. The messages were intended to increase beliefs in susceptibility, seriousness, and benefits of preventive behavior. Manipulation of the three variables resulted in a significantly greater number of physician visits for routine checkups in the experimental group, as opposed to the control group following the intervention.

Extending the concept of susceptibility to include resusceptibility to illness previously experienced, Elling et al.[18] found that mothers' beliefs in the probability of their children contracting rheumatic fever a second time correlated highly with prophylactic administration of penicillin and keeping clinic appointments. Becker et al.[19] found that mothers who believed that their children were highly susceptible to the recurrence of otitis media were more likely to give medication appropriately and keep follow-up appointments than were mothers who did not exhibit such beliefs.

Other studies have found no relationship between perceived susceptibility and preventive behavior. For example, Howe[20] did not find that the level of breast self-examination among high-risk women was related to reported perceptions of susceptibility. Some studies have found negative relationships between susceptibility and health actions. Weisenberg, Kegeles, and Lund[21] reported negative relationships between measures of susceptibility and participation of seventh-grade children in a preventive dental program.

In summary, the preponderance of evidence supports the importance of susceptibility beliefs to taking preventive health actions. Some studies have shown that augmenting perceived susceptibility through intervention may increase the incidence of preventive behavior. Other studies have shown no relationship or a negative relationship between susceptibility and preventive actions. Thus, further studies are needed to determine what factors confound or modulate the relationship between perceived susceptibility and behaviors to avoid disease.

Perceived Seriousness. Perceived seriousness or severity of a given health problem can be judged either by the degree of emotional arousal created by the thought of the disease or by the difficulties that individuals believe a given health condition would create for them. Perceived seriousness may include the broad implications of the illness for work, family life, or social relationships and commitments. A number of studies have shown a relationship between perceived seriousness and preventive behaviors, while some studies have failed to support such a relationship.[22]

In one of the supporting studies, the relationship of perceived seriousness to obtaining genetic screening for Tay-Sachs disease was studied. The study was conducted in a Jewish population in the Baltimore–Washington area. Individuals from the population were invited to participate in screening, and all adults who appeared for screening were asked to complete a brief questionnaire. Approximately 500 participants and 500 nonparticipants were selected at random for inclusion in the study group. Severity or seriousness was measured by the reported impact of learning about being a carrier on family planning in the future. Interestingly, participation in the screening program was negatively rather than positively correlated with perceived seriousness. It appeared that perceived severity was so high that it became an inhibiting rather than facilitating factor for action. Severity appeared to produce overwhelming threat and subsequent avoidance of the screening program.[23] This finding is consistent with other studies that have shown very low levels of seriousness are not sufficiently motivating, while high levels of perceived seriousness thwart constructive actions.[24]

Evidence for the role of perceived seriousness in motivating preventive behavior is unclear. In some studies perceived seriousness has been positively related to taking preventive action; in others, negatively related; and in still other studies, no relationship has been evident at all. It is possible that very high or very low levels of perceived seriousness inhibit preventive behavior, while a moderate level of perceived seriousness facilitates preventive behavior. Further research is needed to clarify the contribution of perceived seriousness to motivation to engage in health-protecting behaviors.

Perceived Threat. According to Becker,[25] perceived susceptibility and perceived seriousness combine to determine the total perceived threat of an illness to a specific individual. Theoretically, the extent of threat represents the negative valence of illness and predisposition to avoidance. A number of studies have explored the impact of these factors in combination. Fink et al.[26] found that perception of personal susceptibility to breast cancer and belief in the serious nature of the disease augmented participation in a cancer screening program for detection of breast abnormalities. Champion,[27] in examining the potential of susceptibility and seriousness to explain breast self-examination in a convenience sample of 301 women, found that neither variable accounted for a significant amount of variance in self-examination behavior.

Tash et al.,[28] in exploring the relationship between attitudes and preventive dental visits, found a significant negative relationship between perceived susceptibility to dental problems and dental visits and a significant positive correlation between perceived seriousness of dental disease and visits. The negative relationship was explained as reflecting the low level of perceived susceptibility to dental disease as a result of frequent preventive visits. While initial beliefs in susceptibility may have been high, repeated visits decreased such beliefs because appropriate preventive measures had been taken.

It is apparent that the combined effects of perceptions of susceptibility and seriousness on the performance of various preventive actions need further study. The nature of the relationship between the two variables in determining perceived threat needs to be clearly specified.

Modifying Factors. Modifying factors proposed in the Health Belief Model as affecting predisposition to take preventive action include a variety of demographical, sociopsychological, and structural factors. However, they have had little specific testing in research based on the model.

Demographic Factors. While some demographic factors, such as sex, age, income, and education, have been clearly shown to be correlated with use of health services, their relationship to the use of preventive services in the absence of symptoms is much less clear. Sex is the demographic variable most predictive of preventive behaviors, and women exhibit a predisposition to engage in those behaviors more frequently than men. Education as a determining factor is supported by some studies in which the level of formal education correlated positively with the frequency of preventive actions. In other studies, years of formal education does not emerge as a significant predictor variable. Race and ethnicity appear to be factors in use of preventive services only when they are associated with socioeconomic level. Socioeconomic status appears to exert an effect only when significant cost or time is required to carry out preventive actions. Further exploration of demographic variables can yield information about users or preventive services and identify low-use populations for special motivational or programmatic efforts. However, such information provides little assistance to health professionals in structuring meaningful interventions to increase the incidence of health-protecting actions.

Sociopsychological Variables. Social pressure or social influence appear to play a role in stimulating appropriate health actions even when low levels of individual motivation exist. Reference groups can affect health behavior by changing attitudes and beliefs or by forcing conformity with group behavior norms. Bond[29] found that women involved in discussion groups regarding techniques for early detection of breast cancer (breast self-examination) were more likely to report continued use of early detection measures than women who were taught breast self-examination in lecture sessions with little opportunity for peer interaction. It appeared that group support and pressure provided motivation to adopt the new health practice.

In another study, Lambert[30] noted the importance of support and encouragement from family members and friends in use of dental clinics offered by public health personnel within the community. Endorsement of dental services by significant others and "word of mouth" advertising affected incidence of use by individuals of differing age, ethnicity, and socioeconomic background.

The importance of normative beliefs (expectations of significant others) concerning health-related behaviors has been further supported by the work of Ajzen and Fishbein.[31,32] Normative beliefs are defined as the perceived behavioral expectations of others and motivation to comply with those expectations.[33] In predicting intentions to participate in an influenza immunization program, normative beliefs (expectations of others) emerged as a meaningful variable. However, it is important to note that the impact of expectations of significant others was weak compared to the effects of beliefs about possible outcomes or consequences of the target behaviors.

In studying the incidence of polio vaccinations among children, Gray et al.[34] found that expectations of friends were powerful sources of motivation for parents to obtain immunizations for their children. Parents appeared to seek polio vaccination for their children not only to prevent the occurrence of disease but also to fulfill the expectations of friends and family members concerning what "good parents should do." Meeting the behavioral norms of important reference groups appeared to play a significant role in this study in promoting use of preventive measures.

Structural Variables. Two such variables presumed by the model to influence preventive behavior include knowledge about the target disease and prior contact with it. Few studies address these variables. In one study, Heinzelmann[35] found that continuation of penicillin prophylaxis among college students was directly related to the history of past bouts of rheumatic fever and expectations of recurrence. Becker[36] found higher compliance rates with the treatment regimen for otitis media when mothers reported that their child was often ill and that illness was a major threat to their child. Becker et al.[37] also found that the number of asthma attacks that children had experienced previously affected mothers' compliance with a medical regimen for control of asthmatic symptoms. Further research is needed to clarify the extent to which knowledge about a disease or previous experience with it contribute to motivation for preventive actions.

Cues to Action. Cues, while proposed as affecting the incidence of health behavior by triggering appropriate overt actions, have not been systematically studied. This may be due to the transient nature of cues and the difficulties of retrospectively recalling stimuli that initiated specific behaviors.[38] The intensity of cues needed to trigger preventive actions given a certain level of readiness to engage in such activities is unknown. The general assumption is made that the higher the level of readiness to act, the lower the intensity of the cue needed to trigger behavior. In other words, a negative relationship is postulated between intensity of cue and level of readiness to engage in preventive actions. Cues can be either internal or external. Examples of internal cues include uncomfortable symptoms, feelings of fatigue, or recall of the condition of affected individuals to whom the individual is close. External cues include, for example, mass media, advice from others, posters, billboards, newspaper or magazine articles, or a reminder postcard from health professionals who have previously provided services. There is a need for further research that addresses the relationship between cue configurations, cue intensity, cue-use patterns, and health-related behaviors.

Likelihood of Action. Two additional factors identified in the model as affecting the probability of action are perceived benefits and perceived barriers. In the model, it is proposed that benefits minus barriers determine the likelihood of taking recommended preventive health actions.[39] A number of studies have shown a significant positive relationship between perceived benefits and preventive behavior, while in a smaller number of studies a significant positive relationship has not been shown. In several studies where an attempt was made to measure the effect of perceived barriers on preventive actions, the majority showed a significant relationship, with greater barriers resulting in fewer preventive actions.[40]

Perceived Benefits. Beliefs about the effectiveness of recommended preventive actions appear to be important determinants of health-protecting behavior. Kegeles,[41] in a field experiment to identify factors associated with participation in a screening program for cervical cancer, found that women who obtained a Pap smear were more likely than nonparticipants to believe that the test could detect cervical cancer, that such a test could reveal cancer prior to the occurrence of symptoms, and that early detection would lead to a more favorable prognosis. Other studies also support the relationship between beliefs in benefits and use of cancer-screening programs. Haefner and Kirscht[42] found a higher incidence of physician visits for routine checkups to detect cancer and other health problems by a group exposed to a communication that addressed the benefits of early detection than by a group not exposed to the communication. In another study, belief that accidents could be prevented among sugarcane field workers by use of a protective glove resulted in greater frequency of use of the glove as a safety device.[43]

Battistella[44] reported that "perceived chances of recovery" (that is, perceived benefits from medical care) were inversely related to the length of delay before seeking care. The lower the perceived chances of recovery, the longer individuals waited before seeking medical attention. In a study of follow-up care of school-age children referred for a medical problem, Gabrielson et al.[45] found that belief in the effectiveness or potential success of follow-up care was positively associated with the frequency with which parents complied with follow-up recommendations.

Perceived Barriers. The barriers to obtaining preventive care can take many forms and can be perceived or real. Cost, inconvenience, unpleasantness, or extent of life change required are only a few of the possible blocks to engaging in preventive behaviors. Fear of pain or discomfort from dental procedures and anticipated costs for such care have been shown to be negatively related to the frequency of obtaining preventive dental services.[46,47] A study by Antonovsky and Kats[48] indicated that the expense of preventive dental care was a significant factor in frequency of use. Champion[49] found that perceived barriers to preventive action was the most important variable out of the entire model in explaining breast self-examination behavior. When barriers were perceived as formidable, the frequency of examination behavior was low.

A limited number of studies have been conducted focusing on the barriers component of the Health Beliefs Model. With emphasis on long-term lifestyle change for the prevention of chronic disease, it appears critical to examine the extent to which duration, complexity, and frequency of preventive behaviors may serve as barriers to their practice. Research efforts must not only be directed toward the identification of barriers but also toward identifying effective strategies for decreasing or compensating for such blocks to action.

Critique of Health Belief Model

Wallston and Wallston[50] have provided insight into some of the problems inherent in the current version of the Health Belief Model. They propose that the model is essentially a catalog of variables rather than a well-articulated model specifying the nature of the relationship among variables. In addition, they point out the lack of consistent operationalization and measurement of the variables across studies. Such inconsistency makes it impossible to compare results across multiple investigations. Further refinement of the model and development of instrumentation is critical in future research efforts.

OTHER PROPOSED MODELS FOR HEALTH-PROTECTING BEHAVIOR

In addition to the Health Belief Model, a number of other models have been proposed for explaining preventive behavior. Two of these models will be described in brief here. Since the models are relatively new, additional research is needed before their usefulness can be determined.

Resource Model of Preventive Health Behavior

The Resource Model of Preventive Health Behavior has been proposed by Kulbok.[51] According to the model, people act in ways that maximize their "stock in health." The model hypothesis is that the greater the social and health resources of the individual, the more frequent the performance of preventive behaviors. The major variables in the resource model are defined as follows:

1. Social resources are education level and family income
2. Health resources are perceived health status and energy level, concern about health and feelings about capability of taking care of one's own health, participation in social groups and religious services, number and closeness of friends and relatives, and general psychologic well-being
3. Preventive health behaviors are diet, physical activity, sleeping, smoking, drinking alcoholic beverages, drinking caffeinated beverages, dental hygiene, use of seat belts, use of professional health services for prevention of disease, and behavior with respect to high blood pressure
4. Control variables are age, sex, and race

The source of data for the original test of the model was the National Survey of Personal Health Practices and Consequences (NSPHPC) Wave 1, which was conducted in the spring of 1979 by the Office of Health Information, Health Promotion, Physical Fitness and Sports Medicine and the Division of Environmental Epidemiology of the National Center for Health Statistics. The number of successfully completed interviews was 3025. Secondary analyses of the data by Kulbok revealed that health resources factored into Activity Level, General Well-being and Health Comparison (evaluation of health in relation to others). Preventive practices factored into dental, physical fitness, health protection, harmful consumption, and checkup factors. Social and health resources explained the dental and physical fitness factors but did not satisfactorily explain other preventive practice factors. Favorable dental behavior was related to higher education, higher income, higher activity level, better health comparison, and being younger, female, and white. Favorable fitness behavior was related to higher education, higher income, higher activity level, better health comparison, and being younger, male, and white.

The model was retested on Wave II data of the NSPHPC. The sample consisted of 2436 individuals who were reinterviewed a year after the initial survey. This study demonstrated the stability and replicability of the preventive health behavior factors. It is interesting to note that comparison of Wave I and Wave II data indicated that physical fitness was the least stable preventive health behavior over time and the most difficult behavior to maintain.[53]

Results of these studies indicated the potential usefulness of the Health Resource Model in explaining some preventive health behaviors. Further conceptual refinement and empirical testing of the model is needed.

Model of Multiple Risk Factor Behavior

The Model of Multiple Risk Factor Behavior proposed by Kar, Schmitz, and Dyer[53] is a multidimensional, psychosocial model of determinants of risk-taking behavior. The model proposes that in populations with comparable ethnicity, socioeconomic, and biological status, risk-taking behavior is a function of the following categories of variables: (1) behavioral intentions, (2) social support from significant others, (3) accessibility of information and services, (4) personal autonomy, and (5) action situation. The model is based on a systems approach that integrates elements of Lewin's field theory and Fishbein's theory of reasoned action.[54] Behavioral intentions and personal autonomy are internal determinants of behavior, while the other variables exert external influence on actions.

The model has been tested in three cultures, Venezuela, Kenya, and the Philippines, through surveys of the psychosocial determinants of contraceptive behavior among married women in reproductive age groups. The factors exerting the strongest influence on contraceptive use in the three target countries were: behavioral intention, social support from significant others, accessibility of information and services, communication and decision-making power, social network communication about family planning, and number of living children. Intention to use contraceptives had the strongest relationship of all the variables to contraceptive behavior in all three countries. When all communication and social support factors were combined, this variable was the second most powerful influence on contraceptive behavior. While differing patterns of impact for intention, social support, and accessibility emerged across cultures, the combined impact of these variables resulted in a contraception use rate of 74 percent in Venezuela, 61 percent in the Phillippines, and 44 percent in Kenya. The number of living children was the single most important nonpsychological determinant of contraceptive use. This factor was proposed as a part of the action situation or behavioral context in which the risk behavior took place.

The cross-cultural studies conducted by these investigators provide empirical support for the model. A strength of the model is its potential transcultural applicability. The validity of a model across cultures is often given little attention in attempts to understand preventive behavior. In future research, the model needs to be tested in terms of its ability to explain and predict a variety of other preventive behaviors in addition to use of contraceptives.

SUMMARY

The Health Belief Model is most frequently cited in the literature as an explanatory framework for preventive behavior. However, serious problems persist in the clarity with which the model relationships are articulated and in the reliability and validity of the measures used to assess component variables. New models are being proposed for preventive health behavior. The Resource Model of Preventive Health Behavior and the Model of Multiple Risk Factor Behavior were described briefly in this chapter. The reader is referred to the references cited in the text for more in-depth coverage of each of these models. Further research will provide important information regarding the models most useful in explaining and predicting various health-protecting behaviors among individuals. Models that describe preventive behaviors of family units[55] and community systems are also needed.

REFERENCES

1. Shamansky, S. L., & Clausen, C. L. Levels of prevention: Examination of the concept. *Nursing Outlook*, 1980, *28*, 104–108.
2. Harris, D. M., & Guten, S. Health-protective behavior: An exploratory study. *Journal of Health and Social Behavior*, 1979, *20*, 17–29.
3. *Healthy People: The Surgeon General's Report on Health Promotion and Disease Prevention.* U. S. Department of Health, Education and Welfare Publication No. (PHS) 79–55071, U. S. Public Health Service, 1979.
4. Robischon, P. Prevention and chronic illness. In B. W. Spradley, (Ed.), *Contemporary community health nursing.* Little, Brown, 1975, pp. 39–40.
5. Strauss, A. L. *Chronic illness and the quality of life.* St. Louis: C. V. Mosby, 1975, p. 133.
6. Becker, M. H. (Ed.). The Health Belief Model and personal health behavior. Thorofare, N. J.: Charles B. Slack, 1974.
7. Rosenstock, I. M. Why people use health services. *Milbank Memorial Fund Quarterly*, July 1966, *44*, 94–127.
8. Hochbaum, G. M. Public participation in medical screening programs: A sociopsychological study. Public Health Service Publication (No. 572). Washington, D. C.: U. S. Government Printing Office, 1958.
9. Kegeles, S. S., Kirscht, J. P., Haefner, D. P., et al. Survey of beliefs about cancer detection and taking Papanicolaou tests. *Public Health Reports*, September 1965, *80*, 815–823.
10. Lewin, K., Dembo, T., Festinger, L. & Sears, P. S. Level of aspiration. In J. Hunt (Ed.), *Personality and the behavioral disorders: A handbook based on experimental and clinical research.* Ronald Press: New York, 1944, pp. 333–378.
11. Davidhizar, R. Critique of the health-belief model. *Journal of Advanced Nursing*, *8*, 1983, 467–472.
12. Rosenstock, 1966, op. cit., p. 104.
13. Becker, 1977, op. cit., p. 35.
14. Becker, M. H., & Maiman, B. A. Sociobehavioral determinants of compliance with health and medical care recommendations. *Medical Care*, January 1975, *13*, 10–24.
15. Hochbaum, G. M. Why people seek diagnostic x-rays. *Public Health Reports*, 1956, *71*, 377.
16. Kegeles, S. S. Why people seek dental care: A test of a conceptual formulation. *Journal of Health and Human Behavior*, 1963, *4*, 166 ff.
17. Haefner, D. P., & Kirscht, J. P. Motivational and behavioral effects of modifying health beliefs. *Public Health Reports*, 1970, *85*, 478.
18. Elling, R., Whittemore, R., & Green, M. Patient participation in a pediatric program. *Journal of Health and Human Behavior*, 1960, *1*, 183.
19. Becker, M. H., Drachman, R. H., & Kirscht, J. P. A new approach to explaining sick-role behavior in low income populations. *American Journal of Public Health*, 1974, *64*, 205–216.

20. Howe, H. Social factors associated with breast self-examination among high risk women. *American Journal of Public Health*, 1981, *71*, 251–255.
21. Weisenberg, M., Kegeles, S., & Lund, A. Children's health beliefs and acceptance of a dental preventive activity. *Journal of Health and Social Behavior*, 1980, *21*, 59–74.
22. Becker, 1977, op. cit.
23. Becker, M. H., Kaback, M. M., Rosenstock, I. M., & Ruth, M. V. Some influences on program participation in a genetic screening program. *Journal of Community Health*, 1975, *1*, 3.
24. Leventhal, H. Fear communications in the acceptance of preventive health practices. *Bulletin of the New York Academy of Medicine*, 1965, *41*, 1144 ff.
25. Becker et al., 1977, op. cit., p. 30.
26. Fink, R., Shapiro, S., & Roester, R. Impact of efforts to increase participation in repetitive screenings for early breast cancer detection. *American Journal of Public Health*, 1972, *62*, 328 ff.
27. Champion, V. L. Instrument development for health belief model constructs. *Advances in Nursing Science*, 1984, *6* (3), 73–85.
28. Tash, R. H., O'Shea, R. M., & Cohen, L. K. Testing a preventive-symptomatic theory of dental health behavior. *American Journal of Public Health*, 1969, *59*, 514.
29. Bond, B. W. *Group discussion-decision: An appraisal of its use in health education.* Minneapolis: Department of Health, 1965.
30. Lambert, C., Jr. Interpersonal factors associated with the utilization of a public health dental clinic (Doctoral dissertation, Brandeis University, 1962). *Dissertation Abstracts International*, 1962, *23*, 609–610. (University Microfilms No. 62–3071).
31. Ajzen, I., & Fishbein, M. The prediction of behavior from attitudinal and normative variables. *Journal of Experimental Social Psychology*, 1970, *6*, 466–487.
32. Ajzen, I., & Fishbein, M. Attitudinal and normative variables as predictors of specific behaviors. *Journal of Personality and Social Psychology*, 1973, *27*, 41–57.
33. Fishbein & Ajzen, 1975, op. cit., p. 302.
34. Gray, R. M., Kesler, J. P., & Moody, P. M. The effects of social class and friends' expectations on oral polio vaccination participation. *American Journal of Public Health*, December 1966, *56*, 2028–2032.
35. Heinzelman, F. Factors in prophylaxis behavior in treating rheumatic fever: An exploratory study. *Journal of Health and Human Behavior*, 1962, *2*, 73.
36. Becker, M. H., Drachman, R. H., & Kirscht, J. P. Predicting mothers' compliance with pediatric medical regimens. *Journal of Pediatrics*, 1972, *81*, 843–854.
37. Becker, M. H., Radius, S. M., Rosenstock, I. M., et al. Compliance with a medical regimen for asthma: A test of the Health Relief Model. *Public Health Reports*, May–June 1978, *93*, 268–277.
38. Rosenstock, I. M. Historical origins of the health belief model. In M. H. Becker (Ed.), *The Health Belief Model and personal health behavior.* Thorofare, N. J.: Charles B. Slack, 1974, p. 5.
39. Ibid., p. 4.
40. Becker et al. 1977, op. cit., p. 35.
41. Kegeles, S. S. A field experiment attempt to change beliefs and behavior of women in an urban ghetto. *Journal of Health and Social Behavior*, 1969, *10*, 115.
42. Haefner & Kirscht, op. cit.
43. Suchman, E. A. Preventive health behavior: A model for research on community health campaigns. *Journal of Health and Social Behavior*, 1967, *8*, 197.

44. Battistella, R. M. Factors associated with delay in the initiation of physicians' care among late adulthood persons. *American Journal of Public Health*, 1971, *61*, 1348.
45. Gabrielson, I. W., Levin, L. S., & Ellison, M. D. Factors affecting school health follow-up. *American Journal of Public Health*, 1967, *57*, 48.
46. Tash et al., op. cit.
47. Kegeles, op. cit.
48. Antonovsky, A., & Kats, R. The model dental patient: An empirical study of preventive health behavior. *Social Science and Medicine*, 1970, *4*, 367.
49. Champion, 1984, op. cit.
50. Wallston, B. S., & Wallston, K. A. Social psychological models of health behavior: An examination and integration. In A. Baum, S. Taylor, & J. E. Singer (Eds.), *Handbook of Psychology and Health, Volume IV: Social Psychological Aspects of Psychology*, Hillsdale, N. J.: L. Erlbaum Assoc., 1984.
51. Kulbok, P. P. Social resources, health resources, and preventive health behavior: Patterns and predictions. *Public Health Nursing*, 1985, *2* (2), 67–81.
52. Kulbok, P. P. The resource model: Toward a theory of health promotion. Paper presented at the American Public Health Association Annual Meeting, Washington, D. C., November 1985.
53. Kar, S. B., Schmitz, M., & Dyer, D. A psychosocial model of health behavior: Implications for nutrition education, research and policy. *Health Values: Achieving High Level Wellness*, 1983 7 (2), 29–37.
54. Kar, S. B. Psychosocial environment: A health promotion model. *International Quarterly of Community Health Education*, 1983–84, *4* (4), 311–341.
55. Duffy, M. E. Primary preventive behaviors: The female-headed one-parent family. *Research in Nursing and Health*, 1986, *9*, 115–122.

CHAPTER 3

A Proposed Model for Health-Promoting Behavior

In Chapter 2, three models were presented as proposed descriptions of the determinants of preventive or health-protecting behavior. Health protection is directed toward *decreasing* the probability of experiencing illness by active protection of the body against pathological stressors or detection of illness in the asymptomatic stage. The Health Promotion Model proposed in this chapter is intended to be a complementary counterpart to models of health protection. Health promotion is directed toward *increasing* the level of well-being and self-actualization of a given individual or group. Health promotion focuses on movement toward a positively valenced state of enhanced health and well-being. The negatively valanced states of illness and disease, while relevant to motivation for health-protecting behavior, appear to have little, if any, motivational significance for health-promoting behavior. Desire for growth, expression of human potential, and quality of life provide the motivation for health-promotive behaviors.

The Health Promotion Model, as revised since it appeared in the first edition of this book, is presented in Figure 3–1. The model is based on a synthesis of research findings from studies of health promotion and wellness behavior and serves three important functions: (1) introduces order among concepts that may explain the occurrence of health-promoting behavior, (2) provides for the generation of hypotheses to be tested empirically, and (3) integrates disconnected research findings into a coherent pattern. The Health Promotion Model meets a major criteria for theoretical models, that is, it is consistent with knowledge to date yet remains flexible and subject to change

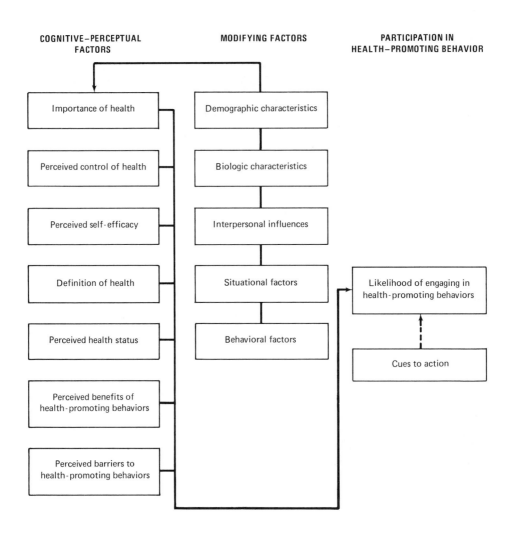

Figure 3–1. Health Promotion Model.

as new knowledge is generated. Thus, testing of the proposed model is more appropriately described as model discovery, since modifications will need to be made as new empirical evidence becomes available regarding the determinants of health-promoting behaviors and their interrelationships. The extent to which the Health Promotion Model can explain life style patterns or specific behaviors that are health-promoting remains to be determined.

At present, a federally funded research program is being conducted by the author of this book and three of her nursing colleagues at Northern Illinois University* to test the power of the model in explaining patterns of physical exercise and health-promoting life styles in three different populations. The 3-year research program grant,[1] entitled "Health-Promoting Behavior: Testing a Proposed Model," is funded by the National Center for Nursing Research, NIH, USPHS under Grant No. P01 NR 01121.

The four research projects in the program focus on working adults, older adults, ambulatory cancer patients and cardiac rehabilitation clients. Collectively, the projects address the following specific aims:

1. To determine to what extent cognitive–perceptual and modifying factors identified in the Health Promotion Model explain the occurrence of health-promoting behaviors in adult populations
2. To determine if cognitive–perceptual factors and modifying factors identified in the Health Promotion Model differ in their ability to explain the occurrence of health-promoting behaviors in adult populations of varying ages and populations with and without a recent catastrophic illness

Health-promoting behaviors almost without exception are continuing activities that must be an integral part of an individual's life style. Examples of behaviors that persons may engage in for the promotion of health include physical exercise, nutritional eating practices, development of social support, and use of relaxation or stress management techniques. Frequently, old patterns of behavior must be extinguished and new patterns of behavior learned to enhance health and well-being.

Health-promoting behaviors are an expression of the actualizing tendency. Such behaviors are directed toward maximizing positive arousal such as increased self-awareness, self-satisfaction, enjoyment, and pleasure. For example, jogging is almost always a health-promoting behavior for the child, adolescent, or young adult, since the source of motivation is a desire to approach a positively valenced state of increased physical endurance, greater psychomotor competence, enhanced physical energy, and improved personal appearance. Seldom do children or adolescents exercise primarily to avoid the risk of cardiovascular problems in middle age. In fact, there may be

---

* Dr. Marilyn F. Stromborg (Ambulatory Cancer Patient Project), Dr. Susan N. Walker (Older Adult Project), and Dr. Karen R. Sechrist (Cardiac Rehabilitation Project).

minimal awareness within this age group that a relationship exists between physical fitness and the incidence of such illness. While many middle-aged or older adults may begin jogging because they are "at risk" for cardiovascular disorders (avoidance motives), as the positive internal sensations and feelings engendered by running become more salient, approach tendencies often assume greater dominance in the motivation of behavior. Thus, jogging, which began as a preventive action, may become primarily a health-promoting effort.

Health-promoting behaviors represent man *acting* on his environment as he moves toward higher levels of health rather than *reacting* to external influences or threats posed by the environment. Persons seek to increase the complexity, variation, and meaningfulness of stimuli within their environment in order to increase positive tensions that promote maturation and expression of human potential.[1]

THE HEALTH PROMOTION MODEL

The Health Promotional Model is derived from social learning theory, which emphasizes the importance of cognitive mediating processes in the regulation of behavior. Structurally, the Health Promotion Model is organized similarly to the Health Belief Model. That is, determinants of health-promoting behavior are categorized into cognitive–perceptual factors (individual perceptions), modifying factors, and variables affecting the likelihood of action. The nature of interrelationships among the variables, additive or multiplicative, will be tested in the research program currently underway.

Cognitive–Perceptual Factors

Cognitive–perceptual factors are identified within the model as the *primary motivational mechanisms* for acquisition and maintenance of health-promoting behaviors. Each factor is proposed as exerting a direct influence on the likelihood of engaging in health-promoting actions. Cognitive–perceptual factors that influence health-promoting behavior have been identified within the model as (1) importance of health, (2) perceived control of health, (3) perceived self-efficacy, (4) definition of health, (5) perceived health status, (6) perceived benefits of health-promoting behavior, and (7) perceived barriers to health-promoting behavior.

The Importance of Health. The impact of valuing health on the frequency of health-promoting behaviors received support from a study of 88 college students conducted by Wallston, Maides, and Wallston.[2] They found that individuals who held a high health value, that is, ranked health within the top 4 out of 10 value positions, chose more health-related pamphlets to read when they were made available to them than did individuals with a low health value. The data support the notion that placing a high value on health results in information-seeking behavior. Thus, individuals engage in actions directed toward becoming more knowledgeable on health-related topics.

Christiansen studied a national probability sample of adults to determine factors that differentiated those engaged in health-promoting activities from those who were not. The importance of health as measured by the Health Value Scale was a significant differentiating factor between persons reporting a moderate to high level of health-promoting behavior and those reporting little health-promoting behavior.[3]

In studying the relationship between value placed on health and participation in physical activity during leisure, Laffrey and Isenberg did not find a significant relationship. The perceived importance of physical exercise per se rather than the value of health was the most powerful variable in explaining exercise behavior.[4]

The role of values in motivating and directing health-promoting behavior needs further study. A person's global value hierarchy may affect the performance of some health behaviors but not others. On the other hand, so many variables may mediate the impact of values on behavior that the relationship is obscured. Behavior-specific values may be more effective predictors of health actions than global life values.

Perceived Control. The effect of perceived personal control on health behavior has been supported in a number of studies. Williams[5] found that individuals who were internally controlled reported more frequent use of seat belts than individuals who were externally controlled. James, Woodruff, and Werner[6] found that nonsmokers were more likely to be internally controlled than smokers, although this finding has been questioned as a result of additional research.[7]

Wallston et al.[8] found that success in weight loss depended on structuring the weight-loss program according to each person's locus of control, either internal or external. Individuals who were externally controlled achieved greater weight loss than internally controlled persons in a group program relying on social pressures as motivation. "Internals" achieved greater weight loss than externally controlled individuals in a self-directed program. Perceived control of health appears to influence the effectiveness of differing strategies for inducing or facilitating continued practice of health-promoting behaviors.

Brown, Muhlenkamp, Fox, and Osborn investigated the relationship between health locus of control, health values, and positive health practices in a sample of 63 middle-class adults in a southwestern metropolitan area. Health locus of control and health values explained 20 percent of the variance in health behaviors. Of the three health locus-of-control dimensions—internality, externality (powerful others), and externality (chance)—only chance explained a significant amount of variance (14 percent) in health practices.[9]

Laffrey and Isenberg, in their study of participation in physical activities during leisure among 75 women between the ages of 24 and 65, found no significant relationship between internal health locus of control and frequency of exercise.[10] Saltzer found that perceptions of health locus of control did not differentiate between persons completing a weight loss program and those who dropped out. However, these groups were distinguished by specific beliefs concerning their ability to control weight.[11] Thus, general health beliefs may be less predictive of health-promoting actions than behavior-specific beliefs.

Desire for control of health and perceived probability of control of health status need to be conceptually and empirically differentiated. Perceiving oneself to be in control as well as having a strong desire for control should result in overt health-promoting behaviors. However, having a strong desire for control but little perceived probability of control may result in helplessness, frustration, and behavioral inhibition. The interactive effects of desire for control and perceptions of control on the occurrence of health-promoting behaviors needs further study.

The importance of cross-cultural investigations on health locus-of-control beliefs is described by Stein, Smith, and Wallston.[12] They pose questions regarding the characteristics of varying cultural environments that may lead to different control desires and expectancies and thus to differential effects of these perceptions on health behaviors.

Perceived Self-efficacy. Within the revised Health Promotion Model, *desire for competence* has been replaced by *perceived self-efficacy*. While competence represents the generalized ability of an individual to interact or transact effectively with the environment, perceived self-efficacy is a more specific concept that refers to individuals' convictions that they can successfully execute the required behavior necessary to produce a desired outcome.[13]

DiClemente[14] and Condiotte and Lichtenstein[15] found that perceived self-efficacy was an important factor in the maintenance of smoking cessation. They found that perceived inefficacy increased vulnerability to relapse following a period of cessation. At the end of treatment, relapsers as compared to abstainers expressed lower self-efficacy about their ability to resist smoking under subsequent instigating conditions. The higher the perceived self-efficacy, the more successfully smoking cessation was maintained during the follow-up period. Condiotte and Lichtenstein also noted that the highly self-efficacious individuals reinstated control following a slip, whereas the less self-efficacious ones displayed a marked decrease in perceived self-efficacy and relapsed completely. When beset with difficulty, people who have serious doubts about their capabilities often decrease their efforts and give up, while those with a strong sense of efficacy exert greater effort to master problems or challenges.[16,17]

Chambliss and Murray[18] used persuasion to promote behavior that would increase self-efficacy among persons attempting weight loss. Attribution of efficacy to self had a greater influence on extent of weight loss than perceived locus of control. Atkins, Kaplan, Timms, et al.[19] developed cognitive and behavioral interventions to increase self-efficacy. They used the interventions to determine if the incidence of walking could be increased among persons with chronic obstructive pulmonary disease. Those persons who received the experimental interventions increased in exercise tolerance, reported general health status, and self-efficacy judgments.

Dishman, Sallis, and Orenstein, in reviewing multiple studies on the determinants of physical activity and exercise, concluded that in studies of spontaneous physical activity, there were mixed findings concerning the impact of self-efficacy on exercise frequency.[20] The role of perceptions of self-efficacy in motivating initiation and continuation of health behaviors remains to be demonstrated.

Individuals of all ages are beginning to assume increased responsibility for their own health and to expect greater mastery of personal and environmental factors that impinge on health. It is possible that those people with positive perceptions of their health promotion skills may be more likely to initiate actions that enhance health.

Definition of Health. The definition of health to which individuals subscribe may influence the extent to which they engage in health-promoting behaviors. It is possible that defining health as adaptation or stability would predispose individuals toward health-protecting behaviors directed toward avoiding illness and disease. Defining health primarily as self-actualization should result in self-initiated activities directed toward attaining higher levels of health and well-being. Since how goals are defined often determines the means used to achieve them, differences in definitions of health should result in differing patterns of health behaviors.

The prevailing definition of health within the medical community is "absence of illness." As the public redefines health as a positive construct rather than a negative one, the nature of behaviors directed toward maintaining health should also change.

The definition of health to which individuals subscribe was found by Christiansen[21] to vary greatly from absence of illness to a state of optimum health and well-being. While Christiansen did not find a significant relationship between definition of health and frequency of health-promoting behaviors in the sample she studied, the relationship approached significance. Laffrey[22] developed the Health Conception Scale to measure individuals' definition of health. The scale is based on the work of Smith,[23] who described four models of health: clinical, role-performance, adaptive, and eudaimonistic. These models were discussed in Chapter 1. Laffrey found that defining health as high-level wellness as opposed to absence of illness was positively correlated with reported participation in health practices for the purpose of promoting health. Laffrey did not relate health conception (definition) to the actual frequency of health behaviors in the sample she studied.

Few studies have focused on the impact of definition of health on health behaviors. Since personal definitions of health and well-being appear to be changing in our culture, this area warrants further study.

Perceived Health Status. Perceived health status appears to play a role in the frequency and intensity of health-promoting behaviors. Sidney and Shephard,[24] in studying a group of older adults engaged in physical training classes for 14 weeks, found that individuals who exhibited more physical complaints or symptoms on the Cornell Medical Index Health Questionnaire had a lower frequency and lower intensity of participation in the exercise program than individuals who reported fewer symptoms on the index. All individuals had been examined by a physician prior to the program, and any overt clinical symptoms of illness had been ruled out. The prolonged experience of uncomfortable symptoms even in the absence of identifiable illness may represent a threat, induce fear and avoidance, and reduce personal capacity to engage in positive health behaviors. "Feeling good" may be a source of motivation for taking actions that increase personal health status. Kaplan and Cowles[25] have suggested that an appropriate approach for smoking cessation may be initially to encourage health-promoting behaviors through which individuals experience rapid and noticeable changes in well-being, e.g., exercise and relaxation. Experiences of increased well-being and improved health status can then be used to reinforce the value of good health and promote more extensive changes in life style that individuals perceive as difficult.

In a study of 502 individuals between 45 and 69 years of age, Palmore and Luikart[26] found that self-rated health correlated more highly with life satisfaction than did activity level, organizational or social activity, productivity, or career anchorage. Either individuals who are healthy perceive themselves as more satisfied, or self-perceptions of health result in behaviors directed toward achieving increased satisfaction.

Christiansen,[27] in studying a national sample of 378 adults, found that individuals who perceived their health status to be good reported a higher frequency of health-promoting behaviors than individuals who perceived their health status to be poor. Pender and Pender,[28] in studying 377 adults, found that perceived health status was a significant determinant of behavioral intentions to attain or maintain recommended weight. Individuals who perceived themselves to be in good health reported more frequent intentions to control weight than persons reporting that their health status was fair or poor. Dishman et al.[29] concluded from review of studies focused on the determinants of participation in supervised exercise programs that perceptions of being in good health are repeatedly associated with an increased probability of continuing exercise behavior.[29]

Perceived Benefits of Health-Promoting Behaviors. A number of studies have provided evidence that perceived benefits of health-promoting behaviors affect level of participation in such behaviors. In comparing 30 middle-aged males with low-frequency participation in a program of physical activity with 30 males with high-frequency participation, Brunner[30] found marked differences in perceived personal benefits. High-frequency participants ranked keeping fit physically as the most important benefit, while low-frequency participants ranked keeping physically fit fifth in importance. The low-frequency participants ranked the short-term benefit of relaxation at the end of the day as the major benefit of the physical activity program. The data suggest that the perception of long-term benefits rather than short-term benefits from health-promoting behavior may determine frequency of participation and predisposition to continue health-enhancing behaviors.

Sidney and Shephard,[31] in studying 42 elderly men and women participating in supervised physical training, found that individuals who participated more frequently and more intensively than others showed greater awareness of the importance of health and fitness as a benefit and greater appreciation of physical activity as an aesthetic experience. Perception of benefits from health-promoting behavior appears to facilitate continued practice. In addition, repetition of the behavior itself appears to strengthen and reinforce beliefs about benefits.

Perceived Barriers to Health-Promoting Behavior. Within the revised Health Promotion Model, *perceived barriers* has been identified as a cognitive–perceptual factor which, parallel to perceived benefits, exerts a direct influence on predisposition to engage in health-promoting behavior. Barriers to health-promoting behaviors may be imagined or real and consist of perceptions concerning the unavailability, inconvenience, or difficulty of a particular health-promoting option.

A number of studies have supported the importance of barriers as a determinant of frequency of health-promoting behaviors. For instance, inaccessibility of or distance from an exercise facility has been found by a number of investigators to decrease involvement of adults of varying ages in physical fitness activities.[32–34] Still other investigators[35] found that high intensity of exercise early in physical fitness programs appeared to be a barrier to continuing participation in the program for some individuals who considered the activity too strenuous. Dishman et al.[36] concluded that perceived available time and easy access to facilities were important environmental characteristics that promoted exercise adherence.

Potential or actual barriers to engaging in health-promoting behaviors should be identified for persons of varying ages as well as for families and other aggregates. In addition, the extent to which barriers inhibit specific health behaviors and the adoption of a healthful life style needs further clarification.

Additional Refinements of Cognitive–Perceptual Factors Within the Model. Both self-awareness and self-esteem, components of the Health Promotion Model as originally proposed, have been deleted from the revised model. Self-awareness is a general and rather ambiguous personal characteristic that is not well operationalized. Thus, problems of measuring such a concept are formidable. While the positive impact of self-esteem on physical performance has received some support, there is only limited empirical evidence that self-esteem affects level of participation in health-promoting behaviors. While it may be that individuals who regard themselves highly are more likely to set aside time to nourish personal health than people with low self-esteem, the general rather than specific nature of self-esteem as a personal characteristic may weaken its potential for predicting specific health actions.

Summary. Cognitive–perceptual factors that are proposed in the Health Promotion Model as directly affecting predisposition to engage in health-promoting behaviors include: importance of health, perceived control of health, perceived self-efficacy, definition of health, perceived health status, perceived benefits of health-promoting behaviors, and perceived barriers to health-promoting behaviors. Research is in progress to determine the extent to which the cognitive–perceptual factors identified in the model singly or in additive or multiplicative combination explain exercise habits and life style patterns among adults.

Modifying Factors

Demographic Factors. Characteristics such as age, sex, race, ethnicity, education, and income are proposed within the model as affecting patterns of health-promoting behavior indirectly through their impact on cognitive–perceptual mechanisms. For instance, Sidney and Shephard[37] found that only women identified psychological well-being as an important outcome of exercise, while both men and women believed that improved fitness was a major benefit. Also, when older adults were compared to middle-aged individuals on perceived value of exercise, older adults valued exercise as an aesthetic experience more than the other age group.[38]

In studies of use of preventive services, women rather than men, highly educated versus less well educated, and high-income rather than low-income individuals show more frequent utilization. The extent to which demographic characteristics influence participation in health behavior and the similarities and differences between demographic influences on health-protecting versus health-promoting behavior need to be determined. A closer look at demographic variables and their impact on health actions will clarify critical differences among age, sex, or ethnic groups that must be considered in structuring appropriate health promotion programs.

Biological Characteristics. A number of biological factors have been found to be related to exercise adherence. Pender and Pender[39] found weight to be a significant predictor of intention to engage in exercise. The higher the total body weight, the lower the intention to exercise regularly. In several studies,[40-42] percent body fat and total body weight discriminated consistently between exercise program adherers and dropouts, with overweight people finding it more difficult to continue with regular exercise when compared to individuals with less body fat or lower weight.

Interpersonal Influences. Interpersonal factors that are proposed within the model as modifying influences on health-promoting behaviors include expectations of significant others, family patterns of health care, and interactions with health professionals. The impact of these factors on health behavior has received support from research findings.

In studying the responses of 239 men to a physical activity program, Heinzelmann[43] found that the expectations of significant others—in this case, the spouses—were important in the men's continuing participation in the program. Although few men reported joining the program primarily as a result of pressure from their wives, positive attitudes toward the program on the part of their wives were critical to continuing participation and program adherence. Eighty percent of those men with wives exhibiting positive attitudes had excellent or good adherence patterns. Only 40 percent of men with wives exhibiting neutral or negative attitudes had excellent or good adherence.

In a study to determine the relative impact of personal attitudes and expectations of others on the occurence of health-promoting behaviors, Pender and Pender[44] found that exercising regularly was significantly influenced by both factors. Family members, but spouses in particular, exerted an important influence on exercise behavior. Further research is needed to determine the mechanisms through which family members influence participation in health behaviors. The dynamics of family impact on the emergence and continuation of health-enhancing life styles is also an important area for investigation.

Interactions with health professionals constitute another source of interpersonal influence on health-promoting behavior. Sidney and Shephard[45] found that an important reason for participation of the adults that they studied in a physical activity program was the instruction and guidance offered by health professionals. In fact, competent direction of the program by health professionals ranked second in the reasons for participation.

Cox[46] has developed an interactional model of client health behavior that focuses on the interpersonal influence of health professionals on client actions. Empirical testing of the model has indicated its potential usefulness in explaining the occurrence of health behaviors.

Situational Factors. Important situational or environmental determinants of health-promoting behavior appear to include health-promoting options available and ease of access to health-promoting alternatives. The availability of a range of behavioral options increases the opportunity to make responsible choices. For example, if low-cholesterol, low-calorie, or low-sodium meals are not available when one is dining out, there is little opportunity in that situation to behave in a healthful way. Also, if vending machines are stocked with foods high in refined sugars and low in nutritional value, options for healthy behavior by school-age children, industrial workers, and office personnel are limited. Individuals may wish to behave in ways that promote health, but environmental constraints prevent access to healthful options.

Behavioral Factors. Previous experience with health-promoting actions increases the ability of people to carry out various behaviors to promote well-being. Some of the cognitive and psychomotor skills necessary to plan nutritious meals, maintain an exercise program, and deal with stress may have been learned previously from participation in similar activities. Previously acquired knowledge and skills can facilitate the implementation of complex health-promoting behaviors. Dishman et al.[47] identified past physical fitness program participation as a major factor positively influencing current involvement in exercise activities.

Summary. A number of modifying factors are proposed as indirectly influencing patterns of health behavior. These factors include: demographic characteristics, biological characteristics, interpersonal influences, situational factors, and behavioral factors. According to the Health Promotion Model, modifying factors exert their influence through the cognitive–perceptual mechanisms that directly affect behavior.

Cues to Action

The likelihood of taking health-promoting action is hypothesized also to depend on activating cues either of internal origin or emanating from the environment. Personal awareness of the potential for growth or increased feelings of well-being from beginning health promotion efforts may serve as important internal cues for behavior. For example, "feeling good" as a result of physical activity can serve as a cue for continuing exercise behavior.

Conversations with others regarding their patterns of exercise, nutrition habits, rest and relaxation, management of stress, and interpersonal relationships can serve as external cues for health promotion. The mass media are a source of cues for action through programs about personal health, family health, and environmental concerns. The intensity of the cues needed to trigger action will depend on the level of readiness of the individual or group to engage in health-promoting activity.

STAGES OF HEALTH BEHAVIOR

A review of health-promotion literature, especially in the areas of exercise and weight loss, suggests there is a distinction between the period of initial involvement in a health-promoting behavior and continuing involvement. A number of health-enhancing behaviors are characterized by a rapid dropout rate within the first 3 to 6 months of initial involvement and a plateau or stabilized dropout rate after that point.[48] This pattern is consistent with a distinction between short-term (1 to 6 months) and long-term (more than 6 months) behavioral stages. Dishman[49] has postulated the existence of distinct adherence stages of health behavior based on several studies suggesting that determinants of health behavior may be different when an expanded time frame is considered. The initial stage of health behavior is referred to by Dishman as the *acquisition stage* and the period of continuation as the *maintenance stage.*

The validity of stage theory is being tested in the research program grant, "Health-Promoting Behavior: Testing a Proposed Model," that was described earlier in this chapter. If differing constellations of cognitive–perceptual factors influence health-promoting behavior during the acquisition and maintenance stages, interventions for facilitating behavior during each stage may differ considerably.

SUMMARY

The Health Promotion Model described in this chapter provides an organizing framework for theory development and research in the area of health-promoting behavior. Literature supporting inclusion of various factors in the revised model is presented. Research that tests the explanatory potential of the Health Promotion Model is in progress. The research program extends over 3 years and consists of projects focusing on working adults, older adults, ambulatory cancer patients, and cardiac rehabilitation clients. Stage theory as proposed by Dishman provides a temporal framework for considering the development and stabilization of health-promoting behaviors. The Health Promotion Model is proposed as an explanation of why individuals engage in health actions. Models to explain health-promoting behaviors of families and communities must yet be developed.

REFERENCES

1. White, R. W. Motivation reconsidered: The concept of competence. *Psychological Review*, 1959, *66*, 297–333.
2. Wallston, K. A., Maides, S., & Wallston, B. S. Health-related information seeking as a function of health-related locus of control and health value. *Journal of Research in Personality*, 1976, *10*, 215–222.
3. Christiansen, K. E. *The determinants of health promoting behavior*. Unpublished doctoral dissertation, Rush University, Chicago, 1981.
4. Laffrey, S. C., & Isenberg, M. The relationship of internal locus of control, value placed on health, perceived importance of exercise, and participation in physical activity during leisure. *International Journal of Nursing Studies*, 1983, *20*(3), 187–196.
5. Williams, A. F. Factors associated with seat belt use in families. *Journal of Safety Research*, 1972, *4*, 133–138.
6. James, W. H., Woodruff, A. B., & Werner, W. Effect of internal and external control upon changes in smoking behavior. *Journal of Consulting Psychology*, 1965, *29*, 184–186.
7. Best, J. A., & Steffy, R. A. Smoking modification tailored to subject characteristics. *Behavior Therapy*, 1971, *2*, 177–191.
8. Wallston, B. S., Wallston, K. A., Kaplan, G. D., & Maides, S. A. Development and validation of the health locus of control (HLC) scale. *Journal of Consulting Clinical Psychology*, 1976, *44*, 580–585.
9. Brown, N. J., Muhlenkamp, A. F., Fox, L. M., & Osborn, M. The relationship among health beliefs, health values, and health promotion activity. *Western Journal of Nursing Research*, 1983, *5*, 155–163.
10. Laffrey & Isenberg, op. cit.
11. Saltzer, E. B. *Causal beliefs and losing weight: A study of behavioral intention theory and locus of control in the prediction of health-related behavior*. Unpublished doctoral dissertation, 1979, University of California at Irvine.
12. Stein, M. J., Smith, M., & Wallston, K. A. Cross-cultural issues of health locus of control beliefs. *Psychological Studies*, 1984, *29*(1), 112–116.
13. Bandura, A. Self-efficacy: Toward a unifying theory of behavioral change. *Psychological Review*, 1977, *84*, 119–215.
14. DiClemente, C. C. Self-efficacy and smoking cessation maintenance: A preliminary report. *Cognitive Therapy and Research*, 1981, *5*, 175–187.
15. Condiotte, M. M., & Lichtenstein, E. Self-efficacy and relapse in smoking cessation programs. *Journal of Consulting and Clinical Psychology*, 1981, *49*, 648–658.
16. Brown, I., & Inouye, D. K. Learned helplessness through modeling: The role of perceived similarity in competence. *Journal of Personality and Social Psychology*, 1978, *36*, 900–908.
17. Weinberg, R. S., Gould, D., & Jackson, A. Expectations and performance: An empirical test of Bandura's self-efficacy theory. *Journal of Sport Psychology*, 1979, *1*, 320–331.
18. Chambliss, C. A., & Murray, E. J. Efficacy attribution, locus of control, and weight loss. *Cognitive Therapy and Research*, 1979, *3*, 349–354.
19. Atkins, C. J., Kaplan, R. M., Timms, R. M., et al.: Behavioral exercise programs in the mangement of chronic obstructive pulmonary disease. *Journal of Consulting and Clinical Psychology*, 1984, *52*(4), 591–603.

20. Dishman, R. K., Sallis, J. F., & Orenstein, D. R. The determinants of physical activity and exercise. *Public Health Reports*, March–April, 1985, *100*(2), 158–171.
21. Christiansen, op. cit.
22. Laffrey, S. C. Health behavior choice as related to self-actualization, body weight, and health conception. *Dissertation Abstracts International*, 1982, *43*, 3536B (University Microfilms No. 83-06904).
23. Smith, J. A. *The idea of health.* New York: Teachers College Press, 1983.
24. Sidney, K. H., & Shephard, R. J. Attitudes toward health and physical activity in the elderly: Effects of a physical training program. *Medicine and Science in Sports*, 1976, *8*, 246–252.
25. Kaplan, G. D., & Cowles, M. A. Health locus of control and health value in their prediction of smoking reduction. *Health Education Monographs*, 1978, *6*, 129–137.
26. Palmore, E., & Luikart, C. Health and social factors related to life satisfaction. *Journal of Health and Social Behavior*, 1972, *13*, 68–80.
27. Christiansen, op. cit.
28. Pender, N. J., & Pender, A. R. Attitudes, subjective norms and intentions to engage in health behaviors. *Nursing Research*, 1986, *35*, 15–18.
29. Dishman, Sallis, & Orenstein, op. cit.
30. Brunner, B. C. Personality and motivational factors influencing adult participation in vigorous physical activity. *Research Quarterly*, 1969, *40*, 464–469.
31. Sidney & Shephard, op. cit., pp. 250–252.
32. Andrew, G. M., & Parker, J. O. Factors related to dropout of post myocardial infarction patients from exercise programs. *Medicine and Science in Sports and Exercise*. 1979, *11*, 376–378.
33. Andrews, G. M., Oldridge, N. B., Parker, J. O., et al.: Reasons for dropout from exercise programs in post coronary patients. *Medicine and Science in Sports and Exercise*, 1981, *13*, 164–168.
34. Morgan, W. P. Involvement in vigorous physical activity with special reference to adherence. In L. I. Gedvilas, & M. E. Kneer (Eds.), *National College Physical Education Association Proceedings*, 1977, Chicago: University of Illinois.
35. Pollock, M. L., Gettman, L. R., Milesis, et al. Effects of frequency and duration of training on attrition and incidence of injury. *Medicine and Science in Sports*, 1977, *9*, 31–36.
36. Dishman, Sallis, & Orenstein, op. cit.
37. Sidney & Shephard, op. cit., 247–249.
38. Massie, J. F., & Shephard, R. J. Physiological and psychological effects of training. *Medicine and Science in Sports*, 1971, *3*, 110–117.
39. Pender & Pender, op. cit.
40. Dishman, R. K., & Gettman, L. R. Psychobiologic influences on exercise adherence. *Journal of Sport Psychology*, 1980, *2*, 295–310.
41. Dishman, R. K. Biologic influences on exercise adherence. *Research Quarterly for Exercise and Sport*, 1981, 52, 143–159.
42. Pollock, M. L., Foster, C., Salisbury, R., & Smith, R. Effects of a YMCA starter fitness program. *The Physician and Sports Medicine*, 1982, *10*, 89–102.
43. Heinzelman, F., & Bagley, R. W. Response to physical activity programs and their effects on health behavior. *Public Health Reports*, 1970, *85*, 905–911.
44. Pender & Pender, op. cit.
45. Sidney & Shephard, op. cit.

46. Cox, C. An interaction model of client health behavior: Theoretical prescription for nursing. *Advances in Nursing Science*, 1982, *5*, 41–56.
47. Dishman, Sallis, & Orenstein, op. cit.
48. Dishman, R. K. Compliance–adherence in health-related exercise. *Health Psychology*, 1982, *1*, 237–267.
49. Dishman, ibid., 254–258.

PART II

Prevention and Health Promotion: Establishing Client Relationships

The purpose of this section is to familiarize the nurse with the many contexts in which health promotion services can be offered to clients of all ages. In Chapter 4, an overview of traditional and nontraditional settings for health promotion is presented. In Chapter 5, the dimensions of the nurse–client relationship for health promotion are described. Many new practice opportunities in worksites, schools, nursing centers, and other community agencies are becoming available to creative and innovative professional nurses.

CHAPTER **4**

Settings for Health Promotion

If health professionals are going to address the challenges inherent in health promotion, individuals, families, communities, and the environment must be targets for wellness activities.[1] In this chapter, the family, schools, work-sites, hospitals, nursing centers, and the community at large will be discussed as settings for the development of self-care competencies and health-promoting life styles among people of all ages.

HEALTH PROMOTION IN FAMILIES

Health values, attitudes, and behaviors are learned in the family context. The place of health in the family value structure and the extent to which health-promoting knowledge and skills are transmitted to offspring determine the degree of impact that families have on the health potential of future generations. While the family provides a context for individual health actions, it is a unit of health behavior analysis in its own right.[2] Just as individuals must assume increased responsibility for their own health status, so families must assume similar responsibilities for the family structure as a whole. Structural and functional features of the family that must be considered when attempting to influence health practices include value structure, role structure, power structure (decision-making patterns), communication patterns, affective function, socialization function, health care function, and coping function. Specific questions that should be explored in relation to family values, beliefs, and life style include:[3]

1. How does the family unit define health?
2. What health-promoting behaviors does the family engage in regularly?
3. Are these behaviors characteristic of all family members or are patterns of health-promoting behavior highly variable throughout the family system?
4. Is there consistency between family health values as stated and their health actions?
5. What are the explicit or implicit goals of the family in the area of health?

In analyzing the family as a setting for health promotion, variant family forms in addition to the traditional nuclear family must be taken into consideration. Some of the variant family forms are: one-parent families (most often mother only), blended families (parts of two pre-existing families), extended families (nuclear plus a relative, often older), augmented families (additional members, not blood relations), married adult dyads, and unmarried adult dyads (blood and nonblood relations).

Duffy,[4] in studying one-parent families headed by women, a family form found increasingly in Western society, noted a number of differences from other family constellations: the resources of only one adult are available, children must assume a greater number of family-oriented roles, and sources of stress differ both quantitatively and qualitatively from those found in other family types. While the one-parent family is sometimes considered a transitional stage ended by remarriage, an increasing number of single parents are remaining single and raising children to adulthood.

The nurse working with families in the area of health promotion must be sensitive to both the commonalities and differences across varying family forms. Qualitative studies of family form and related life styles are critical to the formulation of theories helpful in understanding the milieu for the promotion of health in families of varying types.

Unfortunately, little is known about the dynamics of health in families. Reutter[5] has proposed integration of Friedman's[6] structural–functional approach to the family with Orem's[7] self-care nursing framework as a basis for a theory of family health that can be applied to all family forms. Friedman's framework was suggested because it views the family in the context of subsystems (triads, dyads, or individuals). Orem's framework was chosen because self-care actions on the part of families are critical to the health promotion process. According to Orem, the appropriate nursing system to meet families' needs for health-promotive care is the supportive–educative system in which families are assisted by the nurse in overcoming their self-care limitations through education and supportive counseling. Synthesis of existing theories and their subsequent testing may be a fruitful approach for the development of new theories undergirding the promotion of health in families.

The patterns of communication established in a family can either facilitate or block cohesive and purposeful family functioning. When a family can articulate shared goals, plan together to achieve goals, implement plans, evaluate goal attainment, and revise goals as necessary, families maintain their evolution as a dynamic and effective group.

A sense of togetherness or cohesion within the family provides the support and feedback necessary for growth. In addition, family support appears to act as a buffer against the hurts and challenges of daily life. Effectively functioning families provide members with a sense of belonging, security, and encouragement.[8]

Most nursing care is delivered to families during transition periods such as transition to parenthood or developmental transitions of children. Nursing care directed at health promotion is no exception. However, the transitions of interest to nurses focused on health promotion are life-style transitions. Important steps in life-style transitions in the family unit include: evaluating current life style, planning for behavior change, implementing changes to enhance family health, evaluating family outcomes. Through supportive–educative care, family members can be encouraged to perceive themselves as competent and in control of family health status.

The well family demonstrates a spectrum of abilities, insights, and strengths. It is a dynamic unit whose members are engaged in tasks aimed at both personal development and continuation of the family system.[9] The challenge for the nurse is to assist the family unit in identifying relevant health goals and in planning for life-style changes that will not only begin but continue as an ongoing family commitment.

HEALTH PROMOTION IN THE SCHOOL

With approximately 46 to 48 million students enrolled in elementary and secondary schools across the nation, school-based health promotion programs can exert a major influence on the acquisition of health-promoting behaviors among children and adolescents. Critical functions of such programs include:

1. Promote acquisition of knowledge and skills for competent self-care and informed decision making about health
2. Reinforce positive health attitudes
3. Structure environment and social influences to support health-promoting behaviors
4. Facilitate growth and self-actualization
5. Sensitize students to aspects of the environment and Western culture that are detrimental to health and well-being

Health-promoting behaviors are acquired more readily in childhood, when routines and habits are less stabilized. In addition, habits or behaviors developed in childhood and adolescence are more likely to persist as an integral part of life style than changes made in health behaviors later in the adult years.

In 1974, the President's Committee on Health Education reported that school health programs were hindered by antiquated laws, indifferent parents, passive school boards, poorly prepared teachers, lack of governmental leadership, lack of funds, lack of scientifically sound knowledge on which to base programs, and lack of sound plans for evaluation.

Few studies evaluating school health programs have measured behavioral outcomes; most have focused on changes in knowledge and attitudes. Lack of evidence that health education in the schools can modify the behaviors and life styles of children and adolescents and current economic constraints have led to the widespread reduction of financial support for school health programs.[10] This is an ironic state of affairs, given the increasing national emphasis on prevention and health promotion for citizens of all ages. While numerous articles in the national press lament the toll that unhealthy life styles take on individuals throughout the life span, little attention is given to the critical period for health promotion that the childhood and adolescent years represent.

Kolbe and Iverson,[11] in emphasizing the important role of schools in the development of health-promoting behaviors among youth, commented:

> Having completed their high school education, no adult should be ignorant about the consequences of individual decisions and social actions that ultimately will influence the health of their families and the communities in which the families reside. To the extent that the educational system fails to gain pace in disseminating and accumulating the complex understandings about health and human actions that influence it, we can expect that our people will be considerably less healthy than they could be.

According to Bartlett,[12] successful school health programs have the following characteristics:

1. Based on an in-depth understanding of behavioral science principles and theories
2. Exhibit a high level of student, peer group, and family involvement
3. Coordinate with and utilize other community resources
4. Contribute to community health promotion efforts

Health-promoting life styles can best be achieved by the school-age population when families, health professionals, and community organizations support school health programming goals and efforts. A supportive environment for health-promoting life styles creates a favorable climate for continuing growth and self-actualization on the part of children of all ages.

Perry and Murray[13] stress the importance of considering the developmental stages of children and adolescents in structuring school health-promotion programs. They identify four environmental structures of influence that affect the health behaviors of the school-age population. The most important is the *model structure*, which includes the actual behavior of significant others. Children are greatly influenced by the food selections, exercise habits, coping methods, smoking habits, and alcohol use of parents, teachers, and friends. The *network structure* consists of loosely organized groups that interact regularly with one another, such as peer groups, neighborhoods, and organizations to which children or adolescents may belong. Establishing health promotion programs in existing support networks may lead to more successful development of health behaviors than randomly grouping the school-age population for purposes of behavior change. The *social system structure* of which the child or adolescent is a member plays a critical role in health. For instance, the school as a social system regulates to a considerable degree the options and choices available to the school-age population for a considerable portion of each day. Schools can have psychologically, socially, and ecologically unhealthy environments that pose threats to students' well-being. The *community message structure* is the fourth influence on health behaviors of school-age children. Television programming, advertisements, community resources, and government regulations shape attitudes toward health behaviors.

Several models for school health education have been described in the literature. Dennison[14] described activated health education as a behaviorally based instructional model that focuses on the active involvement of participants in personal health assessment, awareness of health values in decision-making, and the assumption of personal responsibility for health and self-care. This approach to health education for children and adolescents consists of three phases: the experiential phase, in which students engage in self-assessment, including measurement and recording of indicators of personal health status; the awareness phase, during which students assess positive and negative influences on personal health and evaluate their susceptibility to various illnesses; and the responsibility phase, during which students clarify their personal health values, determine actual and ideal health behaviors, identify barriers to establishing ideal behavior, establish personal behavioral goals, and develop a self-management program of illness prevention and health promotion.

Rustia[15] proposes a school health-promotion model in which an interdisciplinary school health team is constituted with the goal of working together to maximize the potential for learning and participation in the educational process by promoting optimal health. Within the model, the targets for intervention are students, families, teachers, and supportive personnel, as well as the community as a whole. The following behavioral outcomes are identified for students:

1. Make responsible and informed decisions on health care
2. Differentiate between concepts of health and illness
3. Recognize individual health status characteristics
4. Know how to locate and utilize resources to achieve optimal health status
5. Recognize potential health and safety hazards

The model focuses on utilization of the education, service, and environmental maintenance personnel within schools to create a milieu for health promotion that is comprehensive and integrated.

Igoe[16] describes still another model for school health education that is focused on preparing children and adolescents for a participatory and assertive health consumer role. In a comprehensive program entitled Project Health PACT, school-aged children are encouraged to practice the following five approaches to getting the most out of encounters with health personnel:

1. Ask questions
2. Personally communicate information about themselves to the health professional
3. Encourage the health professional to provide them with health instruction
4. Participate with the health professional in making decisions about their health: express their opinions about the acceptability of the health professional's advice so that the health plan developed meets their special needs
5. Clarify what responsibilities they are to assume for their own health on a day-to-day basis before leaving the health facility

Manuals, workshops, and training programs are provided to school districts who desire to institute the program. Unique program materials are available, such as health history forms written at the appropriate grade level, filmstrips depicting the assertive consumer role, a special appointment book in which children can schedule appointments with the school nurse, anatomical models, health books, charts, and games. Project PACT, because of its targeted focus, supplements health courses in most of the schools in which it is introduced.

The program was developed by school nurse-practitioner faculty at the University of Colorado after a review of children's literature revealed the passive role depicted for children in interaction with health professionals. The program is flexible and can be offered in school settings or adapted to clinics or physician offices. The emphasis of the program on the assertive consumer who utilizes health professionals as consultants on personal health matters is philosophically in harmony with current illness-prevention and health-promotion efforts that focus on individual responsibility for health status.

School health programs should familiarize students with the importance of both individual and societal responsibility for health. Not only should experience with health-promoting life styles be offered, but sources of environmental pollution and sociopolitical strategies available to consumers to address such problems should be discussed. A comprehensive school health program can provide: (1) support for healthful living on the part of children and adolescents, (2) enhanced quality of life in the adult years, and (3) a life style conducive to successful aging and extended longevity.

HEALTH PROMOTION AT THE WORKSITE

Over the past decade, employers have accepted increased responsibility for the health of their employees. With concern about the high cost of health insurance benefits, employers have been attracted to prevention and health-promotion initiatives. While limited information is currently available on the impact of health-promotion programs in industry, data suggest that such programs may increase productivity, decrease absenteeism, decrease use of expensive medical care, and lower disability claims.

A 1983 survey of 424 companies in California revealed that 78 percent offered some type of prevention or health promotion program to employees. The program provided most frequently, that is, by 65 percent of the companies surveyed, focused on accident prevention. Other programs reported were: cardiopulmonary resuscitation (53 percent), alcohol and drug abuse (19 percent), mental health counseling (18 percent), stress management (13 percent), fitness (12 percent), hypertension screening (10 percent), and smoking cessation (8 percent).[17] A 1983 survey of 300 companies in Colorado indicated that the vast majority of health-promotion and disease-prevention programs in the state were less than 5 years old. Fifty-five percent of the programs were started between 1980 and 1983. Improved employee morale was perceived as the most frequent benefit among companies surveyed (81 percent). Other benefits perceived by the companies were: improved employee health (52 percent), improved productivity (46 percent), reduced illness and injury on the job (46 percent), reduced employee turnover and absenteeism (40 percent), reduced medical care utilization (30 percent), and attracted better-caliber applicants (17 percent).[18] It is predicted that by 1990, over half of all companies in the United States will offer some aspect of wellness programming for their employees.[19]

All businesses share a dependency on human resources. Today, when corporations in the United States are working to improve their competitiveness in the world marketplace, a healthy labor force is especially important. Employers are realizing that every dollar spent on prevention and health promotion today may save $10 or $100 in the future.[20]

The major benefits of workplace health-promotion programs as identified by O'Donnell[21] are shown in Figure 4–1. However, more data is needed concerning the impact of employer-sponsored health-promotion programs on employee health, quality of life, longevity, and corporate costs and profits.

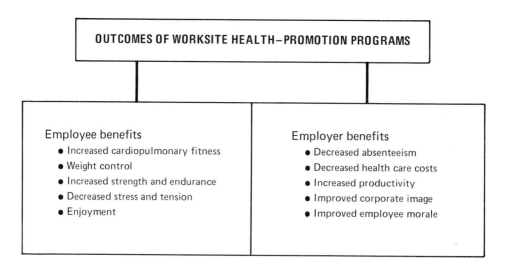

Figure 4–1. Projected outcomes of worksite health-promotion programs.

A definite advantage of health-promotion activities at the worksite is that they create a cultural milieu that supports and rewards health-promoting behaviors. The social and physical environments of corporations can be altered to increase their health-enhancing potential. As behaviors of employees and characteristics of the work environment change, new social norms emerge that positively influence health.[22]

Golaszewski and Prabhaker,[23] in emphasizing the importance of applying marketing strategies to health-promotion efforts in the workplace, stress the need to seek employee input in planning health-promotion programs. The employee input phase involves an analysis of the concerns, beliefs, attitudes, and priorities of employees. Surveys, interviews, or group meetings can be used to obtain employee input.[23] Initiating a pilot health promotion program on a small scale allows "debugging" and refinement of program initiatives and an opportunity for additional employee input before beginning program efforts corporation-wide.

Offering a variety of health-promotion programs at the worksite, using differing approaches, increases the appeal of the program to employees of varying cultural backgrounds and of differing ages. Considerations in marketing health-promotion programs include: (1) the programs should be well-defined and priced to sell, (2) immediate personal benefits from participation should be publicized, (3) barriers to participation should be minimized, and (4) programs should be individualized for all participants.[24]

Reward or incentive programs also play a crucial role in motivating employees to begin and sustain health promotion efforts. Various approaches to incentives include: a point system with prizes for point accumulation, team competition, return of membership fee in installments based on level of participation, and monthly employee profiles reporting miles run and caloric expenditure. Other motivational devices include a kickoff health party, development of an employee health committee, posters, slogans, and T-shirts. In addition to tangible rewards, social rewards such as group reinforcement and team spirit contribute to employee motivation to make health-enhancing changes in life style.

Worksite health-promotion programs offer many advantages. These include:[25]

1. Most employees go to the workplace on a regular schedule, facilitating regular participation in the programs
2. Contact with co-workers can provide reinforcing social support, a primary force in sustaining life style change
3. The workplace offers many opportunities for environmental supports, such as healthy food in the cafeteria, office policies regarding smoking, and aesthetic work space
4. Opportunities abound for positive reinforcement for employees participating in the program
5. Programs in the workplace are generally less expensive for the employee than comparable programs in the community
6. Programs in the workplace are conveniently located

Evaluation of the impact of worksite health-promotion programs is complicated by several factors such as: lack of uniform methods for measuring cost savings across departments and corporations, inadequate systems to measure short-term outcomes, insufficient time to measure long-term impact, the synergistic effect of unhealthy life style and exposure to hazardous substances, and employee mobility.[26] However, epidemiological studies indicate that worksite health-promotion programs may result in cost savings. If all employees in the country were of average fitness, it is estimated that the cost of insurance plans could be reduced by $45 million per year. Disability following retirement might also be reduced considerably by corporate health-promotion programs.[27]

Health-promotion initiatives at the worksite will continue to grow and expand into the twentieth century. Since the majority of adults spend many of their waking hours at their places of employment, corporations and industries will play an increasingly vital role in maintaining the health of the nation. For a comprehensive review of issues related to health-promotion and disease-prevention programs at the worksite, the reader is referred to Fielding.[28]

Despite the progress that has been made to date in the development of worksite health programs, many of these efforts are geared primarily to white-collar workers. Little attention has been given to developing health-promotion programs in heavy industry, where there is a preponderance of blue-collar workers. The challenge of tailoring health-promotion programs to industrial workers remains largely unmet. This should be a primary focus of health-promotion efforts in the workplace within the next decade.

HOSPITAL-BASED HEALTH-PROMOTION PROGRAMS

Over the last decade, community hospitals have become increasingly involved in health-promotion efforts. Some hospitals have incorporated health-promotion concepts into ongoing programs such as cardiac rehabilitation. Realizing that persons who have experienced a recent catastrophic illness such as a heart attack may have a high degree of readiness to learn, fitness, nutrition, stress management, and smoking cessation programs often are an integral part of cardiac rehabilitation. Also, diabetic education programs are increasingly incorporating strategies such as exercise, good nutrition, and management of stress as a means of health enhancement and disease control. Since the historical mission of the hospital has been treatment of disease, illness prevention and health promotion represent new directions for provision of services.

Many hospitals began their health-promotion efforts with programs for their employees. Despite the responsibility that hospital personnel assume for the care of others, knowledge about health is often not applied to personal life styles. Health promotion for health care providers can improve the role-modeling capabilities of health professionals. Hospital employee programs for health promotion have focused most heavily on nutrition and weight control, stress management, and fitness. Unfortunately, little research is reported in the literature concerning the impact of wellness programs on the behaviors and life styles of hospital employees or on their viability as healthy role models for patient populations.

Another area in which health-promotion efforts of hospitals have expanded tremendously is community-oriented programming. Emphasis by hospitals on community programs to promote health has occurred for a variety of reasons:

1. Interest in serving the community as a comprehensive health center
2. Decreased income from inpatient services
3. Search for new sources of revenue
4. Pressure from the public to provide health services in addition to illness care
5. Interest in attracting new patients
6. Need for increased visibility and a more positive image

The economic climate for hospitals has shifted drastically. According to recent statistics, the rate of increase in health care costs has begun to taper off, the average length of hospital stay has declined by one day, and the number of admissions has decreased dramatically. Decreasing lengths of stay and decreasing revenues per admission mean less total income. Layoffs of hospital personnel are widespread. Some hospitals have closed, and many others are projected to close.[29] These multiple forces have caused hospitals to re-examine their mission. Frequently, the result of such examination is the reapportionment of efforts and resources toward health-promotion efforts within the community.

While some hospitals have mounted stellar health-promotion programs employing an interdisciplinary team of health-oriented professionals, others have utilized personnel employed in illness care without efforts to resocialize such personnel into the "culture of health promotion." Quality illness care characteristic of many hospitals does not automatically translate into quality prevention and health-promotion services for the general population. The expertise and skills needed in the respective areas of illness care and health promotion are quite different. While there is some overlap, the degree of overlap is small. Thus, hospitals run the risk of failure with health-promotion endeavors unless they carefully assess the expertise needed to plan and implement such programs. Hospitals that have achieved success in health-promotion programming realized the importance of hiring community health nurses rather than acute-care nurses, nutritionists rather than therapeutic dietitians, and exercise physiologists as opposed to rehabilitation therapists.

The American Hospital Association's policy on health promotion supports such programming as a critical strategy on the part of hospitals to optimize their long-term success and viability. The policy states:

> Hospitals have a responsibility to take a leadership role in helping ensure the good health of their communities. In addition to the primary mission of providing health care and related education to the sick and injured, the hospital has a responsibility to work with others in the community to assess the health status of the community, identify target areas and population groups for hospital-based and cooperative health promotion programs, develop programs to help upgrade the health in those target areas, ensure that persons who are apparently healthy have access to information about how to stay well and prevent disease, provide appropriate health education programs to aid those persons who choose to alter their personal health behavior or develop a more healthful lifestyle, and establish the hospital as an institution in the community that is concerned about treating illness.[30]

The Center for Health Promotion at the American Hospital Association focuses on encouraging the development of hospital-based health-promotion–wellness programs among its member hospitals. The Center provides newsletters, reports, consultations, and conferences to advance the health-promotion concept and to provide a networking mechanism for hospital administrative personnel incorporating wellness into the mission of their respective hospitals. In 1978, the Swedish Medical Center in Englewood, Colorado was one of the first hospitals to establish a wellness center staffed with full-time personnel. The program was highly successful and has since served as a model for the development of similar programs by other hospitals. With the economic potential of the health-promotion market and the increasing motivation on the part of hospitals to change their image to a more positive one, the development of health-promotion activities as an integral part of hospital services will gain momentum in the coming years.

HEALTH PROMOTION IN NURSING CENTERS

Nursing centers represent an ideal setting for health-promotion activities. While many nursing centers are relatively new, there are approximately 100 centers throughout the United States. Such centers offer a spectrum of services, from health promotion and primary care to counseling and support for the chronically ill.

The goals of most nursing centers incorporate both health promotion and health protection services. For example, the goals of one nursing center for ambulatory, well, older adults are described as follows:

1. Prevention and health maintenance through health teaching for biophysical and psychological concerns
2. Early detection of disease through individual health histories and examinations, as well as screening sessions
3. Health maintenance for persons with chronic conditions through teaching, monitoring health status, and mobilizing resources[31]

The philosophy of the same nursing center notes the following:

> The intradisciplinary nursing wellness center is a health clinic dedicated to preventive health care. As such, its services are designed to promote an optimal level of wellness for each individual, to explore both developmental and situational events that affect the individual's ability to carry out activities of daily living, and to assist in maintenance of the highest possible level of functioning, preserving dignity and independence.... The staff is dedicated to a belief in holistic, humanistic care. The individual is an active participant in the process of health care and interacts with community and with health care providers. Care should be facilitative rather than intrusive or overly directive. Care should capitalize on individual potential, not deficit.... [32]

The center seeks to support client coping mechanisms and mobilize client resources and supports by nursing care that is person-centered and holistic. A major emphasis is clients' assumption of responsibility for their own care. To accomplish this goal, group sessions are offered in areas such as developmental tasks of aging, obesity, and foot care. Screening sessions and outreach programs are also offered to older adults.

Neighborhood nursing offices (NNOs) provide another interesting example of the application of the nursing center "concept" by community health nurses in a city health department. In an effort to be creative and at the same time provide for the needs of the community, the city of Baltimore established over 35 nursing offices in neighborhoods throughout the city.[33] The primary focus of the NNOs is to "provide information for people seeking help in matters of health, in order to prevent serious illness."[34] Each NNO is staffed by one community health nurse and one community health aide. Some offices also have volunteer helpers. Services provided include health assessment, health screening, individual and group teaching, counseling and referral, and crisis intervention. News of the NNOs was spread about through neighborhood newspapers, organization newsletters, posters, fliers, and church bulletins. The NNOs coordinate their work with other community health programs such as the city's High Blood Pressure Program, the Risk Reduction Program, and the Cancer Prevention Program. The program is serving groups in the community with whom community health nurses had limited contact prior to the establishment of NNOs: the elderly, young adults (including males), and the homeless. Nursing personnel report that they are seeing more people in less time and at less cost than by the traditional home visit.

The nurse-managed center in Milwaukee, Wisconsin, affiliated with the School of Nursing, University of Wisconsin-Milwaukee, offers family-oriented care. The center offers services such as family life style assessment, education in role management for working mothers, instruction in child stimulation and child development for new parents, and parenting skills for teenage mothers. The center has a full-time director responsible for planning and coordinating the program and a center nurse scientist who works with staff in planning and implementing practice-focused research projects.[35] The center is staffed by nurse faculty and nursing students. Thus, the missions of education, practice, and research are combined in an innovative way. The concept of a "center scientist" is a creative approach to structuring research projects in settings that are managed by nurses and where staff have autonomy in establishing nursing care protocols for clients at all stages of the life span. In addition, having nurse researchers affiliated with nurse-managed centers provides the opportunity for planning multisite research and demonstration projects across a number of centers. Such projects can have considerable impact on the acceptance of nurse-managed centers as feasible, economical, and effective approaches to the provision of health promotion and prevention services to the public.

Lang provides an interesting overview of the issues and concerns related to nurse-managed centers.[36] Issues such as the nature of nursing services—substitutive or additive—approaches to collaboration with physicians as partners in health care, appropriate preparation for practice in nurse-managed centers, and equitable plans of reimbursement for services are critical concerns that must be addressed if nurse-managed centers are to thrive and become an integral part of the health care system.

THE COMMUNITY AT LARGE AS A SETTING FOR HEALTH PROMOTION

Community-based health-promotion programs have many advantages over programs directed toward smaller aggregates. Weiss[37] has cited a number of benefits of the community-based intervention model:

1. It enhances opportunities for information exchange and social support among members of the target community
2. It reduces the unit cost of health promotion programming because large groups rather than individuals are the recipients of services
3. It allows for observation of the efficacy of health-promotion efforts and related health outcomes that may have policy implications

Other advantages of community-wide programming include:

4. Societal norms regarding health behavior are amenable to change over time as a result of community-wide programming
5. Comprehensive rather than piecemeal approaches to promotion of health can be implemented
6. Powerful interorganizational systems within the community can be used to facilitate health-promotion efforts

The Stanford three-community survey[38] conducted in 1971 through 1977 is one of the best known community-wide prevention projects. While the project focused on a specific disease, that is, lowering risk factors associated with cardiovascular disorders, it provided a model or prototype for community-based programs focused on health promotion. Within the study, mass media were used in one community for educational intervention. In a second community, intensive face-to-face counseling was used in addition to mass media education to lower risk factors. A third community served as a control, receiving no intervention.

Results from the study revealed that the health education intervention utilizing mass media resulted in a 20- to 40-percent decrease in cholesterol and saturated fat consumption among both men and women. Intensively counseled men decreased risk to a greater extent than men exposed to mass media alone. Women responded equally well to both interventions. Improvement in eating patterns appeared to be maintained over a 2-year period, indicating the potential of community interventions for producing long-term behavior change.

Following the three-community survey, the Stanford Heart Disease Prevention Program has initiated a second trial of community interventions, The Five City Project.[39] Two cities will receive educational interventions, while three cities will be used as controls. The major aim of the project is to determine if a significant decrease in risk for the experimental communities will lead to a decline in morbidity and mortality from cardiovascular disease that is greater than the current national downward trend. A 6-year education program to stimulate and maintain changes in life style will be implemented. The three goals of the community-based program are: to achieve a change in knowledge and skills of individuals and educational practices of schools and other institutions such that risk factor reduction and decreased morbidity and mortality are achieved; to carry out the intervention program in a way that creates a self-sustaining health-promotion structure within the organizational network of the community; and to derive a model for cost-effective community health promotion.

The Pawtucket Heart Health Project[40] is another example of community-wide prevention efforts that can serve as a prototype for approaches to community health-promotion programming. The goal of the project is to lower risk for cardiovascular disease by modifying life style. The community program focuses on reduction of the following factors: high blood pressure, smoking, high-cholesterol diet, obesity, sedentary life style, and high stress. The unique feature of the experimental program is that volunteers from the community lead the behavior change seminars and also design approaches for achieving supportive changes in organizations within the community. The goal of the project is a self-sustaining health-promotion effort within the community run with minimal reliance on health professionals.

Healthstyles[41] is an innovative health promotion demonstration project in Ottawa, Canada, funded by the W. W. Kellogg Foundation. The overall objective of the project is to promote the abandonment of unhealthy habits and the adoption of health-enhancing behaviors through intensive workshops and long-term follow-up of community residents.

The first component of the program, Healthstyle Basics[42] is a $2\frac{1}{2}$ day workshop that provides the opportunity for adults to assess the impact of their current life styles on personal health. Workshops are offered to 15 to 20 people who through group activities gain an understanding of what they can do to improve their health. The Healthstyles workshop focuses on four areas: nutrition, physical activity, stress management, and habits. The need to assume self-responsibility for acquiring and maintaining a healthy life style is emphasized. Workshop participants learn that the change process depends on *awareness* of changes that are needed, development and *acceptance* of a plan for change, and *adjustment* to the demands that changes in life style require.

After attendance at weekend workshops, the Healthstyles Support[43] program begins. Five sources of encouragement to maintain healthful changes in life style are provided: telephone support calls, follow-up group sessions to facilitate peer support and exchange of ideas, bimonthly health awareness sessions on a variety of topics, dissemination of health information, and individual counseling sessions as needed.

The project will compare 660 individuals participating in the program with 1320 nonparticipants to determine if there are differences between the groups on: (1) food choices, (2) physical activity, (3) stress management methods, (4) use of tobacco, alcohol and drugs, (5) weight control, (6) attitudes toward health, and (7) exercise of self-responsibility for health.

The potential of community-based health-promotion programs to improve the health of the public has not yet been determined. Few programs like Healthstyles exist to offer services or to allow for systematic evaluation of the concept in operation. Communities should be encouraged to develop such programs and to make well-planned program evaluation an integral part of their efforts.

SUMMARY

Multiple settings offer the opportunity for provision of health-promotion services. Nurses, particularly nurses with an understanding of community health issues and problems, are ideally suited to provide leadership in the design, development, implementation, and evaluation of health-promotion programs in schools, worksites, hospitals, nursing centers, and other community settings. Financial support for such programs should be sought from a variety of public and private sources. Consumers are becoming increasingly supportive of the development of health-promotion programs and facilities. Quality as well as length of life is emerging as a public concern. The health-promotion effort in many communities is a consumer-driven initiative. Nurses can help community residents capitalize on their interest in wellness by assisting them to identify their health-promotion needs. Secondly, nurses can provide leadership for health-promotion programming efforts in a wide array of community settings.

REFERENCES

1. Dunn, H. L. *High-level wellness*. Arlington, Va.: Beatty, 1973.
2. Gilliss, C. L. The family as a unit of analysis: Strategies for the nurse researcher. *Advances in Nursing Science, 5* 1983, (3), 50–59.
3. Pender, N. J. Health promotion: Implementing strategies. In B. Logan & C. Daw kins (Eds.), *Family-centered nursing in the community*. Menlo Park, Calif.: Addison-Wesley, 1986, 295–334.
4. Duffy, M. E. Transcending options: Creating a milieu for practicing high-level wellness. *Health Care for Women International*, 1984, *5*, 145–161.
5. Reutter, L. Family health assessment—an integrated approach. *Journal of Advanced Nursing*, 1984, *9* (4), 391–399.
6. Friedman, M. M. *Family nursing: Theory and assessment*. New York: Appleton-Century-Crofts, 1981.
7. Orem, D. E. *Nursing: Concepts of practice* (3rd ed.). New York: McGraw-Hill, 1985.

8. Petze, C. F. Health promotion for the well family. *Nursing Clinics of North America,* *19* (2), 229–237.
9. Ibid.
10. Green, L. W. Health promotion and research development. *Alabama Journal of the Medical Sciences,* 1984, *21*(2), 271–279.
11. Kolbe, L. J., & Iverson, D. C. Comprehensive school health education programs. In D. Matarazzo, S. Weiss, J. A. Herd, et al. (Eds.), *Behavioral health: A handbook of health enhancement and disease prevention.* New York: Wiley, 1984, 1094–1116.
12. Bartlett, E. E. The contribution of school health education to community health promotion: What can we reasonably expect. *American Journal of Public Health,* 1981, *71* (12), 1384–1391.
13. Perry, C. L., & Murray, D. M. Enhancing the transition years: The challenge of adolescent health promotion. *The Journal of School Health,* 1982, *5,* 307–311.
14. Dennison, D. Activated health education: The development and refinement of an intervention model. *Health Values: Achieving high-level wellness,* 1984, *8* (2), 18–24.
15. Rustia, J. Rustia school health promotion model. *The Journal of School Health,* 1982, *2,* 108–114.
16. Igoe, J. B. Project Health PACT in action. *American Journal of Nursing,* 1980, 2016–2021.
17. Fielding, J. E., & Breslow, L. Health promotion programs sponsored by California employers. *American Journal of Public Health,* 1983, *73,* 538–542.
18. Davis, M. F., Rosenberg, K., Iverson, D. C., et al. Worksite health promotion in Colorado. *Public Health Reports,* 1984, *99,* 538–543.
19. Toohey, J. V., & Shirreffs, J. H. Future trends in health education. *Health Education,* 1980, *2,* 15–17.
20. Gray, H. J. The role of business in health promotion: A brief overview. *Preventive Medicine,* 1983, *12,* 654–657.
21. O'Donnell, M. P. The corporate perspective. In M. P. O'Donnell & T. Ainsworth (Eds.), *Health promotion in the workplace.* New York: John Wiley, 1984, pp. 10–35.
22. Richard, E. A rationale for incorporating wellness programs into existing occupational health programs. *Occupational Health Nursing,* 1984, *32,* 412–415.
23. Golaszewski, T., & Prabhaker, P. Applying marketing strategies to worksite health promotion efforts. *Occupational Health Nursing,* 1984, *32,* 188–192.
24. Wilbur, C. S. The Johnson and Johnson Program. *Preventive Medicine,* 1983, *12,* 672–681.
25. Cohen, W. S. Health promotion in the workplace: A prescription for good health. *American Psychologist,* 1985, *40,* 213–216.
26. Richard, op. cit., p. 414.
27. Shephard, R. J. Employee health and fitness: The state of the art. *Preventive Medicine,* 1983, *12,* 644–653.
28. Fielding, J. E. Health promotion and disease prevention at the worksite. *Annual Review of Public Health,* 1984, *5,* 237–265.
29. Smith, J. P. Is bad health good business? *Optimal Health,* 1984, *1,* 14–16.
30. American Hospital Association. *Policy and statement: The hospital's responsibility for health promotion.* Chicago: American Hospital Association, 1979.
31. Hawkins, J. W., Igou, J. F., Johnson, E. E., & Utley, Q. E. A nursing center for ambulatory, well, older adults. *Nursing and Health Care,* 1984, *5* (4), 209–212.
32. Ibid., p. 210.

33. Grimes, R. E. Developing neighborhood nurse offices. *Nursing and Health Care,* 1983, *4* (3), 138–139.
34. Ibid.
35. Riesch, S. Nurse-scientist, Nurse-managed Center, University of Wisconsin-Milwaukee, School of Nursing, personal communication, April 1984.
36. Lang, N. Nurse-managed centers: Will they thrive? *American Journal of Nursing,* September 1983, 1291–1296.
37. Weiss, S. Community health promotion demonstration programs: Introduction. In J. D. Matarazzo, S. M. Weiss, J. A. Herd, et al. (Eds.), *Behavioral health: A handbook of health enhancement and disease prevention.* New York: Wiley, 1984, 1137–1139.
38. Stein, M. P., Farquhar, J. W., Maccoby, N., & Russell, S. H. Results of a two-year health education campaign on dietary behavior: The Stanford Three Community Study. *Circulation,* 1976, *54,* 826–832.
39. Farquhar, J. W., Fortmann, S. P., Maccoby, N., et al. The Stanford Five City Project: An overview. In J. D. Matarazzo, S. M. Weiss, J. A. Herd, et al. (Eds.), *Behavioral health: A handbook of health enhancement and disease prevention.* New York: Wiley, 1984, 1137–1139.
40. Abrams, D., & Elder, J. *Pawtucket Heart Health Program general theoretical model.* PHHP Technical Report, 1981.
41. Black, A., & McDowell, I. Healthstyles: moving beyond disease prevention. *Canadian Nurse,* 1984, *80,* 18–20.
42. O'Hagen, M. Healthstyles Basics: Lifestyle and behavior change. *Canadian Nurse,* 1984, 80, 21–23.
43. Kort, M. Support: An important component of health promotion. *Canadian Nurse,* 1984, 80, 24–26.

CHAPTER 5

Establishing Nurse–Client Relationships for Prevention and Health Promotion

The nature of the nurse–client relationship for illness prevention and health promotion will be explored in this chapter. The various settings in which nurses can establish health-promotive relationships with individuals and families have been described in Chapter 4. Unfortunately, only limited knowledge is currently available concerning the behavioral and biophysical mechanisms that facilitate movement of human beings toward optimal health. Thus, it is important for nurse-researchers and other health scientists to continue their quest to understand human health processes in order to provide a scientific basis for professional practice in prevention and health promotion. While the nurse–client relationship within the context of care in illness may be wholly or partially compensatory, providing care that the clients cannot accomplish for themselves, the nurse–client relationship for prevention and health promotion is educative–supportive in character.[1] In such a helping relationship, the ultimate goal is empowerment of the client for self-determination and self-management in order to enable attainment of high-level health and well-being.

Nurse–client relationships for prevention and health promotion are based on the following assumptions:

1. Individuals and families are ultimately responsible for their own health
2. Clients (individuals or groups) have an inherent capacity for change in constructive as well as destructive directions
3. Clients have a right to health information in order to make informed decisions concerning behavior and life-style choices

4. The health-seeking process occurs in the context of interpersonal and social relationships
5. Clients will engage in health behaviors that they find relevant personally and acceptable in their social context

The nurse–client relationship for prevention and health promotion must be based on a dynamic person–environment interactive model rather than on a traditional medical model. The nurse guides clients in the self-assessment of personal health status and in the exploration of their health situations, helping them "define concerns" rather than "offering solutions." Within a context of mutual respect, by deliberately posturing for less control, the nurse facilitates assumption of more control of their health situation by clients.[2]

The role of the nurse in prevention and health promotion is flexible and multifaceted. The nurse must possess the skills necessary to assist clients in the following activities:

1. Values clarification
2. Self-assessment
3. Goal setting
4. Information acquisition
5. Decision making
6. Planning behavior change
7. Implementing life-style modification
8. Sustaining health-promoting behaviors over time
9. Social support building

Self-directed health initiatives provide clients with a sense of power and control in their lives. As a result, they become "producers of health" rather than passive recipients of health care services.

The control dynamics of the nurse–client relationship described here differ considerably from traditional client–health professional relationships in the illness context, where concession or compliance are the identified goals. Often in illness-focused relationships, clients are given few options and minimal decision-making authority. Their capacities and strengths are ignored. Such relationships take away power from clients, leaving them resentful, guilt-ridden, and helpless. Through supportive relationships with clients in the context of health promotion, nurses can do a great deal to revitalize individuals' and families' faith in themselves, their sense of worth, and their ability to participate actively in the health care process.

In a health context, the nurse focuses on strength building as well as on assisting clients to decrease their limitations for optimizing personal health.[3] Actually, the relationship is that of client and consultant, since the nurse serves as an expert consultant to individuals and families as they determine and control the course of their health experience throughout the life span.

Prevention and health promotion consist of alternating phases of decision-making and action. Decision-making includes: (1) confronting a challenge, (2) identifying a goal and searching for alternatives to goal accomplishment, (3) considering the advantages and disadvantages of each alternative, (4) making a choice and becoming committed to a new course of action, and (5) discounting challenges to decision and renewing commitment to action. The stages of the action phase are acquisition and stabilization or maintenance of new behaviors. Phases of the nurse–client relationship that facilitate client progress through decision making and action will be described.

PHASES OF THE NURSE–CLIENT RELATIONSHIP

Establishment of a helping relationship is a formal or informal contract for services between nurse and client, indicating a mutual commitment on the part of both to work toward identified health priorities. The phases of the relationship can be identified as initial phase, transition phase, working phase, step-down phase, and follow-up. Successful implementation of all phases is necessary to provide continuity of care for clients.

Initial Phase
This phase of the nurse–client relationship begins with the first contact. Early interactions provide an opportunity for the nurse to explore with the client the nature of the services needed and the ways in which such services can be appropriately provided. The nurse's understanding of the client's health goals and expectations from the relationship provide the basis for quality care. It is important to stress that when clients seek services from the health care system, they are asking for assistance, not abdicating their rights as individuals.[4] The orientation of the professional nurse must be one of sustaining and enhancing the independence of clients while facilitating further developing of self-care competencies.

Nurses should be aware of their own "helping style" and evaluate its impact on clients with differing personalities, backgrounds, and life styles. Self-awareness on the part of nurses concerning how they work with clients is critical for meaningful self-evaluation and improvement of helping skills.

A major goal during the initial phase of the relationship is further arousal of the client's interest in improving personal or family health status and life style. The antecedents of decision-making and action begin when clients are confronted with a challenge to their current course of action through events or communications that convey threats or opportunities.[5] In the context of prevention, the challenge may be the threat of illness if action is not taken. In health promotion, the challenge is the opportunity for growth and realization of human potential. The central issue for the client at this point is whether the threat or opportunity is important enough to warrant the effort of making an active decision about it and engaging in the actions required to implement the decision. A low level of motivation results in ignoring or rejecting the challenge and continuing an original course of action without change. Accepting the challenge motivates active decision making and moves the client toward behavior change.[6] The nurse can best enhance the client's motivational level by providing information about the positive consequences of taking action or by arranging contact for the client with others who have successfully undertaken similar changes in life style.

It is during this early phase of the relationship that the nurse comes to understand the many frames of reference of the client: personal, social, cultural, and environmental. Familiarity with the client's life experience is essential in order to provide meaningful assistance to the client in integrating new health practices into current life style. Nurses must seek to appreciate and understand the world view of their clients and be fully aware of the dangers of imposing their world view on the client's reality.[7]

Attitudes developed by the client as a result of previous contacts with the health care system are most apparent during the initial phase. Traumatic experiences or negative reactions from health care professionals in prior encounters can result in hesitancy on the part of the client to establish an open and honest relationship with the nurse. Thus, the client must assess the nurse as a potential professional consultant in terms of expertise, trustworthiness, reliability, and helpfulness.[8] The extent to which the nurse can convey concern, respect, and unconditional positive regard for the client will determine the potential productivity of the helping relationship and the length of the initial phase.

During decision-making, the client sets goals for behavior change. That is, what is to be accomplished through the helping relationship with the nurse is identified. Next, the client searches for alternatives and carefully considers each one in terms of its promise for enabling achievement of the desired health goal. The nurse assists the client in making informed choices concerning actions to take for health protection and promotion through health assessment, values clarification, health education for self-care, and development of a Health Protection–Promotion Plan. As a result of these activities, the client and nurse have a clearer understanding of the competencies of each, the goals to be achieved, and the mutual obligations of each in the nurse–client relationship. During the initial phase, the decision maker, in this case the client, selects a course of action and becomes more and more committed to the new course of action as information about the decision is shared with significant others.[9] The nurse can assist the client at this stage by encouraging frequent verbalization of behavioral commitments to family and friends. This strengthens motivation for performance of the desired behaviors.

Transition Phase

This phase represents a critical period for the client in terms of continuation of the nurse–client relationship. Commitment to the helping relationship as a means of attaining personal health goals may fluctuate. During this period, the client may vacillate between enthusiasm and apathy, between acceptance and rejection, and between open and guarded communication with the nurse.[10] This is particularly true of clients with low self-esteem or of those who have difficulty in establishing close relationships with others. Some suggestions for stabilizing the client's commitment to the helping relationship and to behavior change at this time include focusing on issues important to the client, augmenting contact with the client by phone or mail when face-to-face contact is not possible, including the entire family in the plan of care, and establishing very specific nurse–client contracts to facilitate commitment to prevention and health-promotion activities.[11]

During the transition phase, the client may experience the challenge of maintaining the decision to change despite questioning and doubt by significant others. Getting further into the client's frame of reference can be particularly critical at this point. Questions to be asked by the nurse include: what are the client's perceptions concerning self-competence or ability to change? How does the client view behavior change in the context of social roles, significant others, goals or ambitions? Does the client exhibit persistence despite opposition? Alternative approaches to dealing with opposition to behavior change should be explored by the nurse and client. Challenges, while temporarily threatening the client, frequently result in positive growth and increased decision-making ability. The nurse who is sensitive to the client's world view can help the client in dealing with ambivalency and in moving into the working phase of the relationship.

Working Phase

While the initial and transition phases of the helping relationship take place during the decision-making period of health behavior, the working phase, termination, and follow-up coincide with the action component. In reality, the working phase of the relationship is the most intensive period of action. Considerable energies are expended by both client and nurse in marshalling personal, social, and environmental resources to achieve identified health goals. These goals should be clearly articulated in the Health Protection–Promotion Plan described in Chapter 9.

Self or family exploration begun during the initial phase of the relationship may continue into this phase, with the client developing increased sensitivity to feelings and concerns. In addition, new insights into personal or family assets and attitude–behavior incongruencies may occur. Involvement in initiating health-protecting and health-promoting actions often gives the client new feelings of control, enhanced perceptions of worth, and new opportunities for growth and actualization. Self-discovery is a continuing experience during the working phase of the helping relationship. Such discovery leads to new appreciation of the many dimensions of healthy, happy, and productive living. It may take considerable time for some adults to achieve a better understanding of themselves, their needs, their goals, and their priorities. Yet, unless they experience themselves, their capacity for understanding others and the world around them will be limited.[12] The nurse's role during periods of self-discovery is critical. He or she should be ready to listen, reflect clients' thinking, and accept unconditionally what the clients are learning about themselves.

Sustained contact through regularly scheduled visits is important during the working phase to allow clients to implement various action alternatives and evaluate their success. The support of significant others as well as that of the nurse is particularly important to the client at this time when attempts may be made to develop congruency between values, attitudes, and behaviors, to make major changes in life style, and to maintain consistency in positive health practices. It is critical that there be systematic use and evaluation of the Health Protection–Promotion Plan and modification of the plan as needed to facilitate client progress toward health goals during the working phase of the helping relationship. Knowledgeable use of specific action strategies identified in this book can facilitate client movement toward higher levels of health and well-being. Strategies suggested for the action phase include the implementation of personal or family programs of exercise, improved nutrition (weight control, if needed), stress management, modification of life style, and interpersonal-relationship skill training.

During the working phase of the nurse–client relationship, the time commitment of the client goes far beyond periodic appointments with the nurse. Concerted efforts at self-monitoring, self-management, and evaluation of progress toward valued health goals must take place on a continuing basis within the home setting. Family and significant others should be actively involved whenever possible in providing support and reinforcement during the action phase as well as providing cues for appropriate client behaviors. The crucial role of the family in behavior change is reason to consider working with the family itself as the client. Behavior change for aggregates is more successful and cost effective than dealing with individuals in isolation from meaningful social units.

Progress toward desired change should be well rewarded through tangible or social reinforcements. Lack of progress may signal alterations that need to be made in the plan of care, such as the time frame for implementation or the specific change strategies used.

The working phase is a time of intensive commitment on the part of both nurse and client. The relationship developed should be satisfying to both, providing professional challenge for the nurse and personal challenge for the client.

Step-down Phase

The support and assistance offered in the helping relationship can create a sense of dependency, even when every effort is made to maintain the independence of the client. The satisfaction derived from the relationship may make the experience of terminating the intensive working phase a difficult one. The client and nurse may make attempts to prolong the intensive relationship or express ambivalence, anger, and grief during this phase.

The step-down phase, in which the frequency of contact between nurse and client is decreased, can be handled more easily if, in initial contacts with clients, the length of the working phase can be clearly identified. As an example, this author informs her clients during their first visit that relaxation training and biofeedback sessions will occur over a 13- to 16-week period, with appointments tapering off in frequency during the following 6 months. This not only sets parameters for the working phase but allows gradual rather than abrupt termination of the intensive stage of the relationship. Progressively increasing independence of individuals and families in prevention and health-promotion activities can ease the impact of the step-down period.

During the step-down phase, clients should have a sense of pride in progress made and goals accomplished. Synthesis of information and stabilization of new behaviors that have been learned are the focus of nurse and client actions during this time. Stabilization of behavior through integration into ongoing life style is critical if newly adopted health behaviors are to persist over the years and maximally impact health status. It may be helpful to provide the client with materials to be used in reviewing what has been learned. An example of such materials are the cassette tapes on relaxation that this author provides to clients following completion of the relaxation and biofeedback program. Such materials can be used in the home for "refresher sessions." Working with clients in groups, particularly naturally occurring groups such as co-workers, provides a backup support system for clients as interaction between nurse and client is decreased.

Clients should never feel abandoned after the step-down phase of the helping relationship. The advantages of the intensive relationship with the nurse should outweigh the disadvantages of less frequent contacts. The client should feel free to reactivate an intensive nurse–client relationship at any time that such assistance is needed.

Follow-up Phase

Periodic contacts with the nurse over time can facilitate continued practice of health behaviors. Such contacts can reinforce the progress of the client or provide refresher sessions for review and refinement of positive health practices. The very nature of most health-protecting and health-promoting behaviors require their continued performance throughout the life span. While the intensive phase of nurse–client contact may terminate, the responsibility of the client for self-care remains. Continuity of care can be achieved by the nurse through periodic follow-up visits with clients every 3 to 6 months or at other appropriate time intervals.

Follow-up can be handled by appointments with the nurse in the work, school, or clinic setting, by home visits, by letter, or by telephone. Whenever possible, face-to-face contact between client and nurse is preferred to allow direct communication about further progress toward health goals or about new problems or difficulties encountered. If time allows, the home of the client offers an ideal place for follow-up, enabling the nurse to evaluate progress within the relevant environment. The extent to which there is mutual support for participation in positive health behaviors on the part of family members and a sense of cohesiveness in working toward improved health and well-being can best be determined from a home visit.

Follow-up should be handled systematically, with clients contacted by card or telephone for appointments on a periodic basis. The follow-up phase, while freeing the nurse to work intensively with new clients, also maintains supportive relationships with continuing clients.

SUMMARY

The nurse–client relationship for prevention and health promotion consists of initial, transition, work, step-down, and follow-up phases. The relationship is based on recognition of clients' rights to self-determination and capacities for self-management. It focuses on enhancing clients' strengths for decision making and goal attainment. The client, either individual or group, is viewed as an "active producer" of health rather than as a passive consumer of health care services. Such a relationship is best conceptualized by the nurse as a client–consultant relationship, since the empowered client uses the nurse as an expert consultant in the quest for health and well-being.

REFERENCES

1. Orem, D. E. *Nursing concepts of practice*, 2nd ed. New York: McGraw-Hill, 1980.
2. Chalmers, K., & Farrell, P. Nursing interventions for health promotion. *Nursing Practitioner*, 1983, *8* (10), 62–64.
3. Tatro, S., & Gleit, C. J. A wellness model for nursing: Promoting high level wellness in any setting through independent nursing functions. *Nursing Leadership*, 1983, *6* (1), 5–9.
4. Archer, S. E., & Fleshman, R. *Community health nursing: Patterns and practices.* North Scituate, Mass.: Duxbury Press, 1975, 331.
5. Janis, I. L. The patient as a decision maker. In W. D. Gentrey (Ed.), *Handbook of behavioral medicine.* New York: Guilford Press, 1983, p. 334.
6. Ibid.
7. Keyser, P. Ethics of nurse-patient relationships in the self-care model. In J. Riehl-Sisca (Ed.), *The science and act of self-care.* Norwalk, Conn.: Appleton-Century-Crofts, 1985, 14.
8. Smitherman, C. *Nursing actions for health promotion.* Philadelphia: Davis, 1981, 66.
9. Janis, op. cit.
10. Smitherman, op. cit., p. 67.
11. Archer & Fleshman, op. cit., pp. 329–330.
12. Dunn, H. L. High-level wellness for man and society. In B. W. Spradley (Ed.), *Contemporary community nursing.* Boston: Little, Brown, 1975, 27.

PART III

Strategies for Prevention and Health Promotion: The Decision-Making Phase

The purpose of this section is to assist nurses in identifying appropriate interventions to be used with clients during the decision-making phase of health behavior. Specific strategies described include health assessment, values clarification, development of self-care competencies, and the design of a Health Protection–Promotion Plan. In Chapter 6, a comprehensive approach to health assessment is described. Nurses or students of nursing are encouraged to select those aspects of the assessment that are appropriate for their practice setting. In Chapter 7, numerous approaches to values clarification, an important aspect of health counseling, are presented. Approaches to developing clients' competencies for self-care are discussed in Chapter 8. The process of designing a Health Protection–Promotion Plan is described in Chapter 9. As a whole, Part III offers practical and innovative ideas to nurses concerned with the delivery of prevention and health-promotion services to individuals, families, and community groups.

CHAPTER *6*

Health Assessment

The basis for competent professional care to protect and promote health is a thorough assessment of client health status. The client may be an individual, family, or community. In this chapter, the primary focus will be on individual assessment. However, approaches to assessing families and communities in preparation for developing a Health Protection–Promotion Plan will also be discussed. Comprehensive assessment provides information critical to (1) developing a plan that enhances health status, (2) assisting clients in gaining increased control over their health, and (3) decreasing the probability or severity of chronic disease.

ASSESSMENT OF THE INDIVIDUAL CLIENT

The components of health assessment discussed in this section focusing on individual clients are (1) health history including sexuality, (2) periodic health examination, (3) physical fitness evaluation, (4) nutritional assessment, (5) risk appraisal, (6) life–stress review, (7) life style and health habits assessment, (8) health beliefs review, and (9) spiritual health assessment. Each component of the assessment process except physical examination will be discussed at some length. Where descriptive detail is limited, the reader will be referred to other sources for expanded explanations and illustrations of that aspect of assessment.

Creating a Climate for Assessment

During initial client contact, the nurse should provide clients with an over-view of those areas of health to be assessed during subsequent appointments. This allows clients to be prepared to discuss specific topics or to participate in the varying assessment activities. Before clients will openly share infor-mation about their health concerns and life styles, they must be convinced that the nurse will maintain the confidentiality of information and use it solely for the purpose of promoting their health and well-being. An impor-tant feeling to create during the assessment is one of unconditional accep-tance of the client by the nurse. If clients believe that they are being per-sonally judged by the nurse during the assessment process, the information provided may be what is deemed socially acceptable rather than an accurate description of personal values, beliefs, and behaviors. Such distorted infor-mation thwarts meaningful health evaluation, health planning, and health actions.

Since a considerable amount of time is required for comprehensive as-sessment, this time should be distributed over several visits. The nurse should be flexible in tailoring the content and timing of the assessment to individual needs. The initial phases of the assessment should include those activities least likely to be threatening to the client.

The home of the client may provide a comfortable environment in which to conduct the health assessment. Use of the home setting permits the nurse to observe the family and physical environment as well as the individual client. The setting in which the assessment will occur—work, school, nursing center, clinic, or home—should be mutually determined by nurse and client.

Health History

Learning to collect a meaningful history to assess past and current health and illness experience is an important part of the assessment of clients of all ages. In a study of 104 asymptomatic freshmen at Pennsylvania State Uni-versity, the history was the best case-finding method for existing disease. It was the unit of the comprehensive health screen that was most cost effective.[1]

A suggested format for an adult health history is presented in Figure 6–1. Areas to be explored in history taking are identified. The history can be administered by the nurse, or a self-administered questionnaire format that clients can use for self-assessment can be developed. The reader is also re-ferred to guidelines for both adult and pediatric health histories in *A Guide to Physical Examination* by Barbara Bates.[2] Kopf, Salamon, and Charytan[3] describe a preventive health history form designed to obtain medical and psychosocial information from older adults.

Any health history is incomplete if it does not include items concerning sexuality. A sexual history can be obtained most comfortably within the context of a comprehensive health history. In the adult health history form presented in Figure 6–1, the reader should note that sexuality questions have been placed in the sections on psychosocial history and review of the genito-

Name of client _____

Address _____

Phone number _____

Private physician _____

Place of employment _____

Demographic data on client (age, occupation, marital status, education, religion, and race)

Source of referral, if any

Date of history

Source of history (client or relative)

Chief complaint, if any. Nature and duration of health problem, in client's own words

Present illness, if any. Chronologic narrative on current health problem: initial onset, setting in which it occurred, whether it recurred or was exacerbated, feelings and symptoms, treatments, response to treatments, meaning of illness to patient. Each symptom should be described by location, quality, severity, onset, duration, frequency, and factors that relieve or aggravate it. Relevant risk factors or family history should be included

Past medical history
> General state of health (client's perception)
> Childhood illnesses
> Immunizations (tetanus, pertussis, diphtheria, polio, measles, German measles, mumps, flu, pneumonia)
> Major adult illnesses
> Operations (report complications or sequelae)
> Injuries
> Emergency room visits
> Hospitalizations, not already described
> Obstetrical history (women)
> Current medications being used, including home remedies
> Use of coffee, alcohol, other drugs, and tobacco
> Allergies or drug sensitivities

Family and genetic history
> Age and health or cause of death of immediate family members, i.e., parents, siblings, spouse, children, and grandparents, if known
> Occurrence of chronic health conditions in members of immediate family, such as diabetes, tuberculosis, heart disease, high blood pressure, stroke, renal disease, cancer, arthritis, anemia, headaches, nervous disorders, mental illness, or symptoms like those of the patient

Psychosocial history
> Birth date and places of residence
> Family structure
> Educational history

Figure 6–1. Adult health history (continued on next page).

Significant experiences during childhood and adolescence
Marital history
Personal values and attitudes regarding sexuality
Feelings about self as masculine/feminine
Current life style
Home situation
Significant others and support systems
Religious and cultural beliefs that affect perceptions of health, illness,
   and health care
Job history
Travel and military history
Use of leisure time
Financial status
Sources of satisfaction and distress
Typical day (physical activity, diet, sleep, recreation, and social activities)
(Psychosocial factors are further assessed in the life-style and
   health-habits assessment)
Review of systems
General: usual weight, recent weight change, weakness, fatigue,
   fever, chills, dizziness, sweating, anorexia
Skin: rashes, lumps, itching, dryness, color changes, changes in
   pigmented areas or changes in hair and nails, bruising or bleeding
Head: headache, head injury, syncope
Eyes: vision, glasses or contact lenses, date of last eye examination,
   pain, redness, excessive tearing, double vision, halos around lights,
   color blindness, night blindness, photophobia
Ears: hearing, tinnitus, vertigo, earaches, infection, discharge, itching
Nose and sinuses: frequent colds, nasal stuffiness, chronic discharge,
   obstruction, hayfever, nosebleeds, sinus pain
Mouth and throat: condition of teeth and gums, last dental examination,
   sore tongue, frequent sore throats, hoarseness, halitosis
Neck: lumps in neck, swollen glands, goiter, restricted motion
Breasts: self-examination, lumps, pain, nipple discharge, swelling,
   asymmetry, dimpling, trauma
Respiratory: cough, excessive sputum, hemoptysis, wheezing, asthma,
   bronchitis, emphysema, tuberculosis, tuberculin test, last chest x-ray film
Cardiovascular: palpitations, chest pain, heart murmurs, dyspnea,
   orthopnea, paroxysmal dyspnea, peripheral edema, cyanosis,
   hypertension, varicose veins, intermittent claudication, thrombophlebitis
Gastrointestinal: trouble swallowing, heartburn, belching, bloating, food
   intolerance, nausea, vomiting, hematemesis, indigestion, change in
   bowel habits, rectal bleeding or black tarry stools, constipation,
   diarrhea, abdominal pain, hemorrhoids, jaundice, liver or gallbladder
   trouble, hepatitis
Urinary: frequency of urination, polyuria, nocturia, dysuria, hematuria,
   urgency, hesitancy, incontinence, penile discharge (male), force of
   stream, passage of stones or gravel

Figure 6–1. (continued)

Genitoreproductive
    Male: hernias, scrotal pain or masses, sexual practices, changes in sexual
       functioning, sexual difficulties, history of venereal disease (if any)
    Female: age at onset of menstruation, regularity, frequency, length of pe-
       riods, amount of bleeding, bleeding between periods or after intercourse,
       last menstrual period, dysmenorrhea, amenorrhea, age of menopause,
       postmenopausal difficulties (if any) last Pap smear, itching or discharge,
       sexual practices, changes in sexual functioning, sexual difficulties, birth
       control methods, history of venereal disease (if any)
Musculoskeletal: limitation of movement, trauma, pain, heat, redness, tender
    ness, swelling or crepitus of joints, backache, muscle pains or cramps
Neurologic: fainting, incoordination, seizures, paralysis, local weakness, numb-
    ness, tingling, tremors, pain, unusual reactions to heat and cold
Lymph nodes: enlargement, pain
Endocrine: goiter, exophthalmia, excessive sweating, excessive thirst, excessive
    hunger, polyuria, glycosuria, changes in secondary sex characteristics
Psychiatric: depression, hostility, apathy, phobias, nervousness

Figure 6–1. (continued)

reproductive system. For further information on obtaining a sexual history, the reader is referred to Hogan.[4]

Periodic Health Examination

The value of the routine physical examination has been challenged as a result of the rapid growth of knowledge in the health field. The Canadian Task Force on the Periodic Health Examination has identified a number of deficiencies in current examination practices. These deficiencies include: (1) content and frequency of examinations often are unrelated to the needs of different age groups, (2) tests and procedures are often included in the examination when there is scanty evidence for their effectiveness in case finding, (3) many procedures are conducted annually when they could be performed equally effectively at longer intervals, and (4) the annual physical examination tends to be used by highly educated and affluent individuals who are not necessarily those in greatest need of frequent health monitoring. The Task Force recommended that the routine annual checkup be abandoned in favor of a selective examination approach that is determined by a person's age and sex. The Task Force has recommended specific examination strategies that comprise a lifetime prevention plan. The plan consists of age- and sex-specific health-protection packages. The packages have been developed based on criteria that include: extent of disability, morbidity, and mortality caused by differing illnesses for specific age and sex groups; risks and benefits of procedure, sensitivity, specificity, and predictive value of procedure; and the safety, simplicity, cost, and acceptability to individuals of the test or inter-vention.[5]

The four aspects of the periodic health examination are: history taking and physical examination, immunization, counseling, and laboratory inves-tigations. A different protocol is recommended for each age group. As an example, a woman 55 years of age should have blood pressure checked at each visit, should be tested for occult blood in the stool annually (cancer of colon and rectum), should have mammography plus physical examination of the breast each year (cancer of the breast), should be tested every second year postmenopausally for hypothyroidism, should have a Papanicolaou smear every 5 years (or annually if in high-risk group), and should have visual examination of oral cavity (oral cancer and periodontal disease) and x-rays annually (dental caries).[6] Other tests should be performed on a discretionary basis by the health professional responsible for assessment. Clients may need to be referred to their physicians for certain aspects of testing, further workup, and differential diagnosis. If the client has no existing source of medical care, the nurse can function as an advocate for the client in obtaining services.

Since a comprehensive review of the periodic health examination and physical examination procedures is beyond the scope of this book, the reader is referred to the Canadian Task Force Report[7] and to several excellent texts for explicit guidelines on the physical examination process.[8–11]

The congruency between the findings of the nurse and the client's per-ception of health status should be determined. Dubos[12] has indicated that all too often, although laboratory tests and physical examination findings are normal, the client continues to insist that something is wrong. Perceived health status may be assessed by questioning the client concerning personal perceptions of health status in relation to others of comparable age or eval-uation of current health in relation to previous health experience. Compa-rable views of client health status on the part of nurse and client provide a solid base for collaborative health planning.

Physical Fitness Evaluation

Physical fitness is an important part of personal health status. Methods and procedures have been developed, primarily in physical education, that can be used by the nurse to assess the level of physical fitness of children and adults. As adults continue to stay active into their later years, the need to assess the physical fitness of elderly clients as a basis for recommending appropriate physical activity will increase.

From the physical examination and laboratory tests, the nurse should have available information about the client's height, weight, resting heart rate (beats per minute), resting blood pressure (mm Hg), cholesterol, tri-glycerides, glucose, and high-density lipoproteins. Additional information to be collected as a basis for fitness evaluation is identified in the *adult physical fitness evaluation* format presented in Figure 6–2. The form is an adaptation

Name of Client _____ Date _____

Sex _____ Age _____ Physician _____

<u>Body Composition:</u>

Height _____ inches _____ cm

Weight _____ lbs _____ kg
(1 lb = 0.453 kg; 1 kg = 2.205 lbs)

Percentage Body Fat _____ percent

Lean Body Weight _____ lbs _____ kg

Fat Weight _____ lbs _____ kg

Skinfolds (mm)

Triceps _____ _____ _____
                                           Average

Subscapular _____ _____ _____
                                           Average

Midaxillary _____ _____ _____
                                           Average

Suprailiac _____ _____ _____
                                           Average

Abdominal _____ _____ _____
                                           Average

Thigh _____ _____ _____
                                           Average

Girth Measurements (cm)

Chest _____ Thigh _____ Biceps
                                          (flexed) _____

Abdomen _____ Calf _____ Biceps
(at waist)   (relaxed) _____

Hips _____ Ankle _____ Wrist _____
(1 cm = 0.394 in; 2.54 cm = 1 in)

<u>Step Test:</u>

Number of Minutes _____ Stepping Rate _____

Bench Height _____ inches

Figure 6–2. Adult physical fitness evaluation (continued on next page). *(Adapted from Getchell, L. Adult Physical Fitness Evaluation. Muncie, Ind.: Human Performance Laboratory, Ball State University, 1981. With permission.)*

```
Recoveries (beats)

    1–1½ min _____

    2–2½ min _____

    3–3½ min _____

    Total _____
              (Recovery Index)

Field Tests:

    Bent-Knee Situps _____        (1 min for females, 2 min for males)

    Toe Touch Point in Inches _____
```

Figure 6–2. (continued)

of the approach to fitness evaluation developed by Leroy Getchell, director of physical fitness programs at the Human Performance Laboratory, Ball State University, Muncie, Indiana.[13] The importance of physical fitness evaluation skills for the nurse is stressed by Borgman[14] in her discussion of the nurse's role in structuring an exercise and health-maintenance program.

Measuring Percentage of Body Fat. An important part of measuring body density and percentage of body fat is the accurate measurement of skinfolds. A skinfold caliper is used on the right side of the body. The skinfold (two layers of skin and subcutaneous fat, not muscle) should be grasped between the thumb and forefinger. The calipers should be applied approximately 1 cm below the skinfold grasped and at a depth equal to the thickness of the fold. Skinfolds are picked up in the vertical plane, except for the subscapular and suprailiac, which are picked up at a slight angle. Each skinfold should be measured three times by regrasping the fold. The average value of the two closest readings should be used as the actual measure.[15] The skinfold sites are illustrated in Figure 6–3.

The first step for calculating the percentage body fat is the calculation of body density. This can be done in the following way for men and women:[16]

Men: Body density (g/cc) = 1.1043 − (0.00131 × Subscapula

measure in mm) − (0.001327 × Thigh measure in mm)

Women: Body density (g/cc) = 1.0764 − (0.00088) × Tricep

measure in mm) − (0.00081 × Suprailiac measure in mm)

The computation for the percentage of body fat is as follows:

Percentage body fat = (4.570/body density − 4.142) × 100

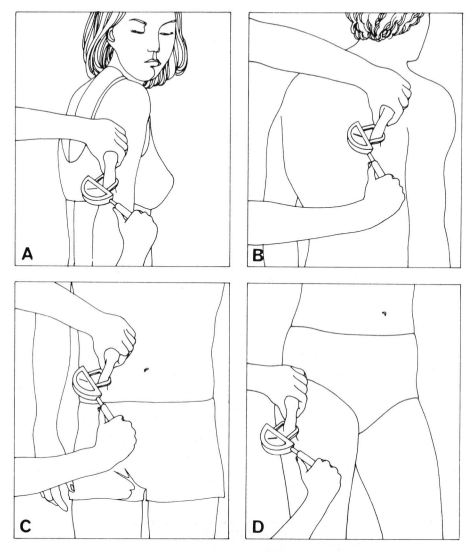

Figure 6–3. Skinfold sites. **A.** Triceps. **B.** Subscapula. **C.** Suprailiac. **D.** Thigh.

The following formula can be used to calculate lean body weight:

$$\text{Fat weight} = \text{Body weight*} \times \frac{\text{Percentage of body fat}}{100}$$

$$\text{Lean body weight} = \text{Body weight} - \text{Fat weight}$$

$$\text{Men: Desired weight} = \text{Lean weight}/0.88 \text{ (12 percent body fat)}$$

$$\text{Women: Desired weight} = \text{Lean weight}/0.82 \text{ (18 percent body fat)}$$

---

* 1 lb = 0.45 kg; kilogram units should be used for body weight.

Girth Measurements. Girth measurements that represent norms serve as rough guidelines for appropriate body proportions:

Men
- Chest and hips: same
- Abdomen (at waist): 13 to 18 cm less than chest and hips
- Thigh: 20 to 25 cm less than abdomen
- Calf: 18 to 20 cm less than thigh
- Ankle: 15 to 18 cm less than calf
- Biceps (upper arm): relaxed, 2 times the size of the wrist

Women
- Bust and hips: same
- Abdomen (at waist): 25 to 26 cm less than bust and hips
- Thigh: 15 cm less than waist
- Calf: 15 to 18 cm less than thigh
- Ankle: 13 to 15 cm less than calf
- Biceps (upper arm): relaxed, 2 times the size of the wrist

The Step Test. The step test is a field version of the laboratory stress test and can be performed when appropriate monitoring equipment and personnel are not available for stress testing. If the step test is conducted in a clinic setting, the electrocardiogram may be monitored. The availability of a physician for emergency backup is suggested if the client is over 40 years of age, obese, or has a history of cardiovascular difficulties. The step test is not as physiologically stressful as the laboratory stress test, but caution should be exercised in testing individuals with high-risk profiles for cardiovascular

TABLE 6–1. THREE-MINUTE STEP-TEST RECOVERY INDEX

	Cumulated Pulse Rate	
	MEN	WOMEN
Excellent	132 or less	135 or less
Good	150–133	155–136
Average	165–149	170–154
Fair	180–164	190–171
Poor	Above 180	Above 190

Adapted from Getchell, B. *Physical fitness: A way of life* (2nd ed.). New York: Wiley, 1979, pp. 72–73. With permission.

disease. While the risk of step testing has not been reported, in a study of 170,000 laboratory stress tests, the mortality rate was 1 per 10,000 and the morbidity rate 2.4 per 10,000.[17]

For the step test, a step 17 to 18 inches high is recommended. The step rate should be 30 steps per minute for men and 24 steps per minute for women. Each step consists of the following sequence: left foot up; right foot up; left foot down; right foot down. Pulse rates are measured after stepping for 3 minutes at the prescribed cadence. Either apical or carotid pulse may be used. Radial pulse may also be checked along with one of the above. With the client comfortably seated in a chair following step testing, pulse rates are counted for 30 seconds at the following intervals.[18]

- 1 to $1\frac{1}{2}$ minutes after cessation of exercise
- 2 to $2\frac{1}{2}$ minutes after cessation of exercise
- 3 to $3\frac{1}{2}$ minutes after cessation of exercise

The sum of the three 30-second pulses is the recovery index. Normative values for recovery for men and women are presented in Table 6–1.

Testing Muscle Strength and Endurance. As a test of muscular strength and endurance, bent-knee sit-ups, as illustrated in Figure 6–4, can be used. For females, the number of sit-ups per minute is counted, while for males, the number of sit-ups in 2 minutes is calculated. Older subjects or those with cardiovascular disorders must be observed carefully for fatigue during strength and endurance testing. Sit-ups should be terminated if signs of distress occur in the client. Normative data for sit-ups for men and women are presented in Table 6–2. For additional tests of strength and endurance, the reader should consult Getchell[19] or other physical fitness and health education references.[20,21]

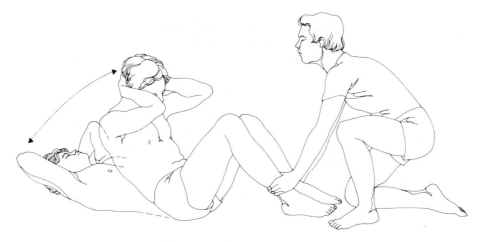

Figure 6–4. Bent-knee sit-ups.

TABLE 6–2. EVALUATION OF BENT-KNEE SIT-UPS

	Women: Number of Sit-ups, 1 min	Men: Number of Sit-ups, 2 min
Excellent	33 or above	69 or above
Good	27–32	60–68
Average	26–20	59–52
Fair	16–21	51–42
Poor	16 or fewer	41 or fewer

Adapted from Getchell, B. *Physical fitness: A Way of Life* (2nd ed.). New York: Wiley, 1979, pp. 56–57. With permission.

Evaluating Flexibility. Flexibility is also an important component of physical fitness. It is the ability to move muscles and joints through their maximum range of motion. Flexibility may decrease with age or as a result of chronic illness. The lack of ability to flex or extend muscles or joints often reflects poor health habits, such as sedentary life style, inappropriate posture, or faulty body mechanics. Loss of flexibility greatly decreases the client's ability to move about with ease and comfort.

As a quick test of flexibility, have the client bend over, keeping legs straight, and touch his or her toes. The continuum that can be used for evaluating extent of flexibility is presented in Table 6–3. Another test of flexibility, trunk flexion, is illustrated in Figure 6–5. Trunk flexion measures the ability of the client to stretch back and thigh muscles. The client sits on the floor with legs fully extended and feet flat against a box extending outward from the wall. Arms and hands are extended forward as far as possible and

TABLE 6–3. EVALUATION OF FLEXIBILITY

	Touch Point (in)
Excellent	+9 or more
Good	+ 4 to 8
Average	+1 to 3
Fair	– 2 to 0
Poor	–12 to –2

+ indicates in front of toes
– indicates above toes
0 indicates at toes

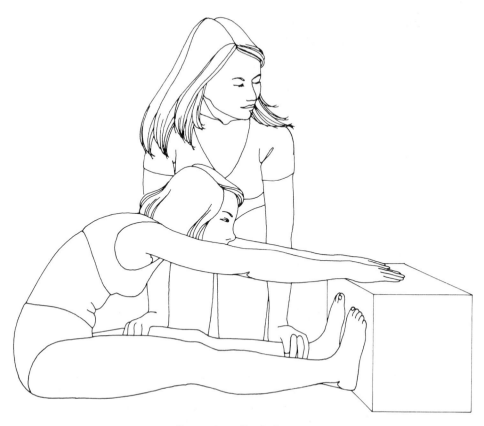

Figure 6–5. Trunk flexion.

held for a count of three. With a ruler, the distance that the client can reach beyond the proximal edge of the box can be measured in inches. If the client cannot reach the edge, the distance of the fingertips from the edge is measured and reported as a negative number. Norms for trunk flexion for men and women are presented in Table 6–4.

TABLE 6–4. NORMS FOR TRUNK FLEXION (inches)

	Women	Men
Range	−4 to +10	−6 to +8
Average (Mean)	+2	+1
Desired range	+2 to +6	+1 to +5

From Getchell, B. *Physical fitness: A way of life* (2nd ed.). New York: Wiley, 1979, p. 59. With permission.

In summary, body composition, girth measurements, cardiovascular status, muscle strength–endurance, and flexibility are critical physiological parameters to consider in a comprehensive fitness evaluation. The data collected during this phase of assessment can be used to assist the client in planning an appropriate exercise or physical activity program. Chapter 11 discusses specific approaches to increase physical fitness of clients.

Nutritional Assessment

Effective planning for health promotion requires evaluation of the nutritional status of clients. Current weight, the percentage of body fat, lean body weight, dietary patterns, and the nutrient composition of the diet should be assessed. Height and weight tables for adults and growth standards for boys and girls from birth to age 18 are presented in Tables 6–5 and 6–6. Height should be measured in 1-inch heels for men and 2-inch heels for women. Weight should be taken with lightweight clothing. In addition to body weight, skinfold measurements provide a simple criterion for obesity.[22] Triceps skinfold thicknesses indicative of obesity for children, adolescents, and men and women of differing age groups are presented in Table 6–7. Procedures for calculating the percentage of body fat and the lean body weight were presented in the previous section under physical fitness evaluation. Deviations from any of the norms on the above measurements should be noted by the nurse and recorded as a part of the nutritional assessment.

Current dietary patterns of clients and percentage of types of nutrients in their usual diet should also be assessed. Clients should be instructed to keep a record a everything eaten for 5 to 7 days during the week prior to their clinic appointment or home visit. The record can be kept on a food diary form that allows the listing of the types of foods and amounts consumed during regular meals and snacks. A simple format for a food diary for one day is illustrated in Figure 6–6. When such a diary is kept accurately, average fat, protein, and carbohydrate intake can be calculated and compared with *Dietary Goals for the United States*.[23] In Figure 6–7, current dietary patterns and recommended dietary goals for adults are presented. The nurse should note that in the *Dietary Goals*, the major changes recommended are a decrease in fat consumption and an increase in consumption of complex carbohydrates and naturally occurring sugars.

In order to convert food intake for each day to grams of fat, protein, and carbohydrates and subsequently to the percentage of total daily diet, a food-consumption chart is needed comparable to the one presented in Suitor and Crowley.[24] Computerized programs are also available. Once the average or usual dietary patterns of the client have been identified, the nurse can provide needed assistance to the client with nutrition and weight control, as described in Chapter 12.

Any signs of malnutrition should also be noted. Physical signs suggestive of malnutrition are described by Caliendo[25] and in other nutrition texts. Laboratory tests in addition to those for cholesterol, triglycerides, glucose,

TABLE 6–5a. WEIGHT TABLE FOR ADULT MALES, ACCORDING TO HEIGHT AND FRAME

Height		Weight in Pounds (Frame)		
FEET	INCHES	SMALL	MEDIUM	LARGE
5	2	128–134	131–141	138–150
5	3	130–136	133–143	140–153
5	4	132–138	135–145	142–156
5	5	134–140	137–148	144–160
5	6	136–142	139–151	146–164
5	7	138–145	142–154	149–168
5	8	140–148	145–157	152–172
5	9	142–151	148–160	155–176
5	10	144–154	151–163	158–180
5	11	146–157	154–166	161–184
6	0	149–160	157–170	164–188
6	1	152–164	160–174	168–192
6	2	155–168	164–178	172–197
6	3	158–172	167–182	176–202
6	4	162–176	171–187	181–207

Derived from data of the Build Study, 1979.

TABLE 6–5b. WEIGHT TABLE FOR ADULT FEMALES, ACCORDING TO HEIGHT AND FRAME

Height		Weight in Pounds (Frame)		
FEET	INCHES	SMALL	MEDIUM	LARGE
4	10	102–111	109–121	118–131
4	11	103–113	111–123	120–134
5	0	104–115	113–126	122–137
5	1	106–118	115–129	125–140
5	2	108–121	118–132	128–143
5	3	111–124	121–135	131–147
5	4	114–127	124–138	134–151
5	5	117–130	127–141	137–155
5	6	120–133	130–144	140–159
5	7	123–136	133–147	143–163
5	8	126–139	136–150	146–167
5	9	129–142	139–153	149–170
5	10	132–145	142–156	152–173
5	11	135–148	145–159	155–176
6	0	138–151	148–162	158–179

Derived from data of the Build Study, 1979.

and high-density lipoproteins, providing additional information concerning nutritional status, include those for protein (creatinine index, serum protein, serum albumin, total lymphocyte count, blood urea nitrogen, and uric acid), those for serum or plasma vitamin levels (water-soluble, fat-soluble), and those for minerals (calcium, sodium, chloride, potassium, iron, phosphorus, and magnesium).

Obesity and malnutrition occur in all socioeconomic classes. In addition, dietary risk factors are widespread in the American population. Therefore, assessment of nutritional status and dietary habits is an important part of holistic assessment.

TABLE 6–6a. GROWTH STANDARDS FOR BOYS, FROM BIRTH TO AGE 18

Age	Height (in), Percentiles		Weight (lb), Percentiles	
	50th	95th	50th	95th
Birth	19.8	21.1	7.5	9.1
1 mo	21.4	22.9	9.4	11.1
3 mo	24.0	25.4	13.4	16.0
6 mo	26.7	28.3	18.0	21.3
9 mo	28.7	30.2	21.4	25.1
1 yr	30.2	32.0	23.3	27.8
2 yr	34.6	27.1	29.3	33.3
3 yr	37.8	40.3	32.5	37.9
4 yr	40.8	43.3	36.1	42.4
5 yr	43.4	46.4	40.3	47.6
6 yr	45.9	49.0	44.7	53.4
7 yr	48.1	51.4	50.9	61.5
8 yr	50.5	54.1	57.4	70.4
9 yr	52.8	56.8	64.4	80.4
10 yr	54.9	59.2	71.4	91.4
11 yr	56.4	60.9	78.9	102.5
12 yr	58.6	63.7	86.0	113.5
13 yr	61.3	67.4	98.6	131.9
14 yr	64.1	70.7	111.8	148.1
15 yr	66.9	72.8	124.3	160.6
16 yr	68.9	74.0	133.8	169.8
17 yr	69.8	74.4	139.8	174.0
18 yr	70.2	74.5	144.8	179.3

From Public Health Service, *Obesity and health* (Publ. 1485).

TABLE 6–6b. GROWTH STANDARDS FOR GIRLS, FROM BIRTH
BIRTH TO AGE 18

Age	Height (in), Percentiles		Weight (lb), Percentiles	
	50th	95th	50th	95th
Birth	19.5	20.7	7.3	8.8
1 mo	21.0	22.5	8.3	9.8
3 mo	23.6	25.0	12.4	14.4
6 mo	26.1	27.6	16.7	19.8
9 mo	27.9	29.5	19.8	24.1
1 yr	29.4	31.2	21.7	26.0
2 yr	33.8	36.0	27.1	31.9
3 yr	37.5	39.7	32.3	38.3
4 yr	40.7	43.3	36.1	43.4
5 yr	43.4	46.2	40.9	49.6
6 yr	45.9	49.0	45.7	55.9
7 yr	47.8	51.1	51.0	63.7
8 yr	50.0	53.6	57.2	72.4
9 yr	52.2	56.2	63.6	82.1
10 yr	54.5	59.1	71.0	95.0
11 yr	57.0	62.1	82.0	108.6
12 yr	59.5	64.9	94.4	124.9
13 yr	62.2	66.8	105.5	138.2
14 yr	63.1	67.7	113.0	144.0
15 yr	63.8	68.1	120.0	150.5
16 yr	64.1	68.4	123.0	150.1
17 yr	64.2	68.3	125.8	153.7
18 yr	64.4	68.7	126.2	156.4

From Public Health Service, Obesity and health (Publ. 1485).

Risk Appraisal

Risk appraisal is a method for attempting to estimate individual risk for disease or death in which information from a client's medical history, physical examination, physical fitness evaluation, and nutritional assessment are used with additional information to quantify personal risk factors. Risk is frequently estimated for the ensuing 5 or 10 years by using probability tables of death from specific causes.[26] The principle behind risk appraisal is that each person is faced with certain quantifiable health hazards as a member of a specific group and that average risks may be applied to a client if the health professional knows the client's characteristics and the mortality experience of a large group of cohorts with similar characteristics.

The usual format for risk appraisal is to collect data relevant to an

TABLE 6–7. TRICEPS SKINFOLD THICKNESS INDICATING OBESITY (mm)

Age (yr)	Males	Females
5	≥12	≥15
10	≥13	≥17
15	≥15	≥20
20	≥16	≥28
25	≥20	≥29
30 and above	≥23	≥30

After Seltzer, C.C., & Mayer, J.A. Simple criterion of obesity. *Post graduate medicine*, 1965. Copyright © 1965, McGraw-Hill, Inc.

individual and match those data against a data bank of actuarial statistics based on mortality rates by cause of death, from information gathered by the U.S. Public Health Service and insurance companies. Since the national data base presently available represents mortality alone, rather than mortality and morbidity statistics, the usefulness of risk appraisal is primarily limited to those diseases that have high resultant mortality rates.

Three important ideas relevant to risk appraisal have been presented by Steinbach:[27]

1. Each risk factor has an independent action of varying intensity*
2. The total risk† for a given individual in developing any disease tends to increase with the number of risk factors present and the intensity of each risk factor
3. Risk factors interact synergistically, according to rules not yet identified from scientific inquiry

Risk factors may replace one another. For instance, a very high blood pressure and normal serum cholesterol may have the same atherogenic effects as a moderate blood pressure and hypercholesteremia. Much research needs to be completed before interaction and replacement rules for risk factors can be accurately identified. It appears that the actual risk from a single factor depends on the number and intensity of other coexisting factors in a given individual. As age advances, more factors accumulate and come into play, thus potentiating one another. This makes risk appraisal of the elderly an important nursing concern.

---

* *Threshold of risk* is the value of a risk factor below which the given factor no longer influences the total risk of a given individual for a specific disease. When all factors are at the threshold of risk, total risk should be at a minimum.

† *Total risk* is the cumulative risk of all risk factors or summed level of risk for a given individual for a specific disease.

Record *all* foods and drinks that you had during the day and during the night.

Day of Week (Mon Tues Wed Thurs Fri Sat Sun)

<u>Breakfast</u>

    Foods and Drinks   Amounts (cups, tbsps)

<u>Lunch</u>

    Foods and Drinks   Amounts (cups, tbsps)

<u>Dinner</u>

    Foods and Drinks   Amounts (cups, tbsps)

<u>Snacks</u>

    Time   Foods or Drinks   Amount (cups, tbsps)

Do you take vitamin or mineral supplements?   Yes _____ No _____
Please list kind and how many per day.

Figure 6–6. Food diary form.

Current Dietary Patterns

42% Fat	16% Saturated
	19% Monounsaturated
	7% Polyunsaturated
12% Protein	
46% Carbohydrates	28% complex carbohydrates and naturally occurring sugars
	18% refined and processed sugars

Recommended Dietary Goals

10% saturated	30% fat
10% monounsaturated	
10% polyunsaturated	
	12% protein
48% complex carbohydrates and naturally occurring sugars	58% carbohydrates
10% refined and processed sugars	

Figure 6–7. Current dietary patterns and recommended dietary goals for adults in the United States. *(From Dietary Goals for the United States. U.S. Senate Select Committee on Nutrition and Human Needs. Washington, D.C.: Government Printing Office, December, 1977.)*

Risk factors can generally be classified according to the categories in Figure 6–8. The purpose of risk appraisal is to provide clients with a realistic evaluation of health threats to which they are particularly vulnerable prior to the development of signs and symptoms of disease. The approach to risk appraisal presented in Figures 6–9 and 6–10 has been developed by the author

Risk Factors

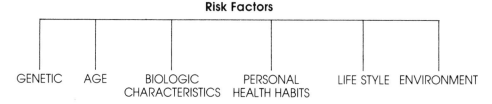

GENETIC   AGE   BIOLOGIC CHARACTERISTICS   PERSONAL HEALTH HABITS   LIFE STYLE   ENVIRONMENT

Figure 6–8. Categories of risk factors.

In each row, place a check in the box that best describes your current life situation or behavior.

Risk for Cardiovascular Disease

RISK FACTOR: ——————————→ INCREASING RISK ——————————→

Sex and age:	Female under 40	Female 40–50	Male 25–40	Female after menopause	Male 40–60	Male 61 or over
Family history (mother, father, brothers, sisters) — High blood pressure	No relatives with condition		One relative	Two relatives	Three relatives	
Heart attack	No relatives with condition	One relative with condition after 60	Two relatives with condition after 60	One relative with condition before 60	Two relatives with condition before 60	
Diabetes	No relatives with condition		One or more relatives with maturity onset diabetes		One or more relatives with preadolescent or adolescent onset	
Blood pressure* — Systolic	120 or below	121–140	141–160	161–180	181–200	above 200
Diastolic	70 or below	71–80	81–90	91–100	101–110	above 110

*Indicates risk factors that can be fully or partially controlled.

Figure 6–9. Risk appraisal form (continued on next page).

In each row, place a check in the box that best describes your current life situation or behavior.

Risk for Cardiovascular Disease

→ INCREASING RISK →

RISK FACTOR:							
Diabetes*	No diagnosis		Maturity onset, controlled	Maturity onset, uncontrolled	Adolescent onset, controlled	Adolescent onset, uncontrolled	
Weight*	At or slightly below recommended weight	10% overweight	20% overweight	30% overweight	40% overweight	50% overweight	
Cholesterol*† level (mg/100 ml)	Below 180	181–200	201–220	221–240	241–260	261–280	Above 280
Serum triglycerides* (mg/100 ml) fasting	150 or below		151–400		401–1000		Above 1000
Percent of fat in diet*	20–30%		31–40%		41–50%		Above 50%
Frequency of exercise* — Recreational	Intensive recreational exertion (35–45 min at least 4 times/wk)		Moderate recreational exertion		Minimal recreational exertion		No recreational exertion
Frequency of exercise* — Occupational	Intensive occupational exertion		Moderate occupational exertion		Minimal occupational exertion		Sedentary occupation

Sleep patterns*	7 or 8 hr sleep/night		More than 8 hr sleep/night		4–6 hr sleep/night	
Cigarette smoking* — No./day	Nonsmoker	1–10/day	11–20/day	21–30/day	31–40/day	Over 40/day
Cigarette smoking* — No. of yr smoked	Nonsmoker	Less than 10 yr	11–15 yr	16–20 yr	21–30 yr	31 yr or more
Stress* — Domestic	Minimal		Moderate	High		Very high
Stress* — Occupational	Minimal		Moderate	High		Very high
Behavior pattern* (particularly males)	Type B — Relaxed, appropriately assertive, not time dependent, moderate to slow speech			Type A — Excessively competitive, aggressive, striving, hyperalert, time dependent, loud, explosive speech		
Air pollution*	Low		Moderate		High	
Use of oral contraceptives* (females)	Do not use oral contraceptives		Under 40 and use oral contraceptives		Over 40 and use oral contraceptives	

*Indicates risk factors that can be fully or partially controlled.

†Serum lipid analysis is also recommended to determine low-density (beta) and high-density (alpha) lipoprotein levels. Evidence suggests that high-density lipoprotein (HDL) carries cholesterol from tissues for metabolism and excretion. An inverse correlation appears to exist between HDL and coronary artery disease.

Figure 6-9. (continued)

In each row, place a check in the box that best describes your current life situation or behavior.

Risk for Malignant Diseases

RISK FACTOR: — INCREASING RISK →

Risk Factor						
Breast Cancer (Women) Age	20–29	30–39	40–49	50 or over		
Race	Oriental	Black	Caucasian			
Family history (grandmother, mother, sister)	None	Mother, sister, or grandmother	Mother and grandmother	Mother and sister		
Onset of menstruation	Over 12 yr of age	Under 12 yr of age				
Pregnancy* — Time	First pregnancy before 25	First pregnancy after 25	No pregnancies			
Pregnancy* — No.	Three or more	One or two	None			
Weight*	0–40% overweight	Above 40% overweight				
Personal history	No evidence of dysplasia or previous breast cancer	Breast dysplasia	Previous breast cancer			
Lung Cancer Cigarette smoking* — No./day	Nonsmoker	1–10/day	11–20/day	21–30/day	21–40/day	Over 40/day
No. of yr smoked	Nonsmoker	Less than 10 yr	11–15 yr	16–20 yr	21–30 yr	31 or more yr

	Less than one yr	1–5 yr	6–10 yr	11–15 yr	Over 15 yr
Occupational exposure to toxic chemicals*‡					
Length of exposure	Less than one yr	1–5 yr	6–10 yr	11–15 yr	Over 15 yr
Frequency and intensity of exposure	Low frequency and low intensity	Low frequency, moderate intensity (or vice versa)	Moderate frequency, moderate intensity	Moderate frequency, high intensity (or vice versa)	High frequency, high intensity
Cervical Cancer					
Onset of sexual activity*	After 28 yrs of age		22–27	16–21	Before 16 yrs of age
No. of sexual partners*	Two	Three		Four or more	
Marital status*	Single			Married	
Sexual partner*	Circumcised			Uncircumcised	
Colorectal Cancer					
Age	Below 45 yr of age			Above 45 yr of age	
Personal history	No history of ulcerative colitis		Ulcerative colitis under 10 yr	Ulcerative colitis more than 10 yr	
Fiber content of diet*	High		Moderate	Low	
Weight* (men)	Less than 40% overweight			More than 40% overweight	
Rectal bleeding or black bowel movement	Never		Occasionally	Frequently	

*Indicates risk factors that can be fully or partially controlled.
‡Chemicals such as asbestos, nickel, chromates, arsenic, chlormethyl ethers, radioactive dust, petroleum or coal products, and iron oxide.

Figure 6–9. (continued)

In each row, place a check in the box that best describes your current life situation or behavior.

Risk for Malignant Diseases

RISK FACTOR:	INCREASING RISK →		
Uterine and Ovarian Cancer Age	Below 45 yr of age		Over 45 yr of age
Weight*	Less than 40% overweight		More than 40% overweight
Vaginal bleeding other than during menstrual period	Never	Occasionally	Frequently
Skin Cancer Complexion	Dark	Medium	Fair
Sun exposure (without protection)	Never or seldom	Occasionally	Frequently

Risk for Auto Accidents

RISK FACTOR:				
Alcohol consumption*	Nondrinker	Occasionally small to moderate consumption	Frequently small to moderate consumption	Occasionally heavy consumption	Frequently heavy consumption
Mileage driven/yr*	Under 5000 miles/yr	5001–10,000 miles/yr	10,001–20,000 miles/yr	Over 20,000 miles/yr
Use of seat belt*	Always	Usually	Occasionally	Never

Use of shoulder harness*	Always	Usually		Occasionally	Never
Use of drugs or medication that decrease alertness*	No use	Occasional use		Moderate use	Frequent use

Risk for Suicide

Family history	No history	One family member			Two or more family members
Personal history*	Seldom experience depression	Periodically experience mild depression	Frequently experience mild depression	Periodically experience deep depression	Frequently experience deep depression
Access to hypnotic medication*	No access	Access to small or limited dosages		Unlimited access to large dosages	

Risk for Diabetes

Weight*	Desired weight	15% overweight	30% overweight	45% overweight	Above 45% overweight
Family history (parent or sibling)	None	Either parent or sibling		Both parent and sibling	

*Indicates risk factors that can be fully or partially controlled.

Figure 6–9. (continued)

Health Problem	(1) Total No. Risk Factors	(2) No. for Which Client Is in Highest Risk Level(s)*	(3) Percent for Which Client Is in Highest Risk Level(s) (Col. 2 ÷ Col. 1)
Cardiovascular disease	21†	_____	_____
Breast cancer	8	_____	_____
Lung cancer	4	_____	_____
Cervical cancer	4	_____	_____
Colorectal cancer	5	_____	_____
Uterine or ovarian cancer	3	_____	_____
Skin cancer	2	_____	_____
Auto accidents	5	_____	_____
Suicide	3	_____	_____
Diabetes	2	_____	_____

* *High risk* is risk within highest level of two to three levels within risk factor, or risk within highest two levels of four or more levels within risk factor.
† All subcategories under a given heading are counted individually. For example, Pregnancy—Time and Pregnancy–Number each count as a separate factor.

Figure 6–10. Profile of total risk.

following extensive review of articles and materials in the field. The approach is practical and useful for the office or clinic setting. More detailed appraisal formats are available from several commercial sources for computerized analysis of individual risk based on comparison with national mortality data for selected health problems.[28–30]

In using risk appraisal, health professionals must recognize that conclusions drawn are highly tentative. Population data in many instances do not accurately reflect the risk profile for a given individual. In addition, risk appraisal in and of itself is unlikely to result in reductions in risk. If clients are to alter behavior significantly, risk appraisal must be linked to behavior-change programs and other appropriate community health resources. At a minimum, persons receiving a personal risk profile should receive an up-to-date list of local resources that can be tapped to assist them in reducing the risks that have been identified.[31] It is unethical to apprise individuals of their risk level without providing supportive education and resources to facilitate behavior change efforts. Weiss[32] has commented on the possible adverse effects of risk appraisal. Predictions of premature death or shortened life expectancy may cause anxiety, depression, guilt, or hypochondriasis, especially in older adults who believe that it is too late to change risk status. Thus, in the decision to use risk appraisal with clients, both the advantages and disadvantages of this assessment tool must be considered.

The nurse should be aware of the differences between risk appraisal and comprehensive life style assessment. Life style assessment and wellness inventories represent a positive approach to appraisal–assessment that is focused on enhancing well-being as opposed to only identifying risk factors for disease. Life style assessment will be discussed later in this chapter.

Life Stress Review

The importance of stress in the direct or indirect causation of illness throughout the life span has been supported in numerous studies. The impact of stress on mental health and physical well-being has been evident in the work of Langer and Michael,[33] Holmes and Rahe,[34] and others. As a part of comprehensive health assessment, life stress review should include use of the following instruments: the Life-Change Index developed by Holmes and Rahe,[35] the State–Trait Anxiety Inventory developed by Spielberger,[36] the Signs of Distress developed by Everly and Girdano,[37] and Stress Charting, developed at the Menninger Foundation by Walters.[38]

Life-Change Index. Holmes and Rahe developed a tool to measure the extent of life change as a predictor of the probability of becoming ill. If enough changes occur within any given 2-year period for the client, the chances of becoming ill are frequently increased. Stressful life events seem to precede many health problems such as tuberculosis, coronary heart disease, accidents, and possibly even malignant diseases. The Life-Change Index is presented in Figure 6–11. Modified forms of this index are available for different age and ethnic groups. The index can be administered to the client in a short period of time and scored by adding up the normative values for all life events checked. The extent of life stress can be evaluated using the scale for scoring presented in Table 6–8.

State–Trait Anxiety Inventory. A second instrument suggested for use as part of the life-stress review is the State–Trait Anxiety Inventory, which consists of 20 items pertaining to the amount of tension or anxiety the client feels at that moment (state), and 20 items concerning the way the client generally feels (trait). Sample questions from the inventory are presented in Figures 6–12 and 6–13. Clients respond by rating themselves on a 4-point scale for each item. The full-length test and test manual can be obtained by contacting Consulting Psychologists Press, Inc., Palo Alto, California. The State–Trait Anxiety Inventory provides an efficient yet reliable means for assessing feelings of tension or stress experienced by clients. Test–retest re-

Please check those life changes that you have experienced personally during the past *two years.*

Life Event	Scale of Impact	
Death of Spouse	100	_____
Divorce	73	_____
Marital separation	65	_____
Jail term	63	_____
Death of close family member	63	_____
Personal injury or illness	53	_____
Marriage	50	_____
Fired at work	47	_____
Marital reconciliation	45	_____
Retirement	45	_____
Change in health of family member	44	_____
Pregnancy	40	_____
Sex difficulties	39	_____
Gain of new family member	39	_____
Business readjustment	39	_____
Change in financial state	38	_____
Death of close friend	37	_____
Change to different line of work	36	_____
Change in number of arguments with spouse	35	_____
Mortgage over $20,000	31	_____
Foreclosure of mortgage or loan	30	_____
Change in responsibilities at work	29	_____
Son or daughter leaving home	29	_____
Trouble with in-laws	29	_____
Outstanding personal achievement	28	_____
Spouse begins or stops work	26	_____

Figure 6–11. Life-change index (continued). *(Reprinted with permission from Holmes, T., & Rahe, E. The social readjustment rating scale. Journal of Psychosomatic Research, 1967, 11, p. 213. Copyright © 1967, Pergamon Press, Ltd.)*

Life Event	Scale of Impact	
Begin or end school	26	_____
Change in living conditions	25	_____
Revision of personal habits	24	_____
Trouble with boss	23	_____
Change in work hours or conditions	20	_____
Change in residence	20	_____
Change in schools	20	_____
Change in recreation	19	_____
Change in church activities	19	_____
Change in social activities	18	_____
Mortgage or loan less than $20,000	17	_____
Change in sleeping habits	16	_____
Change in number of family get-togethers	15	_____
Change in eating habits	15	_____
Vacation	13	_____
Christmas (if approaching)	12	_____
Minor violations of the law	11	_____
Total		_____

Figure 6–11. (continued)

liability of the Trait Anxiety Inventory is reported as 0.73 for males and 0.77 for females.

Signs of Distress. In order to assist clients in understanding how they respond to stress, they must be made aware of the signs that provide personal feedback concerning an elevated stress level. Once clients are aware of their own biological or behavioral responses to stress, they can use stress-management techniques presented in Chapter 13 more effectively. Signs of distress may be in terms of mood and disposition, muscles, bones and joints, or visceral organs. A checklist for signs of distress is presented in Figure 6–14.

Stress Charting The Menninger Foundation Biofeedback Center in their stress management seminar use a stress-charting exercise that allows clients

TABLE 6–8. SCORING THE LIFE-CHANGE INDEX

Score Range	Interpretation
0–150	No significant problems, low or tolerable life change
150–199	Mild life change (approximately 33% chance of illness)
200–299	Moderate life change (approximately 50% chance of illness)
300 or over	Major life change (approximately 80% chance of illness)

Reprinted with permission from Holmes, T., & Rahe, E. The social readjustment rating scale, Journal of Psychosomatic Research, 1967, 11, p. 213. Copyright © 1967, Pergamon Press, Ltd.

to list sources of stress. After listing as many stressors as possible, the client is instructed to write the number associated with each stressor in the section of the circle that describes the area of life in which the stressor occurs. If it is a stressor that is particularly troublesome, the client should place the number closer to the center of the circle. The center of the circle represents

Directions: A number of statements which people have used to describe themselves are given below. Read each statement and then blacken in the appropriate circle to the right of the statement to indicate how you *feel* right now, that is, *at this moment.* There are no right or wrong answers. Do not spend too much time on any one statement but give the answer which seems to describe your present feelings best.

① = **Not at All;** ② = **Somewhat;**
③ = **Moderately So;** ④ = **Very Much So**

I feel at ease	①	②	③	④
I feel upset	①	②	③	④
I feel nervous	①	②	③	④
I am relaxed	①	②	③	④
I am worried	①	②	③	④

Figure 6–12. Sample items from the self-evaluation questionnaire: State Anxiety Inventory. *(Reproduced by special permission from The State–Trait Anxiety Inventory, by Charles Spielberger, Richard Gorsuch, and Robert Lushene. Copyright © 1968, published by Consulting Psychologists Press, Inc., Palo Alto, Calif. 94306.)*

Directions: A number of statements that people have used to describe themselves are given below. Read each statement and then blacken in the appropriate circle to the right of the statement to indicate how you generally feel. There are no right or wrong answers. Do not spend too much time on any one statement, but give the answer that seems to describe how you generally feel.

① = **Not at All**; ② = **Somewhat**;
③ = **Moderately So**; ④ = **Very Much So**

I wish I could be as happy as others seem to be	①	②	③	④
I am "calm, cool, and collected"	①	②	③	④
I feel that difficulties are piling up so that I cannot overcome them	①	②	③	④
I am inclined to take things hard	①	②	③	④
I am content	①	②	③	④

Figure 6–13. Sample items from the self-evaluation questionnaire: Trait Anxiety Inventory. *(Reproduced by special permission from The State–Trait Anxiety Inventory, by Charles Spielberger, Richard Gorsuch, and Robert Lushene. Copyright © 1968, published by Consulting Psychologists Press, Inc., Palo Alto, Calif. 94306.)*

the client. The stress-charting exercise appears in Figure 6–15. Following completion of this portion of the life-stress review, the client should be aware of (1) the stresses that he or she is experiencing in daily living, (2) the areas of life in which multiple stressors are occurring, and (3) the personal closeness or distance of each stressor from the self.

Life-stress review provides the client with an understanding of personal sources of stress, level of stress, and specific responses to anxiety-producing life events. Increased self-awareness resulting from this component of health assessment facilitates the use of stress management and relaxation techniques described in Chapter 13.

The Life Style and Health-Habits Assessment

Clients often have unreal expectations that physicians and nurses can undo the ill that clients have inflicted on themselves through health-damaging styles of living. While a healthy life style does not guarantee freedom from chronic illness, much evidence indicates that there is a great deal that individuals can do to maintain and enhance their health and prevent the early onset of disabling health problems. The Life Style and Health-Habits Assessment is intended to help the nurse assist the client in reviewing personal life style in terms of its impact on health. A thoughtful review and follow-up counseling and education can greatly increase the motivation and competence of clients to care for themselves in a responsible manner.

136

Mood and disposition signs

_____ I become overexcited

_____ I worry

_____ I feel insecure

_____ I have difficulty sleeping at night

_____ I become easily confused and forgetful

_____ I become very uncomfortable and ill-at-ease

_____ I become nervous

Musculoskeletal signs

_____ My fingers and hands shake

_____ I can't sit or stand still

_____ I develop twitches

_____ My head begins to ache

_____ I feel my muscles become tense or stiff

_____ I stutter or stammer when I speak

_____ My neck becomes stiff

Visceral signs

_____ My stomach becomes upset

_____ I feel my heart pounding

_____ I sweat profusely

_____ My hands become moist

_____ I feel light-headed or faint

_____ I experience cold chills

_____ My face becomes "hot"

_____ My mouth becomes dry

_____ I experience ringing in my ears

_____ I get a sinking feeling in my stomach

Figure 6–14. Signs of distress. *(From Girdano, D.A., & Everly, G. S., Controlling stress and tension: A holistic approach. Bowie, Md.: Robert J. Brady, 1979, p. 137. With permission.)*

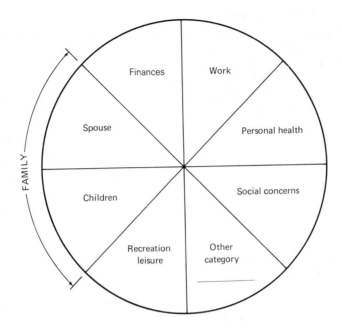

List of stressors:

1. _____
2. _____
3. _____
4. _____
5. _____
6. _____
7. _____
8. _____
9. _____
10. _____
11. _____
12. _____
13. _____
14. _____
15. _____
16. _____

Figure 6–15. Stress charting. *(Adapted with permission from Walters, D., Bio-feedback Center, The Menninger Foundation, Topeka, Kan.)*

The Life Style and Health-Habits Assessment is divided into ten sections: (1) competence in self-care, (2) nutritional practices, (3) physical or recreational activity, (4) sleep patterns, (5) stress management, (6) self-actualization, (7) sense of purpose, (8) relationships with others, (9) environmental control, and (10) use of health care system. Ideas used by the author in constructing the assessment guide have been drawn from many sources.[39-44] The Life Style and Health-Habits Assessment form is presented in Figure 6–16.

The rating in each category of the Life Style and Health-Habits Assessment can provide information useful in developing an individualized Health-Protection–Promotion Program. Even though the percentage of behaviors performed in each category provides the basis for overall evaluation, the response to each behavior should be examined. For instance, if the client is

---

Please place an X before each statement that is true regarding your *present* way of life or personal habits. That is, what you generally do.

General competence in self-care (14)

_____ Take 12–15 deep breaths at least three times daily

_____ Drink 6–8 glasses of water each day in addition to other liquids

_____ Do not smoke

_____ Read articles or books about promoting health

_____ Know my body contours and physical sensations well

_____ Do not take laxative medications

_____ Know what my blood pressure and pulse readings should be

_____ Protect my skin from excessive sun exposure

_____ Know the seven danger signs of cancer

_____ Observe my body monthly for cancer danger signs

_____ Understand how to correctly examine my breasts (women only)

_____ Conduct monthly breast self-examination (women only)

_____ Use soft toothbrush regularly

_____ Dental floss regularly

Total number of items checked _____ Percent checked _____

Figure 6–16. Life style and health habits assessment form (continued)

Nutritional practices (16)

_____ Know about the "basic four" food groups

_____ Plan or select meals to meet nutritional needs

_____ Eat breakfast daily

_____ Eat three meals a day

_____ Avoid between meal snacks

_____ Drink only small amounts (no more than 3 cups/day) of caffeinated beverages (coffees, teas, or colas)

_____ Do not consume alcoholic beverages or do so in very limited amounts

_____ Limit intake of refined sugars (junk foods or desserts)

_____ Frequently use unprocessed foods or foods without preservatives or other additives

_____ Maintain adequate roughage (fiber) in diet (whole grains, raw fruits, raw vegetables)

_____ Read labels for nutrients in packaged food

_____ Eat more poultry and fish than red meats

_____ Chew foods thoroughly and eat slowly

_____ Add little or no salt to my food when cooking or during eating

_____ Keep weight within recommended limits for my height

_____ Avoid frequent consumption of charcoaled foods

Total number of items checked _____ Percent checked _____

Physical or recreational activity (9)

_____ Walk up stairs rather than riding the elevator

_____ Exercise vigorously for 30–40 minutes at least four times per week

_____ Regularly engage in recreational sports (swimming, soccer, bicycling)

_____ Perform stretching exercises at least four times per week to increase flexibility.

_____ Participate in individual sports for the pleasure of movement and physical fitness

Figure 6–16. (continued)

_____ Engage in competitive sports primarily for enjoyment rather than competition

_____ Maintain good posture when sitting or standing

_____ Often elevate my legs when sitting

_____ Seldom sit with legs crossed at knees

Total number of items checked _____ Percent checked _____

Sleep patterns (9)

_____ Get 7 hours of sleep per night (not $1\frac{1}{2}$ hours less or more)

_____ Wake up feeling fresh and relaxed

_____ Take some time for relaxation each day

_____ Fall asleep easily at night

_____ Sleep soundly

_____ Systematically relax voluntary muscles before sleep

_____ Sleep on a firm mattress

_____ Use a small pillow for sleep that maintains head and neck in a natural position

_____ Allow the thoughts and worries of the day to leave my mind, concentrating on passive but pleasant thoughts at bedtime

Total number of items checked _____ Percent checked _____

Stress management (11)

_____ Can laugh at myself

_____ Frequently laugh out loud with others

_____ Maintain adequate vitamin C intake when experiencing high stress

_____ Practice relaxation or meditation for 15–20 minutes daily

_____ Understand the relationship between stress and illness

_____ Create relaxed atmosphere at meal time

_____ Forget my problems and enjoy myself when immediate solutions are not possible

_____ Enjoy spending time in unstructured activities

Figure 6–16. (continued)

_____ Consider it acceptable to cry, feel sad, angry, or afraid
_____ Find constructive ways to express my feelings
_____ Have attended training classes or biofeedback sessions to gain relaxation skills

Total number of items checked _____ Percent checked _____

Self-actualization (12)

_____ Maintain an enthusiastic and optimistic outlook on life

_____ Enjoy expressing myself in hobbies, the arts, exercise, or play

_____ Like myself and enjoy occasional solitude

_____ Continue to grow and change in positive directions

_____ Am happy most of the time

_____ Am a member of one or more community groups

_____ Feel fulfilled in my work

_____ Aware of personal strengths and weaknesses

_____ Am proud of my body and my personality

_____ Respect my own accomplishments

_____ Find each day interesting and challenging

_____ Look forward to the future

Total number of items checked _____ Percent checked _____

Sense of purpose (4)

_____ Aware of what is important to me in life

_____ Have identified short-term and long-term life goals

_____ Am realistic about the goals that I set

_____ Believe that my life has purpose

Total number of items checked _____ Percent checked _____

Relationships with others (11)

_____ Have persons close to me with whom I can discuss personal problems and concerns

Figure 6–16. (continued)

_____ Perceive myself as being well accepted by others

_____ Maintain meaningful and fulfilling interpersonal relationships

_____ Communicate easily with others

_____ Recognize accomplishments and praise other people easily

_____ Enjoy my neighbors

_____ Have a number of close friends

_____ Thoughtfully consider constructive criticism rather than reacting defensively

_____ Enjoy being touched and touching people close to me

_____ Find it easy to express concern, love, and warmth to others

_____ Enjoy meeting new people and getting to know them

Total number of items checked _____ Percent checked _____

Environmental control (6)

_____ When possible, prevent overwhelming changes in my environment

_____ Avoid purchasing aerosol sprays

_____ Seldom listen to loud rock music

_____ Do not permit smoking in my home or car

_____ Provide resources to meet my own personal needs

_____ Maintain safe living area free from fire or accident hazards

Total number of items checked _____ Percent checked _____

Use of health care system (8)

_____ Report any unusual signs or symptoms to a physician

_____ Question my physician or seek a second opinion when I do not agree with the recommended treatment

_____ Expect prompt, helpful, and courteous personalized service from health care personnel

_____ Discuss health care concerns or problems with the health professional most qualified to provide meaningful assistance

_____ Have breasts examined at least once a year by nurse or physician

_____ Have a Pap smear at intervals recommended by my physician

Figure 6–16. (continued)

_____ Have a rectal examination at intervals recommended by my physician

_____ Attend educational classes on personal health care provided within the community

Total number of items checked _____ Percent checked _____

Scoring: Calculate the percentage of items checked in each category by dividing the number of items that you checked by the total number of items listed in the category (total number of items in each category is listed in parentheses by category title). Record below the percentage of items checked from each category.

Category	Percentage of Items Checked	Rating (see below)
Competency in self-care	_____	_____
Nutritional practices	_____	_____
Physical or recreational activity	_____	_____
Sleep patterns	_____	_____
Stress management	_____	_____
Self-actualization	_____	_____
Sense of purpose	_____	_____
Relationships with others	_____	_____
Environmental control	_____	_____
Use of health care system	_____	_____

For each category, the following scale may be used to evaluate the extent to which the client's life style and health habits maintain or promote personal health.

Rating	Percentage of Items Checked
Excellent	Greater than 85%
Good	75–84%
Average	65–74%
Fair	55–64%
Poor	Below 55%

Figure 6–16. (continued)

a female and does not examine her own breasts monthly, then the response to that single item is important for educational and counseling follow-up. Through use of the Life Style and Health-Habits Assessment, the client increases self-awareness of personal patterns of living. Such information can facilitate the behavior change process.

Using the 100 behaviors identified in the Life Style and Health-Habits Assessment as a starting point, Walker, Sechrist, and Pender have developed the Health-Promoting Life Style Profile (HPLP).[45] This 48-item instrument has been designed as a research tool for measuring a constellation of health-promoting behaviors that are considered to be dimensions of a health-promoting life style. The HPLP consists of six sections: nutrition (6 items), exercise (5 items), health responsibility (10 items), stress management (7 items), interpersonal support (7 items), and self-actualization (13 items). The instrument was administered to 1023 volunteer adults recruited from regions of Illinois and North Dakota as a basis for determining its factor structure and reliability.* The instrument focuses on health-promoting behaviors. Interestingly, health-damaging behaviors such as smoking or use of alcohol were not found to fit empirically with the health-promoting behaviors as a singular concept, thus, the health-damaging behaviors had to be deleted. This finding adds credence to the idea that health promotion and prevention are different phenomena.

The Life Style Assessment Questionnaire developed in the Wellness Program at the University of Wisconsin–Stevens Point is another format that can be used for assessing life style. The 11 areas of life style measured in the questionnaire are: physical–exercise, physical–nutritional, physical–self-care, physical–vehicle safety, physical–drug abuse, social–environmental, emotional awareness and acceptance, emotional management, intellectual, occupational, and spiritual. A personal-growth section is also part of the questionnaire. Topics of personal interest to clients can be selected. This provides guidance to the nurse in selecting information for individual counseling or groups sessions. The Life Style Assessment Questionnaire also includes a risk-of-death section and a medical alert section. At the University of Wisconsin–Stevens Point, this questionnaire is used as a basis for health-promotion programming for the college-age population.[46]

A short life style assessment form, the Wellness Index, consisting of 16 items, was developed by John Travis at the Wellness Resource Center in Mill Valley, California. This form provides an overall evaluation of wellness and life style. The Wellness Index and instructions for evaluating the results appear in Figure 6–17. This form provides a less detailed assessment than

---

* Cecelia Volden, Margaret Adamson, Diane K. Langemo, Lois Oechsle, and Jenenne Peter Nelson, University of North Dakota, College of Nursing Faculty, assisted in collection of a substantial portion of the data and are acknowledged for their valuable contribution to development of the HPLP.

the other instruments described previously, but the results are graphically displayed. The Wellness Index may be useful when client contact time is limited or when the attention span of the client is short. Children and adolescents often enjoy completing this assessment tool.

Through review of life style, clients gain an awareness of those behaviors they perform regularly that are health-promoting. Such information can increase self-esteem and provide the momentum for further development of a health-enhancing life style.

Health-Beliefs Review

In this section of the chapter, a Health-Beliefs Review is included for use in clarifying the beliefs of clients concerning personal control of their own health status. The Multidimensional Health Locus of Control (MHLC) Instrument developed by Wallston and Wallston[47,48] is recommended for assessing perceptions of health control. The two forms of the MHLC appear in Figures 6–18 and 6–19. Use of both forms yields more reliable data than use of either alone (one form only, reliability 0.67 to 0.77; two forms, reliability 0.83 to 0.86).

Three important subscales have been identified within the instrument.

Circle the category that most closely answers the question.

1. I am conscious of the ingredients of the food I eat and their effect on me. Rarely, Sometimes, Very Often (R, S, VO)

2. I avoid overeating and abusing alcohol, caffeine, nicotine, and other drugs. R, S, VO

3. I minimize my intake of refined carbohydrates and fats. R, S, VO

4. My diet contains adequate amounts of vitamins, minerals, and fiber. R, S, VO

5. I am free from physical symptoms. R, S, VO

6. I get aerobic cardiovascular exercise. R, S, VO (Very Often is at least 12–20 minutes 5 times per week vigorously running, swimming, or bike riding)

7. I practice yoga or some other form of limbering/stretching exercise. R, S, VO

8. I nurture myself. R, S, VO (Nurturing means pleasuring and taking care of oneself, for example, massages, long walks, buying presents for self, "doing nothing," sleeping late without feeling guilty, etc.)

Figure 6–17. Wellness index (continued). *(Used with permission from Travis, J. W.,* Wellness *Workbook for Health Professionals. Mill Valley, Calif.: Wellness Resource Center, 1977.)*

9. I pay attention to changes occurring in my life and am aware of them as stress factors.   R, S, VO   (See Life-Change Index—a score of over 300 is considered very stressful)

10. I practice regular relaxation.   R, S, VO   (Suggested: 20 minutes a day "centering" or "letting go" of thoughts, worries, etc.)

11. I am without excess muscle tension.   R, S, VO

12. My hands are warm and dry.   R, S, VO

13. I am both productive and happy.   R, S, VO

14. I constructively express my emotions and creativity.   R, S, VO

15. I feel a sense of purpose in life and my life has meaning and direction.   R, S, VO

16. I believe I am fully responsible for my wellness or illness.   R, S, VO

Using your answers above to guide you, you can synthesize a graphic picture of your wellness. Each numbered pie-shaped segment of the circle below corresponds to the same numbered question on the preceding page. (They are divided into quarters representing four major dimensions of wellness.) Color in an amount of each segment corresponding to your answer to the question with the same number. The inner broken circle corresponds to "rarely," the next one to "sometimes," the third to "very often." You don't need to restrict yourself to these categories, however, and can fill in any amount in between. You may use different colors for each section if you like.

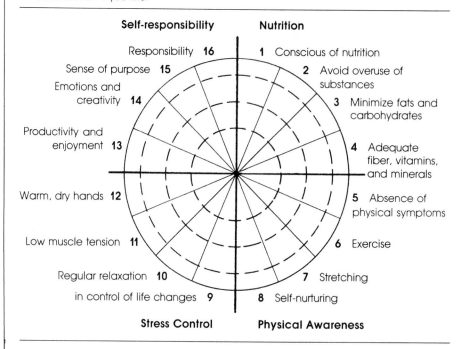

Now look at the shape of your index. Is it lopsided or balanced? This should provide beginning suggestions for improving your lifestyle and health habits.

Figure 6–17. (continued)

The three subscales and the items included in each are as follows for both forms A and B:

- Internal items: 1, 6, 8, 12, 13, 17
- Chance items: 2, 4, 9, 11, 15, 16
- Powerful-others items: 3, 5, 7, 10, 14, 18

The score on each subscale is the sum of the values circled for each item in that subscale. Scores within each subscale using both forms (A and B) can range from 12 to 72.[49] The higher the score on the internal subscale, the more personal control clients believe that they exercise over their own health. The higher the scores on the chance subscale and powerful-others subscale, the higher the beliefs in the importance of chance and others respectively in controlling personal health. Normative means for adults on each subscale are as follows: internal, 50.4; chance, 31.0; power others, 40.9. The reader is

---

This questionnaire is designed to determine the way in which different people view certain important health-related issues. Each item is a belief statement with which you may agree or disagree. Beside each statement is a scale that ranges from strongly disagree (1) to strongly agree (6). For each item we would like you to circle the number that represents the extent to which you disagree or agree with the statement. The more strongly you agree with a statement, the higher will be the number you circle. The more strongly you disagree with a statement, the lower will be the number you circle. Please make sure that you answer every item and that you circle *only one* number per item. This is a measure of your personal beliefs; obviously, there are no right or wrong answers.

Please answer these items carefully, but do not spend too much time on any one item. As much as you can, try to respond to each item independently. When making your choice, do not be influenced by your previous choices. It is important that you respond according to your actual beliefs and not according to how you feel you should believe or how you think we want you to believe.

**1 = Strongly Disagree; 2 = Moderately Disagree;
3 = Slightly Disagree; 4 = Slightly Agree;
5 = Moderately Agree; 6 = Strongly Agree.**

1. If I get sick, it is my own behavior that determines how soon I get well again.	1	2	3	4	5	6
2. No matter what I do, if I am going to get sick, I will get sick.	1	2	3	4	5	6
3. Having regular contact with my physician is the best way for me to avoid illness.	1	2	3	4	5	6

Figure 6–18. Multidimensional health locus of control scale, Form A (continued). *(From Wallston, K. A., Wallston, B. S., & DeVellis, R., Development of the Multidimensional Health Locus of Control (MHLC) Scales. Health Education Monographs, Spring 1978, 6, 164–165. With permission.)*

4. Most things that affect my health happen to me by accident.	1	2	3	4	5	6
5. Whenever I don't feel well, I should consult a medically trained professional.	1	2	3	4	5	6
6. I am in control of my health.	1	2	3	4	5	6
7. My family has a lot to do with my becoming sick or staying healthy.	1	2	3	4	5	6
8. When I get sick, I am to blame.	1	2	3	4	5	6
9. Luck plays a big part in determining how soon I will recover from an illness.	1	2	3	4	5	6
10. Health professionals control my health.	1	2	3	4	5	6
11. My good health is largely a matter of good fortune.	1	2	3	4	5	6
12. The main thing that affects my health is what I myself do.	1	2	3	4	5	6
13. If I take care of myself, I can avoid illness.	1	2	3	4	5	6
14. When I recover from an illness, it's usually because other people (for example, doctors, nurses, family, friends) have been taking good care of me.	1	2	3	4	5	6
15. No matter what I do, I'm likely to get sick.	1	2	3	4	5	6
16. If it's meant to be, I will stay healthy.	1	2	3	4	5	6
17. If I take the right actions, I can stay healthy.	1	2	3	4	5	6
18. Regarding my health, I can only do what my doctor tells me to do.	1	2	3	4	5	6

Figure 6–18. (continued)

referred to publications by Wallston and associates identified previously for more specific information on evaluating test results.

The information available to the nurse following completion of the MHLC provides an indication of the extent to which clients believe that they can influence health status through personal behaviors. If clients perceive themselves to have little control over their own health, beliefs may need to be changed. Another approach is to use behavior change strategies that have been shown to be successful with persons low in internal control but high in external control, e.g., peer pressure groups for weight loss. If clients score high on beliefs concerning personal control of health, they exhibit an important prerequisite for active participation in self-care.

This questionnaire is designed to determine the way in which different people view certain important health-related issues. Each item is a belief statement with which you may agree or disagree. Beside each statement is a scale that ranges from strongly disagree (1) to strongly agree (6). For each item we would like you to circle the number that represents the extent to which you disagree or agree with the statement. The more strongly you agree with a statement, the higher will be the number you circle. The more strongly you disagree with a statement, the lower will be the number you circle. Please make sure that you answer every item and that you circle *only one* number per item. This is a measure of your personal beliefs; obviously, there are no right or wrong answers.

Please answer these items carefully, but do not spend too much time on any one item. As much as you can, try to respond to each item independently. When making your choice, do not be influenced by your previous choices. It is important that you respond according to your actual beliefs and not according to how you feel you should believe or how you think we want you to believe.

1 = Strongly Disagree; 2 = Moderately Disagree; 3 = Slightly Disagree; 4 = Slightly Agree; 5 = Moderately Agree; 6 = Strongly Agree.

1. If I become sick, I have the power to make myself well again.	1	2	3	4	5	6
2. Often I feel that no matter what I do, if I am going to get sick, I will get sick.	1	2	3	4	5	6
3. If I see an excellent doctor regularly, I am less likely to have health problems.	1	2	3	4	5	6
4. It seems that my health is greatly influenced by accidental happenings.	1	2	3	4	5	6
5. I can only maintain my health by consulting health professionals.	1	2	3	4	5	6
6. I am directly responsible for my health.	1	2	3	4	5	6
7. Other people play a big part in whether I stay healthy or become sick.	1	2	3	4	5	6
8. Whatever goes wrong with my health is my own fault.	1	2	3	4	5	6
9. When I am sick, I just have to let nature run its course.	1	2	3	4	5	6
10. Health professionals keep me healthy.	1	2	3	4	5	6
11. When I stay healthy, I'm just plain lucky.	1	2	3	4	5	6
12. My physical well-being depends on how well I take care of myself.	1	2	3	4	5	6

Figure 6–19. Multidimensional health locus of control scale, Form B (continued). *(From Wallston, K. A., Wallston, B. S., & DeVellis, R., Development of the multidimensional health locus of control (MHLC) scales. Health Education Monographs, Spring 1978, 6, pp. 164–165. With permission.)*

13. When I feel ill, I know it is because I have not been taking care of myself properly	1	2	3	4	5	6
14. The type of care I receive from other people is what is responsible for how well I recover from an illness.	1	2	3	4	5	6
15. Even when I take care of myself, it's easy to get sick.	1	2	3	4	5	6
16. When I become ill, it's a matter of fate.	1	2	3	4	5	6
17. I can pretty much stay healthy by taking good care of myself.	1	2	3	4	5	6
18. Following doctor's orders to the letter is the best way for me to stay healthy.	1	2	3	4	5	6

Figure 6–19. (continued)

Spiritual Health Assessment

Beliefs about spirituality, life after death, and purpose in life are important dimensions of high-level wellness. Beliefs to which individuals subscribe affect their interpretations of birth and death as well as their response to other important life events such as marriage, childbearing, and childrearing. Daily interactions with others, goals, and feelings about self-worth are related to spiritual beliefs and life philosophy. For this reason, it is critical to appraise the spiritual health of clients in a holistic approach to health assessment. Thought-provoking reflection as part of the assessment process assists clients in determining the meaning of spirituality and purpose in their lives. Rather than judging the value of life by its length, persons should assess the importance of principles and purposes for which they live.[50] A spiritual assessment guide developed by Young[51] appears in Figure 6–20.

A Basis for Action

The assessment process described in this section of the chapter provides both the client and the nurse with important information from which to develop individually tailored plans for protective–promotive care. Many of the tools presented are appropriate for use with children and adolescents as well as with adults of all ages.

ASSESSMENT OF THE FAMILY

The family is the primary social structure for health promotion within society. It is within the context of the family that health behaviors are learned

Instructions

People's religious beliefs and philosophy about life are important to them. Most recently, nursing has realized that considering the spiritual dimension in planning nursing care is part of what it means to take a holistic approach. Spiritual assessment is particularly important when an individual family member and family are dealing with some important life event, such as birth, marriage, death, or some other crisis. The following guide is designed to determine significant information that can assist the nurse in helping the client meet spiritual needs.

Family member _____

Religious preference _____

Participation in worship and related activities

_____ regularly, usually every week

_____ occasionally, such as on special occasions

_____ rarely, but still identifies with a religious group

_____ never participates in religious worship or activities

Do you have a way of describing *God,* or *deity,* that is meaningful to you? ___
_____

    If yes, what is it? _____
_____

Do you have hope? _____

    If yes, how would you describe the source of your strength and hope? ___
_____
_____

Is there a clergy or religious leader that you find especially helpful to you? ___
_____

    If yes, who? _____

Describe the importance of the following to you

    Symbols used _____

    Rituals used _____

    Religious days observed _____
_____

    Other practices _____
_____

Figure 6–20. Spiritual assessment guide.

Do you have religious beliefs that relate to your dietary practices? _____

    If yes, what are they? _____

_____

_____

What events in your life had an effect on your spiritual beliefs? _____

_____

_____

What are your spiritual beliefs about the following? _____

    God _____

    Birth _____

    Death _____

    Health _____

    Illness _____

    Other _____

_____

_____

As a nurse, is there anything I can do to help you meet your spiritual needs?

_____

_____

Figure 6–20. (continued)

and life styles emerge. The family is a logical unit of intervention for health promotion, since the family has the primary responsibility for: (1) developing competencies of family members to care for themselves, (2) backing members up with the social and physical resources of the family group, and (3) promoting autonomy and individuality.[52] While women generally carry the major responsibility for health education of children, family nutrition, and health care planning, responsibility for health should be "mainstreamed" as an integral part of family life style.

    In assessment of the family, the varying family forms that exist today, such as one-parent families and blended families, must be taken into consideration. The milieu for the promotion of health is likely to differ significantly across families, depending on their composition and structure.

Several approaches to assessment that can be used in all types of families will be described briefly here. Both observation and use of self-report information is critical to the in-depth understanding of the dynamics in any family.

Friedman[53] has described a structural–functional approach to family assessment. Within this framework, the family is viewed as a system with the following features: value structure, role structure, power structure, communication patterns, affective function, socialization function, health care function, and family coping function. This approach to assessment is based on systems theory and provides insight concerning the internal processes of the family as well as the relationship of the family to the environment and larger social system. Family decision-making patterns in relation to health are identified in assessing power structure and health care function. A complete description of the structural–functional approach to family assessment as well as guidelines for use of this approach can be found in Friedman's book, *Family Nursing: Theory and Assessment.*[54]

Wright and Leahey[55] provide a thorough description of the Calgary Family Assessment Model (CFAM), which they have adapted specifically for nurses to use when assessing families. Their model for assessment consists of the following major categories: family structural assessment, family developmental assessment, and family functional assessment.

In structural assessment, the family is appraised in terms of both its internal and external structure. Aspects of the internal structure include family composition, rank order, subsystem, and boundary. Components of the external structure are culture, religion, social class status and mobility, environment, and extended family.

Through family developmental assessment, the nurse appraises the current stage of the family in relation to family developmental history.[56] Wright and Leahey's assessment of family development focuses primarily on the traditional family developmental cycle. However, within their book, *Nurses and Families: A Guide to Family Assessment and Intervention*, the authors also discuss assessment of alterations in the family developmental life cycle brought about by separation, divorce, single parenthood, and remarriage by divorced persons.

Family functional assessment is dichotomized as instrumental functioning and expressive functioning. *Instrumental functioning* refers to the routine activities of everyday living, while *expressive functioning* is elaborated as emotional communication, verbal communication, nonverbal communication, circular communication, problem solving, roles, control, beliefs, and alliances and coalitions.[57] The reader is referred to Wright and Leahey's book for a detailed discussion of the family assessment model that they propose.

Other tools that the nurse may wish to consider for family assessment include The Family Environment Scale[58] and the Evaluation of Family Functioning Scale.[59] The former can be used to assess and compare real and ideal family environments. The latter assesses family functioning specifically in relation to health matters and measures the following family dimensions: knowledge of health and illness, ability to solve health problems and prevent complications, health habits, attitudes toward health and health services, ability to cope with stressful situations, family life patterns, action on the physical environment, knowledge and utilization of community health and welfare resources, and participation in community life. Families are evaluated in each of these areas on a 9-point scale ranging from low level of competence to high level of competence.

In summary, a number of excellent tools and models exist within the literature to guide family assessment as a basis for prevention and health-promotion planning. Family assessment complements individual assessment; thus, the two should be considered as interrelated processes. To provide further guidance to nurses in working with families, a format for developing a family Health Protection–Promotion Plan is presented in Chapter 9.

ASSESSMENT OF THE COMMUNITY

A third essential component of health assessment is community analysis or appraisal. A community is a social system that encompasses the collective human energies of individuals, families, and nonfamilial groups. The community is a system with complex relationships among interdependent subsystems. Hanchett has defined the health of a community as dependent on the ability of individuals and groups to direct the flow of energy within the community by working toward common goals that enhance the quality of life and promote the well-being of the population.[60]

Goeppinger has identified five approaches to collecting data about communities: informant interviewing (directed conversation with community members); participant observation (sharing in community life activities); mobile survey (observation while driving about); secondary analyses (use of preexisting data); and community surveys (organized data collection efforts).[61] Since community citizens constitute a critical, primary data source, informant interviewing should always be used as one approach to data collection. An assessment methodology that combines at least 3 to 4 of the above data collection methods is more likely to provide a holistic picture of the community than an assessment that relies on only one or two approaches.

One approach to community assessment is to collect information about the following community subsystems and their interrelationships: (1) values–culture, (2) politics, (3) education, (4) recreation, (5) transportation, (6) religion, (7) communication, (8) welfare, (9) economics, (10) utilities, (11) social life, and (12) health. In assessing the health subsystem, population growth patterns, functional–activity status, nutritional status, dominant life style patterns, coping ability, community stressors, goal setting and achievement capabilities, and risk factors need to be assessed in addition to traditional indices of morbidity, mortality, and accessibility of health care resources.

The community can also be assessed in terms of hierarchical system levels. Microlevel systems include small groups, families, and individuals.[62] Macrolevel systems within the community include organizations, associations, societies, neighborhoods, and cultural aggregates. Each system can be defined in terms of structure, process, functions, and resources. Braden[63] presents a detailed discussion of this approach to analyzing communities.

West describes a community health assessment tool derived from a synthesis of the unitary man framework and Maslow's hierarchy of needs.[64] She proposes that the assessment tool can be used to assess the developmental stage of a community. Factor I of the tool focuses on the interactive processes of exchanging, communicating, and relating. *Exchanging* refers to the interchange of matter and energy between man and the environment and is evaluated by a series of questions including: What is the interchange of services and goods in the community? *Communicating* is defined as the interchange of information between man and environment. Sample evaluative questions include: How does news travel in the community? What groups have a say in the progress of the community? *Relating* refers to connecting with other persons or objects. An assessment question in this area is: To what groups do the citizens belong?

Factor II, Action, has three subcomponents: valuing, choosing, and moving. A series of questions is presented to assess each action component. Factor III, Awareness, consists of the subcomponents of waking, feeling, and knowing. Maslow's needs of safety, love, esteem, and self-actualization are proposed as blending in this category.

For a complete description of the assessment tool, the reader is referred to West.[65] While the tool has been pilot tested on a small community as a basis for assigning a developmental stage to the community and defining patterns of energy exchange, further work is needed to refine and validate the tool. This community health assessment tool, through in the developmental stage, does present useful ideas for assessing communities within the dynamic framework of man–environment interaction.

Assessment of communities is a complicated and time-consuming task. It requires collaboration on the part of many individuals in the community other than health professionals. However, such assessment is critical to the identification of community strengths and resources as well as to the diagnosis of community problems or deficits. While a detailed description of community assessment procedures is beyond the scope of this book, the reader needs to be aware of the importance of analyzing communities as a basis for planning community-wide prevention and health promotion programs.

SUMMARY

Health assessment can be carried out at the individual, family, or community level. Since methodologies developed to date have focused on the assessment of illness status as opposed to health status of individuals, families, and communities, current health assessment approaches at all levels should be viewed as relatively crude. Future efforts must be directed toward conceptualizing health as a dynamic, multidimensional yet holistic process. This will lead to the development and refinement of assessment models that take into account the multidimensionality of health at all levels and the complex ways in which the health status of individuals, families, and communities is interrelated.

REFERENCES

1. Trautlein, J., et al. How much yield from a health screen? *Patient Care*, 1974, *8*, 65–69.
2. Bates, B. *A Guide to physical examination.* Philadelphia: Lippincott, 1979.
3. Kopf, R., Salamon, M. J., & Charytan, P. The preventive health history form: A questionnaire for use with older patient populations. *Journal of Gerontological Nursing*, September 1982, *8*(9), 519–523.
4. Hogan, R. *Human sexuality: A nursing perspective.* New York: Appleton-Century-Crofts, 1980.
5. Canadian Task Force on the Periodic Health Examination. Task Force Report: The periodic health examination. *Canadian Medical Association Journal*, November 3, 1979, *121*, 1193–1254.
6. Ibid.
7. Ibid.
8. Bates, op. cit.
9. Malasanos, L., Barkauskas, V., Moss, M., & Stoltenberg-Allen, K. *Health Assessment.* St. Louis: C. V. Mosby, 1977.
10. Sauve, M. H., & Pecherer, A. *Concepts and skills in physical assessment.* Philadelphia: Saunders, 1977.
11. Frank-Stromborg, M., & Stromborg, P. *Primary care assessment and management skills for nurses: A self-assessment manual.* Philadelphia: Lippincott, 1979.
12. Dubos, R. Health and creative adaptation. *Human Nature*, 1978, *1*, 74–82.
13. Getchell, L. Adult physical fitness evaluation. Personal communication, 1980.
14. Borgman, M. F. Exercise and health maintenance. *Journal of Nursing Education*, 1977, *16*, 6–10.
15. Getchell, L. *Physical fitness: A way of life* (2nd ed.). New York: Wiley, 1979, pp. 78–79.
16. Ibid, pp. 79–80.
17. Rochmis, P., & Blackburn, H. Exercise tests: A survey of procedures, safety and ligitation experience in approximately 170,000 tests. *Journal of the American Medical Association*, 1971, *216*, 1061.
18. Getchell, op. cit., pp. 70–73.
19. Ibid., pp. 51–57.
20. Larsen, G. A., & Malmboy, R. O. *Coronary heart disease and physical fitness.* Baltimore: University Park Press, 1971.
21. Cooper, K. H. *The new aerobics.* New York: Evans, 1970.
22. Seltzer, C. C., & Mayer, J. A. Simple criterion of obesity. *Postgraduate Medicine*, 1965, *38*, A101.

23. U. S. Senate Select Committee on Nutrition and Human Needs. *Dietary goals for the United States.* Washington, D. C.: Government Printing Office, December 1977.

24. Suitor, C. W., & Crowley, M. F. *Nutrition: Principles and application in health promotion* (2nd ed.). Philadelphia: Lippincott, 1984, Appendix 3, pp. 577–584.

25. Caliendo, M. A. *Nutrition and preventive health care.* New York: Macmillan, 1981, Appendix I, pp. 648–655.

26. LaDou, J., Sherwood, J. N., & Hughes, L. Health hazard appraisal in patient counseling (preventive medicine). *Western Journal of Medicine,* 1975, *122,* 177–180.

27. Steinbach, M. Risk factors and their interaction. *Revue Roumaine de Médecine Interne,* 1973, *10,* 355–363.

28. U. S. Department of Health and Human Services. Public Health Service. Office of Disease Prevention and Health Promotion. *Health risk appraisals: An inventory.* PHS Publication No. 81-50163 (June 1981).

29. Weiss, S. M. Health hazard–health risk appraisals. In J. D. Matarazzo, S. M. Weiss, J. A. Herd, N. E. Miller, & S. M. Weiss (Eds.), *Behavioral health: A handbook of health enhancement and disease prevention.* New York: Wiley, 1984, pp. 275–276.

30. Beery, W. L., Wagner, E. H., Schoenbach, V. J., & Graham, R. M. A shopper's guide to appraisal instruments. *Promoting health,* July–August 1981, 6–10.

31. Fielding, J. Reducing the risk of risk appraisals. *Promoting Health,* July–August 1981, 4–5, 10.

32. Weiss, op. cit., p. 282.

33. Langer, T., & Michael, S. *Life stress and mental health.* New York: Free Press, 1960.

34. Holmes, T., & Rahe, R. The social readjustment rating scale. *Journal of Psychosomatic Research,* 1967, *11,* 213.

35. Ibid.

36. Speilberger, C. D., Gorsach, R. L., Lushene, R., Vagg, P. R., & Jacobs, G. A. *Manual for the State–trait anxiety inventory.* Palo Alto, Calif.: Consulting Psychologists Press, 1983.

37. Everly, G. S., & Girdano, D. A. *The stress mess solution.* Bowie, Md.: Robert J. Brady, 1980.

38. Walters, D. Stress management seminar format. Personal communication. Topeka, Kan.: Menninger Foundation, 1980.

39. Larson, R. Thirty years of research on the subjective well-being of older Americans. *Journal of Gerontology,* 1978, *33,* 109–129.

40. Wan, T. T. W., & Livieratos, B. Interpreting a general index of subjective well-being. *Milbank Memorial Fund Quarterly/Health and Society,* 1978, *56,* 531–556.

41. Oelbaum, C. H. Hallmarks of adult wellness. *American Journal of Nursing,* 1974, *74,* 1623–1625.

42. Travis, J. W. *Wellness workbook for health professionals: A guide to attaining high level wellness.* Mill Valley, Calif.: Wellness Resource Center, 1977.

43. Kaplan, R. M., Bush, J. W., & Berry, C. C. Health status: Types of validity and the index of well-being. *Health Services Research,* Winter 1976, *11,* 478–507.

44. Belloc, N. B., & Breslow, L. Relationship of physical health status and health practices. *Preventive Medicine,* 1972, *1,* 409–421.

45. Walker, S. N., Sechrist, K., & Pender, N. J. The health promoting lifestyle profile: Development and psychometric evaluation. *Nursing Research* (in press).

46. Hettler, B. Wellness: Encouraging a lifetime pursuit of excellence. *Health Values: Achieving High Level Wellness,* July–August 1984, *8*(4), 13–17.

47. Wallston, B. S., & Wallston, K. A. Locus of control and health: A review of the literature. *Health Education Monographs*, 1978, *6*, 107–117.

48. Wallston, K. A., Wallston, B. S., & DeVellis, R. Development of the multidimensional health locus of control (MHLC) scales. *Health Education Monographs*, 1978, *6*, 161–170.

49. Ibid.

50. Tubesing, N. L., & Tubesing, D. A. *Structured exercises in wellness promotion: A whole person handbook for trainers, educators and group leaders, Vol. II*. Duluth, Minn.: Whole Person Press, 1984, p. 86.

51. Young, R. C. *Community Nursing Workbook: Family as client*. Norwalk, Conn.: Appleton-Century-Crofts, 1982, pp. 189–190.

52. Pratt, L. *Family structure and effective health behavior: The energized family*. Boston: Houghton Mifflin, 1976.

53. Friedman, M. N. *Family nursing: Theory and assessment* (2nd ed.). New York: Appleton-Century-Crofts, 1985.

54. Ibid.

55. Wright, L. M., & Leahey, M. *Nurses and families: A guide to family assessment and intervention*. Philadelphia: Davis, 1984.

56. Ibid., p. 38.

57. Ibid., p. 54.

58. Moos, R. H., & Moos, B. S. A typology of family social environments. *Family Process*, 1976, *15*, 357–371.

59. Reidy, M., & Thibaudeau, M. F. Evaluation of family functioning: Development and validation of a scale which measures family competence in matters of health. *Nursing Papers*, 1984, *16*, 42–56.

60. Hanchett, E. *Community health assessment: A conceptual tool kit*. New York: Wiley, 1979.

61. Goeppinger, J. Community as client: using the nursing process to promote health. In M. Stanhope & J. Lancaster (Eds.), *Community health nursing: Process and practice for promoting health*. St. Louis: C. V. Mosby, 1984, pp. 379–404.

62. Braden, C. J. *The focus and limits of community health nursing*. Norwalk, Conn.: Appleton-Century-Crofts, 1984.

63. Ibid.

64. West, M. Community health assessment: The man–environment interaction. *Journal of Community Health Nursing*, 1984, *1*(2), 89–97.

65. Ibid.

CHAPTER 7

Values Clarification

Exploration of values and the valuing process in such diverse fields as psychology, sociology, philosophy, bioethics, education, and communications attests to the centrality of values in understanding human behavior. Rokeach defined a value as an enduring belief that a specific mode of conduct or a particular end state or goal is personally or socially preferable.[1] Values have both cognitive and affective dimensions. They provide a basis for making decisions and choices and are critical mediating variables in human actions and reactions to environmental stimuli. Life experience shapes personal and family values. Values evolve and change as a result of maturation, interpersonal relations, and social circumstances. Values are organized into value systems that persist over time and are resistant to change.[2] Value systems reflect culture, society, and significant reference groups.[3]

Because no two individuals or groups have the same life experiences, no two value systems are exactly the same. However, similarities in value systems may occur within the same culture and across cultures. Rokeach[4] in *The Nature of Human Values* has identified five assumptions about values:

1. The total number of values that a person possesses is relatively small
2. All persons everywhere possess the same values but to differing degrees
3. Values are organized into value systems
4. The antecedents of human values can be traced to culture, society, institutions and personality
5. The consequences of human values will be manifested in virtually all phenomena that social scientists might consider worth investigating and understanding

TABLE 7–1. THE VALUING PROCESS

Choosing:	(1) Choosing values freely (2) Choosing from alternatives (3) Thoughtfully considering the consequences or outcomes of each alternative
Prizing:	(4) Cherishing, being happy with the choice (5) Willing to make values known to others
Acting:	(6) Doing something with the choice (7) Integrating values into life style

From Raths, L.E., Harmin, M., & Simons, S.B. Values and teaching: Working with values in the classroom. Columbus, Ohio: Charles E. Merrill, 1966. With permission.

The process of valuing has been described by Raths, Harmin, and Simon[5] as consisting of three phases and seven distinct steps. The valuing process is depicted in Table 7–1. Two types of values are described by Rokeach: terminal values and instrumental values. Terminal values are concerned with desired end states or goals, while instrumental values focus on desired modes of conduct. A diagram of the two types of values is presented in Figure 7–1.

Health values do not emerge in a vacuum but in the context of life values. All behaviors express values in some way.[6] The Health Promotion Model presented in Chapter 3 proposes importance (value) of health as a key motivational factor for health-promoting behaviors. The significance or importance that an individual or family places on enhancing health status is likely to affect the frequency and intensity with which health-promoting behaviors occur.

In the health care setting, the values of the nurse and client interact. Thus, nurses must be aware of personal values and avoid imposing their own values on the client. With the current emphasis on the importance of re-

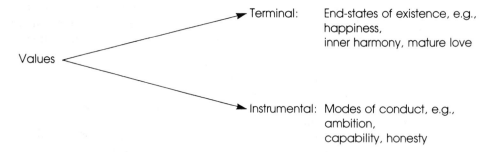

Figure 7–1. Types of values. *(From Rokeach, M. The nature of human values. New York: Free Press, 1973, with permission.)*

sponsible self-care for optimizing health, personal and family health actions should be based on clearly articulated values that direct and organize behavior to accomplish some purpose. The nurse may assist clients with *values clarification* or *values change.*

- Values clarification is increasing personal or group awareness of value priorities and the degree of consistency among values, attitudes, and behavior
- Values-change is the reprioritization of values, abandonment of existing values, or acquisition of new values and subsequent attitude and behavior change

The nurse who utilizes either of these two strategies must clearly understand the differences between them and must possess the requisite knowledge and skills to utilize both interventions appropriately and ethically. Values clarification will be discussed at length in this chapter. Many of the suggested strategies are appropriate for both individuals and families. Some of the strategies are intended for use primarily with individual clients. Values-change strategies will be addressed in Chapter 10.

What should be the role of the nurse in values clarification as she works with individuals of differing ages and families at various stages of the life span? In the view of the author, the nurse can play a critical role in assisting clients to clarify values; understand the personal and social consequences of acting on current values; achieve greater consistency among values, attitudes, and behaviors; and plan health-related experiences that may result in self-initiated changes in value hierarchies. Inadequate decision making on the part of a client may result from lack of clarity about values. By focusing on values clarification, the nurse can increase the capacity of the client for making informed and responsible choices regarding personal, family, and community health. Graham found that persons who had experienced the values-clarification process made more value-based decisions than people without exposure to values clarification.[7]

The consent of the client should be obtained before the nurse initiates values clarification.[8] After an explanation of the values-clarification process, clients have the right of refusal, just as they have with any other intervention. The nurse must respect the right of the client to autonomy and self-determination. Throughout values clarification, the nurse should maintain a nonjudgmental and accepting attitude to facilitate open communication. Values clarification should be used cautiously with persons who have emotional problems or with markedly disorganized families.

STRATEGIES FOR VALUES CLARIFICATION

Modern life offers multiple choices that make selection a bewildering problem. While choices should set paths of action that individuals wish to follow, consistent behavior is required to "act out" the values that clients hold.[9,10]

Values clarification can facilitate decision making and problem solving in the area of health by promoting behavior consistent with health-related values.[11] Values clarification can also serve as a consciousness-raising activity for clients by increasing awareness of personal priorities, identifying ambiguities or confusion in priorities, and determining what major value–behavior conflicts or inconsistencies exist. The notion behind values clarification is that awareness of ambiguities, conflicts, or inconsistencies will result in self-dissatisfaction (dissatisfaction with the self-concept). In an effort to enhance self-esteem, clients will make the changes necessary to decrease inconsistencies.

Many problems throughout the life span stem from not having adequately worked through value issues in the areas of work, school, leisure, religion, health, family, and friends at an early age. The aim of the values-clarifying process is not to impose a value, course of action, opinion, or solution on clients but to encourage them to look at alternatives and their consequences.[12] Nurses are encouraged to review the strategies presented in this chapter and carefully consider the usefulness of each strategy for specific clients within their current caseload.

EXAMINING VALUE HIERARCHIES

A number of instruments have been developed to determine the value hierarchies of individuals. One of the most frequently used instruments for measuring values is the Value Survey developed by Rokeach.[13] It is composed of two parts in which terminal values and instrumental values can be ranked. Wallston and Wallston adapted the Value Survey to include "health" as a value and developed the Health Value Scale.[14] Kavanagh[15] presented helpful reviews on six additional value instruments. He suggested use of the following tools for examining personal values in the counseling setting:

1. The Allport–Vernon–Lindzey Study of Values (SV)[16]
2. The Survey of Personal Values (SPV)[17]
3. The Survey of Interpersonal Values (SIV)[18]
4. The Differential Value Profile (DVP)[19]
5. The Personal Orientation Inventory (POI)[20,21]
6. Ways to Live[22]

Since review of each of the above instruments is beyond the scope of this book, the reader is referred to *The Mental Measurements Yearbook*[23] for further descriptive details. The *Yearbook* will provide information about the scope of the instruments, reliability, validity, qualifications for administration, and publishing source. As examples of value-assessment tools available, the Value Survey and Health Value Scale will be presented and discussed.

Value Survey[24]

The survey consists of two lists, each containing 18 values. The first list contains terminal values; the second list contains instrumental values.

Below are 18 values listed in alphabetical order. Your task is to arrange them in order of their importance to YOU, as guiding principles in YOUR life. Each value is printed on a gummed label that can be easily peeled off and pasted in the boxes on the left-hand side of the page. Study the list carefully and pick out the one value that is the most important for you. Peel it off and paste it in Box 1 on the left. Then pick out the value that is second-most important for you. Peel it off and paste it in Box 2. Then do the same for each of the remaining values. The value that is least important goes in Box 18. Work slowly and think carefully. If you change your mind, feel free to change your answers. The labels peel off easily and can be moved from place to place. The end result should truly show how you really feel.

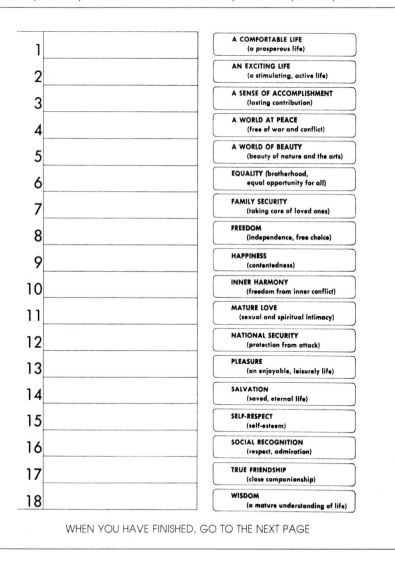

WHEN YOU HAVE FINISHED, GO TO THE NEXT PAGE

Figure 7–2. Value Survey. (continued) *(Distributed by Halgren Tests, 873 Persimmon Ave., Sunnyvale, California 94087. Reprinted from Rokeach, M. The nature of human values. New York: Free Press, 1973, pp. 357–361. With permission.)*

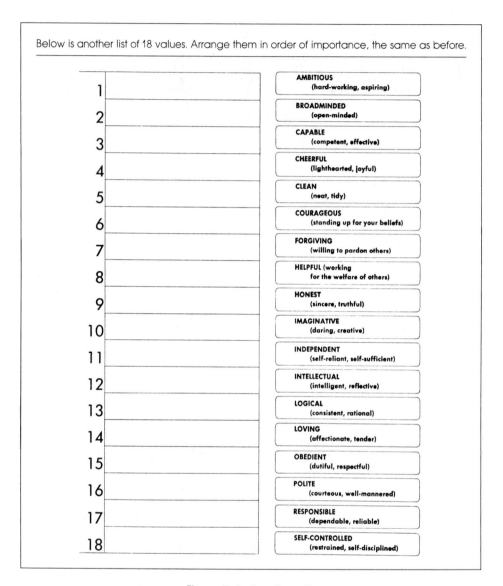

Figure 7–2. (continued)

Test–retest reliability for the survey has been found to be between 0.69 and 0.80 on terminal values and between 0.61 and 0.72 on instrumental values. Reliability data are based primarily on college populations. The Value Survey uses gummed stickers on pressure-sensitive paper so that the stickers can be removed initially and arranged in the preferred order. They can also be rearranged until the client is sure that the order of ranking represents an accurate presentation of values. This instrument provides information on 36 values and can be completed by the client in 15 to 20 minutes. The instructions and survey items appear in Figure 7–2.

A major limitation of the Value Survey for purposes of client counseling is that "health" is not included in the list of 18 terminal values. The author would suggest inclusion of "health" in the list for clinical use but cautions the reader that this change may alter the reliability and validity of the instrument.

The Health-Value Scale presented next is a shortened version of Rokeach's Terminal Value Survey with "health" added as a value. The nurse as health counselor may choose to use the original Value Survey, adapt it by the inclusion of "health," or use the Health Value Scale.

Health-Value Scale[25]

The Health-Value Scale is an adaptation of Rokeach's Terminal Value Survey. The scale consists of ten values that the client is asked to rank in order of importance from 1 to 10. The Health-Value Scale appears in Figure 7–3.

Interpretation of responses to the scale is straightforward. If health appears in the top four positions out of the ten positions possible, the client

---

Below you will find a list of ten values listed in alphabetical order. We would like you to arrange them in order of their importance to YOU, as guiding principles in YOUR life.

Study the list carefully and pick out the one value that is the most important for you. Write the number "1" in the space to the left of the most important value. Then pick out the value that is second-most important to you. Write the number "2" in the space to the left. Then continue in the same manner for the remaining values until you have included all ranks from 1 to 10. Each value will have a different rank.

We realize that some people find it difficult to distinguish the importance of some of these values. Do the best that you can, but please rank all 10 of them. The end result should truly show how YOU really feel.

_____ A COMFORTABLE LIFE (a prosperous life)

_____ AN EXCITING LIFE (a stimulating, active life)

_____ A SENSE OF ACCOMPLISHMENT (lasting contribution)

_____ FREEDOM (independence, free choice)

_____ HAPPINESS (contentedness)

_____ HEALTH (physical and mental well-being)

_____ INNER HARMONY (freedom from inner conflict)

_____ PLEASURE (an enjoyable, leisurely life)

_____ SELF-RESPECT (self-esteem)

_____ SOCIAL RECOGNITION (respect, admiration)

Figure 7–3. Health-Value Scale. *(Adapted with permission from Rokeach, M. Value survey. Halpren Tests, Sunnyvale, Calif. Used with permission, from Wallston, B.S., Personal communication, 1980.)*

places a high value on health. If health appears in any other positions, the value placed on health is moderate (position 5, 6, 7) or low (position 8, 9, 10). In administering the scale, the nurse should encourage clients to rank the items in a way that most accurately reflects their value hierarchy. Care should be taken to avoid biasing the client and thus obtaining an inflated and inaccurate ranking of health as a personal value. Interestingly, health-enhancing behaviors may be based on values other than health, such as inner harmony or self-respect.

CLARIFYING PERSONAL AND FAMILY VALUES

The strategies suggested in this section are directed toward assisting clients in examining priorities, conflicts, or inconsistencies in value systems and congruency or lack of congruency between values and behavior. The strategies are based on the assumption that individuals and families set particular goals and wish to engage in behaviors that move them toward those goals. The purpose and procedure for each strategy will be described, and appropriate materials for use with clients will be presented.

Twenty Favorite Activities[26]

Purpose. An important question for people of all ages to deal with is "Am I getting what I want out of life?" This question can also be posed to families: As a family unit, are we engaging in activities that we enjoy? If living is to be rewarding, it should include activities that are prized and valued. Individuals and families may not know whether they are getting what they really want from life if they have not taken stock of their own needs and feelings. The purpose of this exercise is to help clients decide what activities bring them the most enjoyment.

Procedure. The individual or family should be given the "Twenty Favorite Activities" sheet presented in Figure 7–4 and encouraged to write down as many activities as possible that bring enjoyment or happiness. After the client has listed these activities, the nurse should ask the client to review the list and code all behaviors in the following way:

- A—Activities that the individual or family prefers to do alone
- P—Activities that the individual or family prefers to do with other people
- $—Activities that cost more than $10 each time or require an initial major investment that the individual or family has not made yet
- PL—Activities that require advanced planning.

In the *last time* column, the client should indicate how long it has been since engaging in each of the listed activities, and in the next column the client

Activities	A/P	$	PL	Last Time	Rank Top Five (1–5)	Plan Ahead
1						
2						
3						
4						
5						
6						
7						
8						
9						
10						
11						
12						
13						
14						
15						
16						
17						
18						
19						
20						

Figure 7–4. "Twenty Favorite Activities" sheet. *(Adapted from Simon, S.B. Values clarification—a tool for counselors. Personnel and Guidance Journal, 1973, 51, p. 616. With permission.)*

should rank from 1 to 5 (most enjoyable to less enjoyable) the five activities out of the list that are enjoyed most.

The content of the list can be reviewed with the client to assist in planning more frequent inclusion of enjoyable activities in individual or family life style. If possible, planning should center on the next few weeks or the next month, and encouragement should be given to the client to make concrete plans for engaging in the top-ranked activities in the near future. A projected time plan can be included in the "Plan Ahead" column. If the selected activities are expensive or require an initial outlay of money, the client may need to explore ways in which the necessary funds can be acquired or the cost of the activity decreased.

Real–Ideal Values

Purpose. The purpose of this strategy is to assist clients in comparing their value rankings on the Health-Value Scale with what they picture as the ideal set of values for themselves.

Procedure. Before the client reviews the previous ranking of values, the personal or family ideal set of values should be completed on the scale shown in Figure 7–5. Most important value should be ranked "1" in the space to the

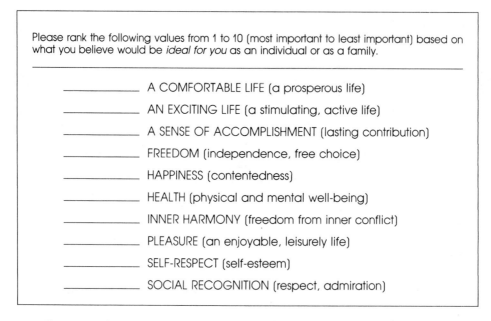

Please rank the following values from 1 to 10 (most important to least important) based on what you believe would be *ideal for you* as an individual or as a family.

_____ A COMFORTABLE LIFE (a prosperous life)

_____ AN EXCITING LIFE (a stimulating, active life)

_____ A SENSE OF ACCOMPLISHMENT (lasting contribution)

_____ FREEDOM (independence, free choice)

_____ HAPPINESS (contentedness)

_____ HEALTH (physical and mental well-being)

_____ INNER HARMONY (freedom from inner conflict)

_____ PLEASURE (an enjoyable, leisurely life)

_____ SELF-RESPECT (self-esteem)

_____ SOCIAL RECOGNITION (respect, admiration)

Figure 7–5. Ideal set of values. *(Adapted from the Health Value Scale developed by Wallston, K.A., & Wallston, B.S., Health locus of control. Health Education Monographs, Spring 1978, 6.)*

left; the client continues ranking the remaining items until values are ranked from 1 to 10. The end result should be a picture of the client's ideal to which rankings on the Health-Value Scale during health assessment can be compared. If discrepancies are apparent between the real and ideal rankings, discussion can follow concerning how the client might move from the real toward the ideal.

Values-Actions Review

Purpose. The purpose of this strategy is to help the client determine how the values of most personal importance are expressed in activities of every day living. Value-action discrepancies are major causes of frustration and conflict in life. Individuals identify goals that they are unable to reach because they do not engage in behaviors that consistently move them toward their desired goals. The consistency of personal values and actions is highly related to the level of satisfaction that a client experiences from a personal life style.

Procedure. The client should use the form presented in Figure 7–6 and list the four most important personal values. Either real or ideal values may be used, or the same exercise can be completed with both if they differ considerably. Following each value, the client can identify those behaviors engaged in regularly that express important values. Upon completion of the Values-Actions Review, additional behaviors that would assist the client in achieving personal goals can be discussed. The possibility of incorporating these new behaviors into personal life style or daily activities can be explored.

Pie of Life[27]

Purpose. This technique allows individual clients to inventory their own life in terms of how time is spent during typical work or leisure days. The Pie of Life can assist the client in identifying value–time inconsistencies. An analysis of how personal time is spent should show that values of highest priority are allocated the most time and effort. As an example, while the client may indicate that a high value is placed on health, review of a typical day may show that little time is devoted to protecting or enhancing personal health.

Procedure. Clients are to indicate on the Pie of Life Form presented in Figure 7–7 how they spend a typical work day (in an occupation or, if a housewife, at home) and a typical leisure day. Each pie is divided into quarters that represent 6-hour segments. The short lines around the circumference of the circle represent 1-hour segments of time. In all, the pie totals 24 hours. The client may work with the categories listed below the circles or add additional categories to describe more appropriately how a typical day is spent.

Top Four Values	Actions I Take to Express These Values in Everyday Living
1.	
2.	
3.	
4.	

Figure 7–6. Values-Actions review. This exercise uses responses from the Health Value Scale or the Value Survey—terminal or instrumental values.

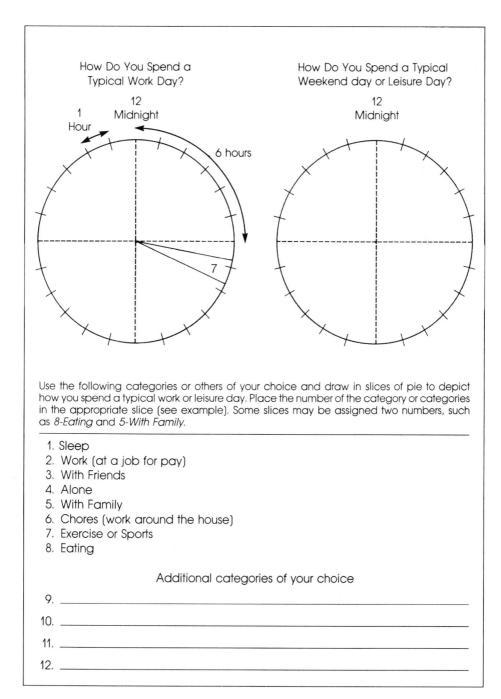

Use the following categories or others of your choice and draw in slices of pie to depict how you spend a typical work or leisure day. Place the number of the category or categories in the appropriate slice (see example). Some slices may be assigned two numbers, such as *8-Eating* and *5-With Family*.

1. Sleep
2. Work (at a job for pay)
3. With Friends
4. Alone
5. With Family
6. Chores (work around the house)
7. Exercise or Sports
8. Eating

Additional categories of your choice

9. _____
10. _____
11. _____
12. _____

Figure 7–7. The pie of life. *(Adapted from Simon, S.B., Howe, L.W., Kirschenbaum, H. Values clarification: A handbook of practical strategies for teachers and students. New York: Hart, 1972. With permission.)*

Following completion of the two pies, the client should be directed to think about the following questions:

1. Are you satisfied with the relative sizes of your slices?
2. Ideally, how big would you want each slice to be?
3. Realistically, is there anything you can do to begin to change the size of some of your slices?

The nurse should stress to the client that there is no right way to section the pie. There is also no need to change if the client is happy with the way personal time is spent. If the client wishes to change, decisions about the direction of change must be made by the client. The nature of changes should be consistent with previously identified values and goals.

Personal–Family Values

Purpose. The purpose of this exercise is to assist families in determining what personal values are shared among family members. Shared values assist families in moving toward mutually desirable goals. If values of family members are very diverse, the exercise may have to be completed for each family dyad.

Procedure. Each individual should work from a hierarchical list of personal values that has been completed. This may be the Value Survey (terminal or instrumental) or the Health Value Scale. The rank order number previously

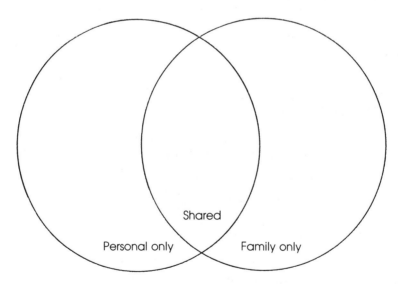

Figure 7–8. Personal-Family Values.

assigned each value should be placed within one of the segments of the two circles in Figure 7–8. Each client can write in additional personal values not shared with the family or, conversely, values considered high-priority by the family but not of high priority for the client. Review of the results will allow each family member to determine whether the highest-ranked personal values are shared with people who are close. This information can be used as a basis for discussion of family interactions, extent of agreement on important values, and ways that families can move together toward shared values and goals. A discussion of the mutuality of health as a value can provide insight into personal and family predisposition to engage in health behaviors. In using this strategy, the nurse should encourage families to focus primarily on shared values and only secondarily on value inconsistencies and disagreements.

Alternatives–Consequences Search[28]

Purpose. The purpose of this strategy is to assist individuals or families in considering alternatives to current life style or ways of dealing with specific problems. Alternatives and the resultant consequences should be carefully considered before making a decision regarding a particular course of action to be pursued. The client is encouraged to identify challenge questions that set the stage for considering various action alternatives. For example: How can physical fitness be enhanced? How can friendships be strengthened or expanded? How can greater control over health status be achieved? Instead of functioning primarily on the basis of habit, life should be lived in consideration of the full range of alternative actions available.

Procedure. At the top of the form presented in Figure 7–9, the client should place a challenge question that represents the dilemma or problem to be addressed. As many alternative actions as possible that address the problem should be listed in the left-hand column of the form. The consequences of each alternative action should be enumerated. The extent to which the client is willing to try each alternative should be based on consideration of the consequences that are most appealing and the practicality of each action for that particular client.

Blocks to Action[29]

Purpose. Acting on beliefs and values is a critical part of the valuing process. Blocks to Action is a strategy that should be used as a follow-up activity to the Alternatives–Consequences search to assist clients in implementing the action alternatives selected. Barriers to action may be perceived or real, internal or external. Regardless of the source of the barrier, action may be inhibited if the barriers are not recognized and removed.

Challenge Question:

Alternatives	Consequences	Place Check in Appropriate Column		
		WILLING TO TRY IT	WILLING TO CONSIDER IT	UNWILLING TO TRY IT
1.	1. 2. 3. 4. 5. 6.			
2.	1. 2. 3. 4. 5. 6.			

3.	1. ____ 2. ____ 3. ____ 4. ____ 5. ____ 6.			
4.	1. ____ 2. ____ 3. ____ 4. ____ 5. ____ 6.			

Figure 7–9. Alternatives/Consequences Search Sheet. *(Adapted from Simon, S.B. Values clarification: A tool for counselors.* Personnel and Guidance Journal 51, *615, 1973. With permission.)*

176

Alternatives to Try Or Consider	Blocks to Action	Source of Blocks W: Within O: Outside	Suggestions for Removing Blocks
1.			
2.			
3.			

Figure 7–10. Discovering blocks to action form.

Alternatives to Try Or Consider	Blocks to Action	Source of Blocks W: Within O: Outside	Suggestions for Removing Blocks
4.			

Figure 7–10. (continued)

Procedure. On the Discovering Blocks to Action Form presented in Figure 7–10, clients should list the action alternatives that they are willing to try or consider as indicated in responses to the Alternatives–Consequences Search. In the second column, barriers to taking action should be listed. Each barrier should be coded in the third column as either within the client (W) or outside the client (O). In the right-hand column, steps that can be taken to remove or reduce barriers should be identified. Following completion of the written exercise, the extent to which perceived barriers actually exist can be discussed. The client is encouraged to look at strengths and potential for dealing with barriers that thwart purposeful health protecting and health-promoting activity.

Value Support System

Purpose. The purpose of this strategy is to allow individuals or families to identify support for important values. This technique expands on the Personal–Family Values exercise presented earlier. Having people available for support is important in encouraging behaviors that move clients toward goals reflecting important values. If individuals or groups who are close to the client do not share similar values, this poses a threat to the personal or family value system and sense of esteem.

Procedure. Clients can use the form presented in Figure 7–11, indicating at the top of the page a specific value that they wish to consider. A different form can be used for each value. In the left-hand column, the client should

Value:

Individual/Group	Support	Neutral	Do Not Support	Emotional Closeness VC: Very Close MC: Moderately Close D: Distant	Frequency of Interaction/Week
Family members					
Friends					

Figure 7–11. Analysis of value support system.

list individual family members, friends, co-workers, and relevant community groups. The client can indicate whether each person or group identified supports, is neutral to, or does not support the target value being considered. Important determinants of the effect of others on the client are emotional closeness and frequency of interaction. The client can include these factors in the analysis in the right-hand column. This exercise allows the client to look at the scope and strength of external support for important personal values.

What did you as an individual or family do this week that was health-promoting or health-damaging?

Health Promoting	Can It Be Done Again?	When?
Health Damaging	What Encouraged It?	What Could Discourage It?

Figure 7–12. Review of health related behavior.

Review of Health-Related Behavior

Purpose. The purpose of this exercise is specifically to encourage the individual or family to focus on health as a value and look at the impact of specific behaviors on health status. Clients should be encouraged to look at health-promoting behaviors that were performed during the previous week, either individually or as a family unit, about which they felt proud or good. Health-damaging behaviors that were undesirable to clients should also be identified.

Procedure. Individuals or families should be provided with a form similar to the one depicted in Figure 7–12. In the left-hand column, the client can list both health-promoting and health-damaging behaviors during the previous 7 days. Each health-promoting behavior should be considered in terms of when it could be repeated again. A specific time commitment should be made. For each health-damaging behavior, factors that encourage the behavior need to be explored and ways of discouraging the behavior identified. This exercise focuses the client on personal or family strengths in the area of health promotion and heightens awareness of behaviors detrimental to health.

RESEARCH ON VALUES AND VALUES CLARIFICATION

Few studies have been conducted by nurses concerning values and the nature of the valuing process as it relates to health. Brink[30] discussed use of the Value Orientation Scale as a tool for assessing cultural diversity in value orientations. Gortner, Hudes, and Zyzanski[31] described development of the Gortner Values in the Choice of Treatment Inventory based on bioethical concepts. Nurse-researchers need to continue efforts to develop and refine instruments for assessing values of clients and families.

Descriptive studies of how individuals and families with differing value profiles make health decisions are critically needed. Experimental studies should be conducted to determine the reactions of different client groups to participation in the values clarification process.[32] Prior to implementing well-designed experimental studies, reliable and valid evaluation instruments for measuring the impact of values clarification on individual and family behavior need to be developed.[33]

SUMMARY

The values-clarification strategies presented in this chapter are directed toward assisting clients to make important decisions about life style. Each individual and family must ultimately choose those values that will serve as standards for actions and interactions with others. Some clients may have given little consideration to their own values and even less attention to whether they hold conflicting values or whether their behavior is supportive of the values that they hold. Gaining insight into values is an important step toward taking action to reinforce and strengthen those behaviors that are consistent with cherished values.

REFERENCES

1. Rokeach, M. *The nature of human values.* New York: Free Press, 1973, p. 5.
2. Rokeach, M., & Regan, J. F. The role of values in the counseling situation. *Personnel and Guidance Journal,* May 1980, 576–583.
3. Rokeach, 1973, op. cit., p. 5.
4. Ibid., p. 3.
5. Raths, L. E., Harmin, M., & Simon, S. B. *Values and teaching: Working with values in the classroom.* Columbus, Ohio: Chas. E. Merrill, 1966.
6. Rokeach & Reagan, 1980 op. cit.
7. Graham, M. D. *The process of teaching decision-making through values clarification and its effects on students' future choices as measured by changes in the self-concept* (doctoral dissertation, St. Louis University, 1976). *Dissertation Abstracts International,* 1976, 37, 1885-A (University Microfilms No. 76-22, 540).
8. Wilberding, J. Z. Values clarification. In G. M. Bulechek & J. C. McCloskey (Eds.), *Nursing interventions: Treatments for nursing diagnoses.* Philadelphia: Saunders, 1985, pp. 173–184.
9. Governali, J. F., & Sechrist, W. C. Clarifying values in a health education setting: An Experimental analysis. *Journal of School Health,* 1980, *50,* 151–154.
10. Raths, Harmin, & Simon, op cit. p. 27.
11. Casteel, J. D., & Stahl, R. J. *Value clarification in the classroom: A primer.* Pacific Palisades, Calif., Good Year, 1975.
12. Glaser, B., & Kirschbaum, H. Using values clarification in a counseling setting. *Personnel and Guidance Journal,* May 1980, 569–575.
13. Rokeach, 1973, op. cit., pp. 357–361.
14. Wallston, K. A., & Wallston, B. S. Health locus of control. *Health Education Monographs,* Spring 1978, 6.
15. Kavanagh, H. B. Some appraised instruments of values for counselors. *Personnel and Guidance Journal,* May 1980, 613–617.
16. Allport, G. W., Vernon, P. E., & Lindzey, G. *Study of values,* (3rd ed.). Boston: Houghton Mifflin, 1960.
17. Ibid.
18. Ibid.
19. Thomas, W. L. *The differential value profile.* Chicago: W. and J. Stone Foundation, 1963.
20. Shostrom, E. L. *The personal orientation inventory.* San Diego, Calif.: Education and Industrial Testing Service, 1963.
21. Shostrom, E. L. *Actualizing therapy.* San Diego, Calif.: Edits, 1976.
22. Morris, C.W. *Varieties of human value.* Chicago: University of Chicago Press, 1956.
23. Buros, O. K. (Ed.). *The mental measurements yearbook* (8th ed.). Highland Park, N.J.: Gryphon Press, 1978.

24. Rokeach, 1973, op. cit., pp. 27–54.
25. Kaplan, G. C., & Cowles, A. Health locus of control and health value in the prediction of smoking reduction. *Health Education Monographs*, Spring 1978, *6*, 129–137.
26. Hawley, R. C., & Hawley, I. L. *Human values in the classroom: A handbook for teachers*. New York: Hart, 1975.
27. Simon, S. B., Howe, L. W., & Kirschbaum, H. *Values clarification: A handbook of practical strategies for teachers and students*. New York: Hart, 1972.
28. Ibid., pp. 198–203, 207–208.
29. Ibid.
30. Brink, P. J. Value orientations as an assessment tool in cultural diversity. *Nursing Research*, 1984, *33* (4), 198–203.
31. Gortner, S. R., Hudes, M., & Zyzanski, S. J. Appraisal of values in the choice of treatment. *Nursing Research*, *33*, (6), 1984, 319–324.
32. Wilberding, op. cit., p. 182.
33. Eddy, J. M., St. Pierre, R. W., & Alles, W. F. A re-examination of values clarification for the health educator. *Health Education*, 1985, *16*, 36–39.

CHAPTER *8*

Promoting Competence For Self-Care

Self-responsibility and self-care are major themes in current health care policy. It is true that individuals spend the vast majority of their lives actively involved in caring for themselves. Self-care is a universal requirement for sustaining and enhancing life and health. The competence with which this task is accomplished determines the quality of life experienced and has a significant impact on longevity. Through health education, a process that informs, motivates, and helps people to adopt and maintain healthful life styles,[1] nurses and other health professionals assist clients in achieving competence in self-care. Self-care can be defined as: "activities initiated or performed by an individual, family, or community to achieve, maintain or promote maximum health."[2] Self-care is both an ongoing activity and a competence to be developed. Conceptually, the term includes much more than ability to carry out activities of daily living. While competence in such activities is part of self-care, care of self also includes actions directed toward minimizing threats to personal health, self-nurturance, self-improvement, and personal growth.

The client serves as the primary resource within the health care system.[3] It has been estimated that informal self-care constitutes 75 percent of all health care within the United States. In addition, at least 25 percent of the health problems seen by physicians could be taken care of by individuals and families themselves without professional help.[4] The goal of the self-care movement is to empower the public for increased control over their own health.[5] While self-care within the medical model has been primarily defined as compliance with therapeutic regimens, self-care for health promotion requires that clients gain knowledge and competencies that can be used to maintain and enhance health in addition to the knowledge and skills required for self-care in illness. Increasing lay competence in health care may be the most effective, safest, and economical way of meeting health needs.[6]

THE ROLE OF THE PROFESSIONAL NURSE

Professional nurses have a major responsibility for enhancing clients' capacity for self-care. Orem describes three types of self-care requisites: universal, developmental, and health-deviation self-care requisites. Universal self-care requisites include:

1. Maintenance of sufficient air
2. Maintenance of sufficient water
3. Maintenance of sufficient food
4. Provision of care associated with elimination processes and excrement
5. Maintenance of a balance between activity and rest
6. Maintenance of a balance between solitude and social interaction
7. Prevention of hazards to human life, human function, and human well being
8. Promotion of human functioning and development within social groups in accord with human potential

Developmental self-care requisites fit into two categories:

1. Maintenance of living conditions that support life processes, promote development, or human progress toward higher levels of organization of human structure and maturation
2. Provision of care either to prevent the occurrence of deleterious effects of conditions that can affect human development or to mitigate or overcome these effects from various conditions[7]

The nurse focusing on health promotion is primarily concerned with universal and developmental requisites, although health-deviation requisites must be promptly attended to if they arise.

Orem has developed a Self-Care Nursing Model that describes three systems within professional nursing practice: a compensatory system, a partially compensatory system, and an educative–developmental system. In compensatory care, the nurse provides total care for the patient. Such care is most common in intensive-, acute-care settings within hospitals during severe illness. Partially compensatory care is implemented when the nurse and the patient share the responsibility for care. Care during rehabilitation from illness or in advanced chronic illness is partially compensatory. In contrast to the preceding two types of care, the educative–developmental nursing system gives the client primary responsibility for personal health, with the nurse functioning in a consultative capacity. It is this third nursing system that is most appropriate for health protection and health promotion.

Major areas of education for self-care that are important in maintaining or enhancing health include exercise and physical fitness, nutrition and weight control, stress management, maintenance of social support systems, and environmental control. All of these areas are addressed within the content of this book.

The public relies heavily on health care personnel as a source of self-care information. In a national sample of 659 adults, Freimuth and Marron[8] found that 71 percent reported receiving self-care information from health personnel, with the reliability of the information estimated to be 91 percent. Fifty-one percent reported getting health information from public-service announcements, with an estimated 77-percent reliability. Forty-nine percent received information from family and friends, with a 50-percent estimate of reliability. Results of the study indicate that health personnel are the most frequent and most trusted sources of health information. The Health Promotion Model presented in Chapter 3 includes interactions with health professionals as an important interpersonal variable in facilitating self-care for health promotion.

Within the past decade, the public has shown increasing concern and motivation to take an active part in its own care. There are, of course, exceptions to this generalization; however, the trend is clearly evident in the proliferation of courses and materials to facilitate self-care. One of the earliest programs was "The Activated Patient: A Course Guide," developed by Sehnert at Georgetown University.[9,10] The major thrust of this and similar programs is to assist clients in becoming knowledgeable partners in maintaining and promoting personal health.

Nurses have long recognized the right of clients of all ages to be both informed and active participants in care. Now as never before, nurses are faced with the exciting challenge of developing the educative–developmental component of nursing practice. Through health education and counseling, positive health practices can be encouraged and the overall impact of the health delivery system greatly improved as clients assume more responsibility for their own care.[11]

Many interesting examples of nurses actively involved in health education for self-care can be cited. As one example, Judy Igoe, a school nurse practitioner in Denver, Colorado, has developed programs for primary care of children of all ages within the school setting.[12] Use of games, such as "Winning at Wellness"[13] and project Health P.A.C.T. (Participatory and Assertive Consumer Training),[14] prepare children and adolescents to engage in health-promoting behaviors and to assume a more active and responsible role in use of existing health care services.

Another nurse, Dolores Alford, has developed ambulatory nursing centers for older adults in which responsibility for self-care is actively promoted.

Each month a program on a health related topic is offered for the centers' clients. Topics can range from promoting healthy feet to how to talk to physicians and utilize the health care system more effectively. As part of self-care, clients are taught to record information in health diaries provided by the nursing centers.

Judy Russell and Barbara Bartlett, nurses employed in the department of Health Services at a large Midwestern corporation, are actively involved in promoting self-care practices of employees. Each employee is seen individually, health goals are assessed, and a tailored program of health promotion activities is developed. The nurses serve as consultants to employees and their families and work collaboratively with the exercise physiologist in the corporation's fitness center.

SELF-CARE EDUCATION THROUGHOUT THE LIFE SPAN

Self-Care for Children and Adolescents

Childhood and adolescence are developmental periods during which social and cognitive skills for autonomous decision making and responsible self-care are developed. Approaches to enhancing self-care behaviors of children and adolescents must focus on both families and peer groups. This dual approach is critical, since values, attitudes, beliefs, and behaviors of families and peers influence children's life style. Parents, in providing physical care for children and promoting cultural adjustment, serve as powerful role models of health and health-related behaviors. They depict family health care functions and various approaches to linking with the broader community. The preschool period is an ideal time to teach preventive and health-promotive behaviors because it is the period when parental influences have the greatest impact on the child.[15]

Healthful habits of eating, exercise, rest, coping, and developing interpersonal relationships can be learned during preschool and early school years. Health-damaging patterns of overeating, sedentary life style, unsafe behaviors, and poor oral hygiene, when developed and reinforced throughout childhood, are difficult to reverse in adults. Self-care education for families can create units within society through which positive self-concept and self-care practices are learned and reinforced.

Peer groups play a critical role in molding life style for school-aged children, particularly adolescents. Developmental capabilities and limitations, enthusiasm for independence, and the fragile egos of adolescents all contribute to ambiguity concerning self-care potential.[16] Socializing school-age children as groups into active participatory roles in school health care can develop future adults who understand self-care and its important role within the health care system.[17] Research findings of Blazek and McClellan[18] suggest that participation in self-care instruction increases the extent to which children view health outcomes as being due to their own actions. When peers reinforce the active health consumer role, peer pressure becomes a positive force. Many school health programs today are giving considerable attention to life style education that teaches children to resist the pressure of peers who encourage them to engage in health-damaging behaviors. Peer discussions and action projects focused on health promotion can create a climate supportive of emerging healthful life styles in school-age youth.

Self-Care for Young and Middle-aged Adults

Young and middle-aged adulthood is the time in the life cycle when many persons are intensely involved in careers and childrearing. The momentum of everyday life and the demands of dependent others may leave little time for focusing on health in the absence of an illness crisis. However, this is the period of life when individuals need to: accept responsibility for modeling and teaching dependent others self-care; refine skills of observation, description, and handling of common illnesses; increase knowledge about health-promotion skills; and learn how to use health care resources for the family appropriately and economically.[19] The strengthening of the intrafamilial support may be particularly important at this time, as the work of Hubbard, Muhlenkamp, and Brown[20] has shown a positive relationship between social support and extent of self-care practices for this age group. Loveland-Cherry[21] found that family cohesiveness was positively correlated at a low but significant level with extent of physical activity and quality of nutritional practices. Caporael-Katz has described self-care education for adults as consisting of the following components:

1. Provision of a period of time for expression of feelings
2. Reinforcement of client self-esteem
3. Provision of open access to health information
4. Practice of self-care skills that could be applied immediately
5. Presentation of alternative views of health issues
6. Critical evaluation of both traditional medicine and alternative therapies[22]

Adults tuned in to their own needs for self-care may be effective in reducing the stress inherent in multiple societal roles that many young and middle-age adults fulfill.

Self-Care for Older Adults

Self-care for older adults focuses on maximizing independence, vigor, and life satisfaction. Adequate self-care education must take into account the physical, sensory, mobility, sexuality, and psychosocial changes that currently characterize the aging process. Interestingly, while not all changes of aging can be slowed or reversed, aggressive self-care can maintain or increase cardiac and pulmonary functioning as well as physical fitness. Weight control can enhance mobility. Research has indicated that exercise can enhance the self-esteem of older adults and in some cases decrease depression and anxiety.

Personality and coping styles do not appear to change significantly with age. Thus, persons who build healthy personalities early in life can meet social demands in later years, find meaning in life, and expend considerable energy in appropriate self-care activities.

Retirement is a significant life event for which appropriate self-care in the form of anticipatory planning must take place to maximize ease of adjustment. Gioella has identified the following self-care actions that facilitate healthy retirement:

1. Planning ahead to insure adequate income
2. Developing friends not associated with work
3. Decreasing time at work in the last years before retirement by taking longer vacations, working shorter days or working part-time
4. Developing routines to replace the structure of the work day
5. Relying on other people and groups in addition to spouse to fill leisure time
6. Developing leisure time activities before retirement that are realistic in energy and monetary cost
7. Preparing for exhilaration followed by ambivalence before satisfaction with one's life style develops
8. Assessing living arrangements, and if relocation is necessary, expending time in developing new social networks
9. Expecting role loss to have a short term impact on self-esteem and one's marital relationship[23]

Older adults often have more discretionary time available for pursuit of personal wellness than younger adults. They should be challenged to use this time productively and counseled concerning resources available within the community to facilitate such efforts.

DOES EDUCATION FOR SELF-CARE WORK?

Health education is currently being challenged on many fronts in regard to its impact on health-related behavior and subsequently on the health status of individuals and groups. However, an increasing number of studies are providing evidence that health education can result in sustained behavioral change. The results of the Stanford Three Community Study are an outstanding example of the impact of health education on individual behavior. The study consisted of a 2-year health education campaign directed at changing dietary behavior among the target populations to decrease the risk of cardiovascular disease. Mass media health education was carried out in two communities, with a third community serving as the control. In one of the experimental communities, mass media health education was supplemented by intensive personal counseling for high-risk individuals.

Analysis of the data on average daily consumption of cholesterol, saturated fat, and polyunsaturated fat revealed that the health-education campaign had resulted in a 20- to 40-percent degree in cholesterol and saturated fat consumption among both men and women. Intensively instructed men tended to out-perform men exposed to mass media alone, while women responded equally well to mass-media and counseling approaches. Mean changes in plasma cholesterol concentration for the various groups under study correlated with those that would have been predicted on the basis of self-reported changes in dietary behavior.

Improvements were maintained over the 2 years of the study, indicating the potential of health education for significantly changing health behaviors.[24] The critical aspect of health education in this study appeared to be the teaching of specific skills to promote the use of the information presented.

Rosenberg[25] reported that patients with congestive heart failure who attended a health-education group had two-thirds less hospital readmission time in days and half the number of readmissions, compared to a control group without health education. The health-education group also complied better with their medical regimen and achieved a lower intake of sodium in their diets than did the control group. Similar results were reported by Levine[26] for patients with hypertension. Individuals who received an educational program reported greater compliance with medical directions, greater weight loss, and more appointments kept than did a control group. In the experimental group, 66 percent had their blood pressure controlled, while only 44 percent showed control in the nonexperimental group. In a study of 88 hypertensive clients over a 5-month period, Given, Given, and Simoni[27] found a significant correlation between the level of knowledge and the extent of patient compliance with the therapeutic regimen.

At the Swedish Wellness Center in Englewood, Colorado, a 6-month pilot wellness program was conducted, with 100 hospital employees as participants. The program included emphasis in the areas of nutrition, stress management, physical fitness, and environmental sensitivity. A battery of tests administered before the program and 6 months later showed that employees who completed all elements of the program experienced significant positive changes in all wellness areas.[28]

While many additional studies are needed to determine the parameters of effective health education and to identify factors affecting population responsiveness, research to date should encourage professional nurses to move ahead in the development and evaluation of health education programs for self-care.

PUBLIC DEMAND FOR HEALTH EDUCATION

With the advent of modern medical technology, self-care fell into disrepute and was essentially ignored or relegated to "folk medicine" or "quackery."[29]

Modern medicine brought with it an "exclusivity of health information" that incapacitated lay people in functioning as effective resources for self-care. People were defined as passive recipients of health care and expected to follow medical orders exactly and unquestioningly. While this philosophy may have worked for acute disease where little follow-through was necessary, the approach failed drastically when applied to chronic disease, prevention, and health promotion. In both prevention and health promotion, self-care is primary, with professional care in the form of education or guidance secondary. Thus, the approach to patient education prescribed within the medical model is fragmented[30] and inappropriate within a self-care framework focused on wellness.

Federal response to public demand for access to health information to enhance competence in self-care is apparent in passage of the National Consumer Health Information Act of 1976. Health education for the public was also listed as one of the ten priorities in the National Health Planning and Resources Development Act of 1974 (P.L. 93-641). Within the federal government, the Office of Disease Prevention and Health Promotion (ODPHP), a unit of the Office of the Assistant Secretary for Health; the Office on Smoking and Health (OSH); and the Center for Health Promotion and Education (CHPE), Centers for Disease Control are examples of major agencies focused on meeting the health-education needs of the public.

The need to move from articulation to implementation of health-education efforts is apparent from the fact that less than 1 percent of the federal budget is currently spent on health-education activities.[31] While education of the public for self-care is an important part of federal policy, it has yet to become a highly viable and visible thrust for federal health expenditures and programs.

GOALS OF HEALTH EDUCATION FOR SELF-CARE

Vuori identified the goals of health education as:

1. To influence an individual's health related behavior either by providing information for decision-making, by changing attitudes or by changing values
2. To change the values of society
3. To create a favorable attitude toward the use of societal means such as legislation, production, and price policies for influencing the health behavior of populations[32]

Similar objectives have been identified by the Task Force on Health Promotion and Consumer Education, sponsored by the John E. Fogarty International Center for Advanced Study in the Health Sciences, National Institutes of Health and the American College of Preventive Medicine. In the

Task Force report, it is proposed that health education is a process that bridges the gap between health information and personal health practices. The ultimate goal of health education is the improvement of the nation's health and the reduction of preventable illness, disability, and death. Health education attempts to influence directly behavioral factors relevant to health. The specific objectives identified for health education within the report are as follows:

1. To improve the health of the people by (A) providing the necessary information to help prevent illness and disability insofar as possible and to maintain the highest possible level of well-being even when ill or disabled and (B) helping them to make the necessary modification in individual life style or behavior when necessary
2. To help restrain inflation in health care costs by relieving some of the preventable demand on health services
3. To involve the consumer–patient positively and constructively in his or her own health maintenance and in responsible effective use of the health care delivery system[33]

Within the context of these objectives, important activities for health-education efforts are as follows:

1. Inform people about health, illness, disability, and ways in which they can improve and protect their own health
2. Inform individuals about relevant risk factors and ways in which they can decrease personal level of risk for specific disease
3. Motivate people to want to change to more healthful practices
4. Help people learn the necessary skills to adopt and maintain healthful practices and life styles
5. Advocate change in the environment that facilitates healthful conditions and healthful behavior[34]

The remaining parts of this chapter will be devoted to an examination of (1) factors that affect the response of individuals to health education, (2) the process of health education for self-care, and (3) potential outcomes of health education. A schema for health education directed toward health protection and health promotion is presented in Figures 8–1 and 8–2.

FACTORS AFFECTING RESPONSE TO HEALTH EDUCATION

Individuals' responses to health education for self-care are multidimensional and thus extremely complex. The client brings to the learning situation a unique personality, established social interaction patterns, cultural norms and values, and environmental influences. Along with these factors, individual learning styles must be considered for effective health education.[35] The

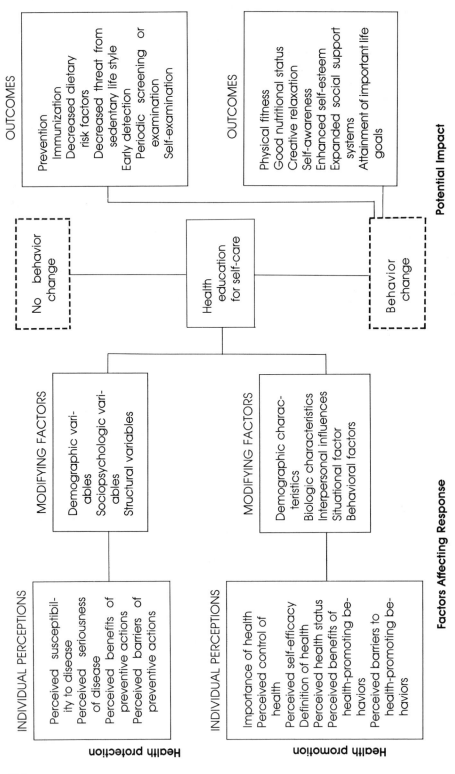

Factors Affecting Response   **Potential Impact**

Figure 8–1. Client education for self-care.

194

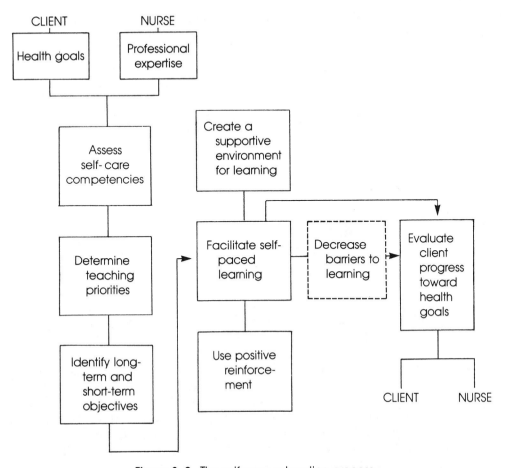

Figure 8–2. The self-care education process.

nurse providing education for self-care must also be aware of characteristic differences that exist between learning patterns of adults and children. Characteristics of the adult learner reported in the literature include:

1. Previous experience that provides a rich background to facilitate learning
2. Self-direction rather than dependency in the learning process
3. Problem-centered or interest-centered rather than subject-centered learning
4. Interest in immediate rather than future applications of knowledge
5. Priority on learning that facilitates mastery of current developmental task[36]

In contrast, health-education experiences for children must be concrete, with emphasis on vivid visual, auditory, tactile, and emotional impact to facilitate learning. Limited experience restricts the extent to which children can call on past events to evoke meaningful feelings and images. Since teenagers represent an intermediate position on the age continuum, their level of maturity and ability to engage in problem solving and futuristic thinking must be carefully assessed. Selection of appropriate teaching strategies and self-care content must take into consideration the chronological, intellectual, and emotional maturity of the client.

Individual perceptions identified in the Health Promotion Model that may affect readiness and motivation to learn self-care include:

- Importance of health
- Perception of health control
- Perceived self-efficacy
- Personal definition of health
- Perceived health status
- Perceived benefits of health-promoting behavior
- Perceived barriers to health-promoting behavior

Wallston, Maides, and Wallston[37] found that both the value placed on health and perceptions of control of health affected the extent to which young adults sought written information (pamphlets) on high blood pressure. Internal control–high health value individuals chose more pamphlets (total) than did internal control–low health value, external control–high health value, or external control–low health value participants. These findings, which have been replicated, would indicate that people who value health and who perceive themselves to be in control of their own health status are more likely to be receptive, motivated, and active in acquiring information about self-care. Clients who place little value on health and do not perceive themselves to be in control of their own lives present a special challenge to the nurse in health education and counseling.

Each client's desire for efficacy or competence in self-care must be taken into consideration by the nurse. The fact cannot be ignored that some individuals do not want to be responsible for their own actions but instead wish to function within society in a highly dependent role. In many instances, the desire for competence has been frustrated by a health care system that makes people feel infantile and helpless. It is critical that the nurse assess very early in interactions with clients the extent to which they desire to assume responsibility for their own care once they are given the requisite knowledge and skills to do so.

Clients' personal definition of health will determine the content that they view as meaningful in health education. When health is defined as maintaining stability or avoiding overt illness, health-protecting behaviors such as immunization, self-examination for signs of cancer, and periodic multiphasic screening may be most important to the client. When health is defined as self-actualization or exuberant well-being, the emphasis of health education can be placed on relaxation, enhancing self-awareness, or appreciating the aesthetics of physical activity. The client's definition of health may change during the self-care education process. If this occurs, the nurse must be sensitive to such changes and readjust the educational plan accordingly.

Perceived health status has also been shown to have an effect on response to health-promotion efforts. Sidney and Shephard[38] reported that those individuals who viewed themselves as very healthy indicated higher motivation to engage frequently and intensively in health-promoting behaviors than did individuals who viewed themselves as only moderately healthy. It appears that the experience of health is in itself a source of motivation for health-information seeking and health action.

Clients' beliefs concerning both the benefits of and barriers to health actions are based on previous life experiences, contact with mass media, and interactions with health professionals. Expected outcomes range from belief in negligible effects to belief in major impact of health behaviors on the quality of life, morbidity, and mortality. Barriers include cost, inconvenience, lack of time, and inaccessibility of appropriate facilities. Assessing the confidence of clients in the benefits of specific health behaviors and their perceptions of barriers will provide the nurse with information important in understanding individual responsiveness to health education interventions.

While individual perceptions that affect responses to self-care education have been considered, demographic factors also influence the health education process. The demographic factor of ethnicity must be given careful consideration in planning for self-care education. Increasingly, health personnel provide care to people from a variety of ethnic backgrounds, including black, Hispanic, Asian, and others. An expanding volume of literature is available to assist health professionals in understanding cultures different from the middle-class, white American culture. Clark[39] and Martinez[40] provide excellent books on the Mexican–American culture, and Hill[41] on black American culture. Spector[42] also offers much helpful information on the impact of culture in health and illness. In working with individuals or families of varying ethnic backgrounds, attempts must be made to incorporate traditional cultural beliefs into health education for self-care.[43]

A word of caution is in order concerning transcultural use of published health education materials. It is often supposed that simply translating materials into the language of another culture provides appropriate audiovisual teaching aids and pamphlets for client education. However, such is often not the case. For example, the sense of modesty in some cultures may make pictures and illustrations of human anatomy offensive to clients. Materials for educational use in specific cultures should be prepared by people within the target culture or in consultation with them.

The process of self-care education may also need to be adapted to cultural beliefs and attitudes. For example, in the Navajo culture, questions directed at finding out information about another's personal problems and habits are considered rude and inappropriate behavior. Thus, assessment of self-care competency has to be approached in an indirect manner or modified to accommodate reluctance for personal disclosure. Within the Navajo culture, the family plays a central role in advice-giving and decision-making. Consequently, failure to involve the family in education for self-care can greatly decrease the impact of such efforts.[44]

In working with black Americans who live in poverty areas, nurses must realize that it is not possible to have effective self-care without altering the environmental factors that affect poverty-level families. These factors include high rates of unemployment, poor housing, inadequate child-care facilities, and prevalence of violent behavior. A major aspect of health initiatives with poverty-level clients is group empowerment to enable change. Within black communities, churches serve as important organizing and support groups. These aggregates, if empowered, can often effect significant environmental changes and provide a milieu conducive to healthier life styles.[45]

Income will affect the health priorities of families and the accessibility of services and materials to follow through with recommended behaviors. As long as access to health care is related to purchasing power, lower-income groups will experience limitations in their potential for acquiring the assistance needed to develop self-care skills.

THE PROCESS OF HEALTH EDUCATION FOR SELF-CARE

Health education consists of teaching and counseling activities in which information is imparted to clients and they are guided in applying what has been learned to everyday living. The components of the health education process for self-care to be discussed in this chapter include: assessing self-care competencies, determining teaching priorities, identifying long-term and short-term objectives, facilitating self-paced learning, using positive reinforcement, decreasing barriers to learning, creating a supportive environment for learning, and evaluating client progress. Figure 8–2 presents an overview of self-care education as a collaborative process between client and nurse.

Assessing Self-Care Competencies

Self-care competencies can be categorized into knowledge, motivation, and skills. Knowledge can be assessed in a variety of ways: through informal discussion, health-knowledge checklists (Fig. 8–3), or structured tests of knowledge in specific content areas. The assessment approach that works best will have to be determined for each client, but, in general, informal discussion or a health-knowledge checklist is less threatening to the client than a structured test. Observation of actual behavior can also provide useful insights. However, frequently, the period available for client observation is too short to allow the nurse to draw reliable conclusions about the level of health knowledge that exists.

Motivation to engage in health education activities in order to develop

In the list below, please check those behaviors that you are comfortable in performing for yourself without assistance from others.

_____ Counting my pulse at the wrist for 1 minute

_____ Counting my pulse at the neck for 1 minute

_____ Selecting comfortable and appropriate shoes for brisk walking or jogging

_____ Selecting appropriate clothing for walking or jogging activities

_____ Planning a progressive schedule of exercise to meet my personal needs

_____ Indicating the ideal weight range for my height

_____ Calculating my maximal heart rate during exercise

_____ Planning time for exercise that is convenient and possible

_____ Describing warm-up exercises that I could do before brisk walking or running

_____ Describing procedures for cooling down after vigorous exercise

_____ Exercising intensively at least four times a week for 30 minutes

_____ Integrating physical-fitness activities with my recreational interests

_____ Maintaining a record of my progress in physical fitness over a period of several months

_____ Eating appropriately before or after vigorous exercise

_____ Explaining how stress is released through physical exercise

_____ Describing how to avoid injuries during exercise

Figure 8–3. Health-knowledge checklist for exercise and physical fitness.

greater expertise in self-care is critical to assess. The activated client shows evidence of motivation in aggressively seeking health information that will assist in self-care. The existence of apathy, lack of interest, and inattention should alert the nurse to a lack of motivation on the part of the client. Reasons for lack of interest should be explored so that the nurse can knowledgeably intervene to increase motivation through appropriate use of reinforcement contingencies or behavioral contracts with the client. These approaches to motivation will be discussed further in Chapters 9 and 10.

Psychomotor skills of the client must also be assessed to determine the extent of fine and gross motor coordination available to carry out the physical aspects of self-care. Assessment of skills allows the client to recognize personal strengths and areas for further skill development.

Determining Teaching Priorities

Deciding where to begin is often a dilemma for the nurse when the client needs information about a variety of different health topics. Futrell et al. have suggested two criteria for determining where to start:

1. Start with the area most important to the client at the time
2. Start with the area of knowledge that will contribute most to the maintenance or enhancement of health[46]

Clients have definite ideas about what they wish to know and what is important to them. Sometimes interest may not lie in the area that poses the greatest threat to personal health. As an example, a client may smoke but be more interested in starting to exercise than in quiting smoking. While the nurse may believe that smoking constitutes a more serious threat to the health of the client than a sedentary life style, it is obviously better to be a physically active smoker than an inactive smoker, since risks are synergistic. If the nurse assists the client to develop an exercise program, the client may also develop a heightened awareness of the negative impact of smoking on lung capacity and physical endurance. At that point, the client may exhibit readiness to discuss approaches to smoking cessation based on concrete experiences with the health-damaging effects of smoking.

Identifying Short-term and Long-term Objectives

Goal setting is important in health education activities. In addition to goal identification, long-term and short-term objectives should be identified. What are the specific knowledge and skills that the client wishes to develop in order to achieve a desired health outcome? Identification of objectives should be cooperatively carried out by the client and nurse. The objectives should be realistic, with each short-term objective fitting under a specific long-term objective so that learning proceeds in a logical sequence toward the desired health goal. An example of a goal-identification form is presented in Figure 8–4.

Long-term objectives guide large segments of learning. Objectives may represent knowledge to be acquired, recalled, or remembered; values, beliefs, and attitudes to be developed; or complex overt behavioral responses to be learned. Short-term objectives identify the specific content or activities that must be progressively mastered to achieve long-term objectives. Recall of information, return demonstration, or practice are some of the activities that may be appropriate as short-term objectives.

Use of the goal-identification form allows the client to identify long-term and short-term objectives, check off each objective as it is attained, and maintain awareness of the desired health outcome. Both the nurse and the client should retain a copy for continuing reference and update. The client should be helped to understand that trying to achieve the final goal immediately is highly likely to lead to frustration and discontinuation of desired behaviors. Good health habits take time to develop, just as health-damaging

Health Goal: Increased Physical Fitness

Long-term Objective: To take a brisk walk for 45 minutes four times a week

Related Short-term Learning Objectives	Objectives Attained
1. Demonstrate how to check my pulse at the neck by counting beats for 10 seconds and multiplying by six 2. State heart rate that I should achieve during exercise 3. Demonstrate two warm-up exercises to use before walking 4. Describe how to cool down after brisk walking 5. Construct a weekly schedule for brisk walking 6. Demonstrate correct diaphragmatic breathing to use during exercise 7. Map out three different and interesting routes to take when walking.	

Figure 8—4. Goal identification form.

habits do. Slowly increasing the time spent on a behavior or the frequency with which the behavior is practiced is likely to result in greater success in changing behavior in the long run than "all-or-none" approaches to behavior change.

Facilitating Self-Paced Learning

The pace at which a client will learn depends on personal motivation, assertiveness, perseverance, skill, and learning style. The pace of learning may also vary with age, health status, and educational level. Self-pacing is important in order to allow the client to be self-directed and maintain control over the learning process. The pace at which the client meets each short-term objective will vary, and expectations of both the client and the health professional should be adjusted accordingly. The important factor is not how rapidly knowledge or skill is attained, but the extent of mastery. The nurse should be attuned to small steps in client progress and use positive reinforcement frequently to enhance the client's feelings of success and sense of forward movement in developing competence in self-care.

The nurse must be realistic about teaching and learning and accept both good and bad days in clients of all ages. Sometimes the nurse and client will be elated with the results, sometimes discouraged. When efforts are less rewarding than anticipated, the pace of learning should be reviewed carefully. It is possible that expanding the time frame for learning will result in increased success for the client. This is especially true for young children, who have less experience to draw on in the learning process than do adults.

Using Positive Reinforcement

In education for self-care, the client, the nurse, and the family of the client all play an important role in reinforcement. Praise should be liberally and meaningfully used to reward client behaviors that indicate progress toward stated goals or objectives. Cues should be used to facilitate successful responses and immediate feedback provided to correct errors in performance. When cues and error feedback are intermingled with positive reinforcement, they are helpful, nonthreatening, and facilitate continued efforts of the client. Immediate and consistent reinforcement facilitates rapid learning and assists the client in deriving satisfaction from learning. Once learning has occurred, intermittent reinforcement of the desired response strengthens the behavior, making it more resistent to extinction.

Clients should be made aware of the importance of self-reward or self-reinforcement in the health education process. It is important that they learn to reward their own efforts and achievements, since much of the time, contingent reinforcement for self-care cannot be supplied by others. A progress-and-reward sheet similar to the one depicted in Figure 8–5 can be helpful in formalizing the reward structure. The client should be discouraged from using foods as reinforcement, since this may encourage between-meal snacks that are undesirable.

Learning Activity	Successful Completion (date)	Reward
Read booklet on tips for safe exercising		30 minutes set aside to read *Vogue* magazine
Review booklet on tips for safe exercising		A telephone visit with Mary
Practice three warm-up exercises		Allow 30 minutes to visit with Jeff, my son
Practice three cool-down exercises		Buy a new perfume
Warm-up for 5 minutes, use stationary bi-cycle for 5 minutes, cool down for 5 minutes		Go to a movie with my husband

Figure 8–5. Developing competence in self-care: progress and reward sheet.

It is important that the client also learn to use self-reinforcement that is internal as well as external. Self-praise, self-compliment, and feeling good about oneself are all forms of internal reinforcement. Learning to use internal self-reward in an appropriate manner permits the client to be less dependent on the availability of tangible objects to facilitate the learning process.

Family members need to learn to serve as sources of support for one another in developing health behaviors. For example, achievement of a specific goal may be rewarded by a family outing in the park or by the family spending time together in a favorite activity at home. By providing mutual support, a sense of healthy interdependence rather than crippling dependence is created within the family.

Identifying Barriers to Learning

Barriers to learning can result from various sources: personal values, beliefs, and attitudes; lack of motivation; poor self-concept; or inadequate cognitive or psychomotor skills. Whatever the source, if the client exhibits lack of progress, barriers within the individual as well as within the family, relevant social groups, and the environment should be explored. Barriers must often be identified and attenuated or eliminated before progress can continue.

Approaches to dealing with obstacles to healthy behavior should be an integral part of the health-education plan. In this way, problems are addressed systematically, and progress in dealing with the barriers can be periodically assessed. The client may be unaware of what is inhibiting progress or reluctant to share such information with the nurse. An open climate of trust and empathy will facilitate communication between the client and the nurse concerning obstacles to learning.

Creating an Optimum Environment for Learning

The environment in which health education for self-care is provided is vitally important to the success of educational efforts. Many clinics or health-center environments intimidate clients, thus making them reticent to participate openly in the learning process. If a clinic is used for health education, the rooms in which self-care is taught should be warm, comfortable, and informal. A desk should not be placed in the room; instead, tables and chairs or sofa and chairs should be placed in a conversational setting. Walls should be wallpapered or painted in pleasant colors, with pictures and textured materials used to create a supportive, nonthreatening climate. Visual aids in flip-chart form and on an easel at a comfortable height for the nurse to use while seated in a chair are ideal for teaching purposes.

Throughout health education, the nurse should avoid use of medical or nursing terminology that is unfamiliar to the client. If very young children are present during the teaching sessions, an area with attractive toys and books may need to be provided for their use. This will minimize distraction of the parents. If children are old enough to be included in the learning sessions, they should be actively involved. Often, use of bright colors and interesting figures or designs on flip charts will amuse children and maintain their interest. Children can play an important role in reinforcing learning or in reminding parents that family members should engage in recommended behaviors.

To the extent possible, actual materials available at home should be used in teaching clients. For instance, if a client is expected to use a booklet on low-cholesterol foods at home in preparing meals, the booklet to be used should be the basis for instruction. If the client is learning relaxation techniques, coaching audiotapes to be used at home should be demonstrated in the clinic, and questions should be answered regarding their use. Well-illustrated materials should be supplied liberally to the client to take home in order to provide reinforcement of knowledge and skills gained during health-education sessions.

Since the minimal time needed for most health instruction is 15 to 30 minutes, the nurse must determine whether individual or small-group teaching methods are to be used. If health education is provided to groups, the groups should be kept small to facilitate interaction and attention to the specific needs of group members. Groups can be formed on the basis of similar health-protection or health-promotion interests or by age, sex, or occupation. Over time, group members can develop a feeling of "esprit de corps" and can serve as sounding boards and support persons for one another in learning new behaviors. A combination of group and individual instruction may also be helpful. The author has found that relaxation techniques can be taught to a small group, but individualization of relaxation methods and use of biofeedback to assist clients in assessing their own progress is handled best in individual appointments. This combined approach allows for efficient use of professional time yet provides for individualization of educative–developmental care to maximize its effectiveness.

Evaluating Client Progress

Evaluation is a process by which the nurse and client in collaboration judge to what degree long-term and short-term objectives and health goals have been attained. Three approaches to evaluation have been described by Green:[47] (1) evaluation of the health-education process, (2) evaluation of impact (changes in knowledge, attitudes, or behavior), and (3) evaluation of resultant morbidity and mortality. While the nurse and client should periodically evaluate the health education process itself, major focus in evaluation should be placed on impact, that is, changes in attitudes, knowledge, or behaviors. Changes in morbidity can also be assessed for a large group of clients over a period of time by evaluating the impact of health education on the occurrence of chronic health problems within the group, compared to a group of cohorts without comparable health education.

All evaluation involves direct or indirect observation of behavior. Actual demonstration of the behaviors learned constitutes direct observation, while client report of participation in health behaviors represents indirect observation. Both approaches are subject to measurement errors of which the nurse should be aware. The major source of error in direct measurement is inadequate sampling of the target behaviors during brief clinic or home visits. If the client is asked to demonstrate specific behaviors in the clinic, the artificiality of the setting may inhibit response. A source of error in indirect measurement is that clients may present a distorted picture of how they actually behave. That is, what they say they do may be different from what they actually do. The client may or may not be conscious of this distortion. Self-observation skills of clients may be inadequately developed, or clients may ascribe a "halo effect" to themselves, seeing performance of health behaviors as more frequent or more intensive than they actually are.

It is the position of the author that a combination of self-report and return demonstration should be used as a means of evaluating client progress. The primary purpose of evaluation is to provide an accurate picture for clients of where they stand in attaining their health goals. Several approaches to evaluation for this purpose will be presented for consideration.

Checklists. A checklist of objectives to be accomplished similar to the one presented in Figure 8–4 can be used for evaluation purposes. As each short-term and long-term objective is attained, it can be checked off on the list. In addition, specific knowledge or skills that the client has acquired can be checked off on a list comparable to the one presented in Figure 8–3. As each objective or behavior is checked off, the client is made aware of his or her own progress in developing positive health practices.

Client Progress Notes. Client progress notes can also be used to chart behavior change. Graphing changes in resting pulse, blood pressure, or electrical muscle activity can visually indicate progress in learning stress management or physical fitness skills. Narrative notes about client progress can also be used to provide more detailed information. Notes should be concise and brief and made by both the nurse and client on the progress forms.

Laboratory Measurements. Certain physiological parameters available through laboratory tests can also be used to measure client progress. Serum cholesterol, triglycerides, blood glucose, lipoproteins, and serum albumin can be used as indicators of biological change. Because of expense, the use of laboratory tests for this purpose should be carefully evaluated.

Testing Devices. Knowledge or performance tests can also be employed to assess client progress. This approach should be used with caution in the case of the client who becomes highly anxious in testing situations. The written test should be concise and provide for ease of response, and the nurse should be able to administer it in a half hour or less. The test should be quickly scored, and, if possible, feedback should be provided immediately to the client. An efficient and interesting approach to testing is through programmed learning. Programs can be written to evaluate the grasp of a particular concept, and immediate feedback and correct information can be provided. Such an approach can decrease the stress of testing and provide reinforcement to the client.

Verbal Questioning. Progress can also be evaluated by questioning the client regarding knowledge of a particular concept or behavior. This is a less formal approach than written testing, yet it allows for feedback from the client that assists both the nurse and the client in evaluating progress. Verbal questioning may be more comfortable for the client than written testing, and it should be done in a nonthreatening manner. Responses to questions can be evaluated and the client further questioned to clarify responses that are initially unclear.

Direct Observation. Direct observation of some health-protecting and health-promoting behaviors is possible. For instance, a client may be observed doing warm-up exercises to determine whether they are being done properly and with correct body alignment. The author asks clients she had trained in relaxation to recline comfortably in a chair in the clinic setting; there they are left alone to achieve relaxation using the approach that they use at home. Following completion of the relaxation sequence, the author quietly enters the room to check pulse, blood pressure, and electrical muscle activity on monitors already comfortably placed on the patient.

Dilemmas of Evaluation. In an insightful article on the dilemmas of evaluating and measuring outcomes of health education, Green[48] has identified potential problems in client evaluation. Conclusions drawn concerning client progress depend on the point in time following health education when observations are made. Curves showing possible trends in performance appear in Figure 8–6. The impact of health education for self-care can be interpreted in different ways, either as successful or unsuccessful, depending on the point in time when outcomes are measured. It is evident that client performance should be evaluated at several different points in time in order to draw accurate conclusions concerning the personal impact of self-care education.

What is desired, of course, is a sustained effect of the health-education intervention that permanently changes life style or behavior. However, clients experiencing decay of effect or backlash effect need to be evaluated carefully to determine why the new behavior patterns were not sustained. It is possible that a prolonged learning period or the development of stronger family or community support systems could have prevented recidivism and the return to earlier, less healthy patterns of behavior.

Potential Outcomes of Health Education
The content of health education for self-care will vary, depending on whether the primary emphasis is health protection or health promotion. Since the

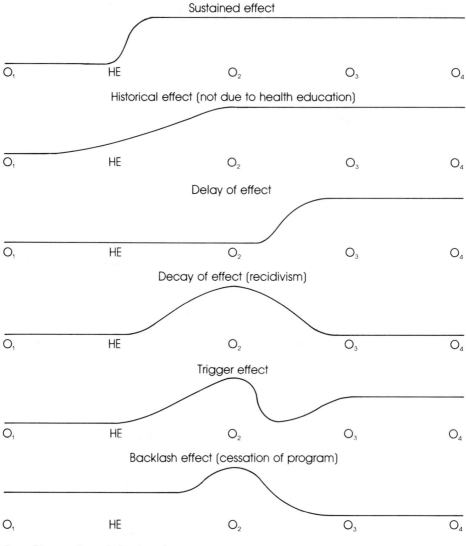

O = Observation of client performance
HE = Health Education

Figure 8–6. Performance trends following client education. *(From Green, L. W. Evaluation and measurement: Some dilemmas for health education.* American Journal of Public Health, *February 1977, 67, 155–161. With permission.)*

emphasis in health protection is on avoidance of disease, risk appraisal, information about specific risk factors, ways of changing behavior or life style to reduce risk, and methods for early detection of disease will most likely be the focus.[49] As a result, specific outcomes to be expected include behaviors such as seeking immunization, changing diet to reduce nutritional risk factors, increasing physical activity to reduce the threat of a sedentary life style, maintaining social support systems as buffers against disease, and use of screening and self-examination methods for early detection of disease.

The emphasis of client education for health promotion is on attaining higher levels of wellness, fulfillment, and life satisfaction. The content of such health education is not disease-specific but holistic in nature. Expected outcomes from education directed toward health promotion include physical fitness, good nutritional status, creative relaxation, self-awareness, enhanced self-esteem, expanded social support systems, and attainment of important life goals. The close relationship between health-protection and health-promotion goals generally results in integrated health education efforts directed toward both ends.

DIVERSITY IN BELIEFS ABOUT PERSONAL RESPONSIBILITY FOR HEALTH

While accumulating research suggests that personal and family behavior have a definite influence on health status, willingness to accept personal causality or responsibility for health differs within the population. From a public survey, Sechrist[50] has noted that, in general, people appear to be willing to accept a higher degree of personal responsibility for being healthy than for illness. People surveyed could be categorized as follows:

1. People who accept relatively high levels of personal responsibility for both health and disease
2. People who accept more personal responsibility for health and less personal responsibility for disease
3. People who reject personal responsibility for both health and disease

The nurse may want clients to assume more personal responsibility for disease prevention and health promotion than they are willing to accept. As the nurse gains insight into clients' attitudes and beliefs, an assessment should be made of self-care interests and motivation.

Sechrist reminds health professionals that for each client, the extent to which genetics, environment, behavior, and other factors singularly or in combination affect health is largely unknown. Thus, while responsible self-care is highly likely to influence health status positively and even prevent or delay the onset of a chronic illness, health professionals cannot give clients any guarantees. The nurse should avoid creating in clients a degree of perceived personal control over health beyond defensible limits.[51] The credibility of the prevention and health-promotion enterprise may be threatened if the causal influence of behavior on health is constantly overestimated.[52]

The best approach may be for the nurse to place major emphasis on the immediate benefits of active self-care such as enhanced quality of life, increased vigor and alertness, less stress, and enhanced feelings of well-being. Possible long-term benefits can be discussed but not precisely defined.

SUMMARY

In health education for self-care, competence of individuals and families, self-direction, and self-responsibility should be emphasized. The content and pace of learning experiences should be controlled by the client. The nurse's primary role is that of consultant. Educative–supportive care provided by the nurse should enable clients to achieve those health goals that they have set for themselves. The nurse in functioning as a resource person enhances the success of clients in acquiring knowledge and skills in self-care.

REFERENCES

1. Preventive Medicine USA: Health promotion and consumer health education. A Task Force Report sponsored by The John E. Fogarty International Center for Advanced Studies in the Health Sciences (NIH) and The College of Preventive Medicine. New York: Prodist, 1976.
2. Steiger, N. J., & Lipson, J. G. *Self-care nursing: Theory and practice.* Bowie, Md.: Robert Brady, 1985, p. 12.
3. Levin, L. S. The layperson as the primary health care practitioner. *Public Health Reports*, May–June, 1976, *91*, 206.
4. Levin, L. S., Katz, A. H., & Holst, E. *Self-care: Lay initiatives in health.* New York: Prodist, 1976, p. 13.
5. Caporael-Katz, B., Health, self-care and power: Shifting the balance. *Topics in Clinical Nursing*, 1983, *5*, 31–41.
6. Levin, L. S. Self-care: Towards fundamental changes in national strategies. *International Journal of Health Education*, 1981, *24* (4), 219–228.
7. Orem, D. E. *Nursing: Concepts of practice*, 3rd ed. New York: McGraw-Hill, 1985.
8. Freimuth, V. S., & Marron, T. The public's use of health information. *Health Education*, July 1978, *9*, 18–20.
9. Sehnert, K. W., & Nocerino, J. T. *The activated patient: A course guide.* Washington, D.C.: Center for Continuing Education, Georgetown University, 1974.
10. Sehnert, K. W., & Eisenberg, H. *How to be your own doctor (sometimes).* New York: Grosset & Dunlap, 1975.
11. Arvidson, E., Connelly, M. J., McDaid, T. , et al. A health education model for ambulatory care. *Journal of Nursing Administration*, March 1979, *9*, 16–21.
12. Igoe, J. B. Changing patterns in school health and school health nursing. *Nursing Outlook*, August 1980, *28*, 486–492.
13. Schodde, G. *Winning at the wellness game.* Seattle: University of Washington Hospital, 1978.
14. *Project Health P.A.C.T.* Denver: University of Colorado School Nurse Practitioner Program, University of Colorado Health Science Center, 1980.
15. Dailey, C. P. Teaching parents and children preventive health behaviors. *Family and Community Health*, 1985, *7* (4), 34–43.
16. Jordan, D., & Kelfer, L. S. Adolescent potential for participation in health care. *Issues in Comprehensive Pediatric Nursing*, 1983, *6*, 147–156.
17. Koster, M. K. Self-care: Health behavior for the school-age child. *Topics in Clinical Nursing*, 1983, *5* (1), 29–40.

18. Blazek, B., & McClellan, M. S. The effects of self-care instruction on locus of control in children. *Journal of School Health*, 1983, *53* (9), 554–556.
19. Sehnert, K. W. Self-care: An educational resource in family practice. *The Journal of Family Practice*, 1983, *16* (6), 1193–1194.
20. Hubbard, P., Muhlenkamp, A. F., & Brown, N. The relationship between social support and self-care practices. *Nursing Research*, 1984, *33* (5), 266–269.
21. Loveland-Cherry, C. J. Relationships between family characteristics and health behaviors. Presentation at the 113th Annual Meeting of the American Public Health Association, Washington, D.C., November 18, 1985.
22. Caporael-Katz, op. cit., pp. 34–35.
23. Gioiella, E. C. Healthy aging through knowledge and self-care. *Aging and Prevention*, 1983, *3* (1), 39–51.
24. Stein, M. P., Farquhar, J. W., Maccoby, N., & Russell, S. H. Results of a two-year health education campaign on dietary behavior: The Stanford Three Community Study. *Circulation*, November, 1976, *54*, 826–832.
25. Rosenberg, S. G. Patient education leads to better care for heart patients. *HSMHA Health Reports*, September 1971, *86*, 793.
26. Levine, D. M., Green, L. W., Deeds, S. G., et al. Health education for hypertensive patients. *Journal of the American Medical Association*, April 20, 1979, *241*, 1700.
27. Given, C. W., Given, B. A., & Simoni, L. E. The association of knowledge and perception of medications with compliance and health states among hypertensive patients: A prospective study. *Research in Nursing and Health*, 1978, *1*, 76–89.
28. Adamson, G. J., Oswald, J. D., & Palmquist, L. E. Hospital's role expanded with wellness effort. *Hospitals*, October 1, 1979, *53*, 121–124.
29. Hentges, K. Health activation: Educating for self-care. *Health Education*, July–August, 1978, *9*, 31–32.
30. Vuori, H. The medical model and the objectives of health education. *International Journal of Health Education*, 1980, *23*, 12–19.
31. Appelbaum, A. L. Who's going to pay the bill? (health promotion), *Hospitals*, October 1, 1979, *53*, 112–120.
32. Vuori, op. cit., p. 18.
33. Preventive Medicine USA, Health Education, op. cit., p. 21.
34. Ibid., p. 3.
35. Mico, P. R. & Ross. H. S. *Health education and behavioral science.* Oakland, Calif.: Third Party Associates, 1975.
36. Knowles, M. S. *The modern practice of adult education.* New York: Association Press, 1970.
37. Wallston, K. A., Maides, S., & Wallston, B. S. Health-related information seeking as a function of health-related locus of control and health value. *Journal of Research in Personality*, 1976, *10*, 215–222.
38. Sidney, K. H., & Shephard, R. J. Attitudes toward health and physical activity in the elderly: Effects of a physical training program. *Medicine and Science in Sports*, 1976, *8*, 246–252.
39. Clark, M. *Health in the Mexican American culture.* Berkeley: University of California Press, 1970.
40. Martinez, R. A. *Hispanic culture and health care.* St. Louis: C. V. Mosby, 1978.
41. Hill, R. *The strengths of black families.* New York: Emerson Hall, 1971.
42. Spector, R. E. *Cultural diversity in health and illness.* New York: Appleton-Century-Crofts, 1979.

43. Faick, V. Planning health education for a minority group: The Mexican Americans. *International Journal of Health Education*, 1979, *22*, 113–121.

44. Hammonds. T. A. Self-care practices of Navajo Indians. In J. Riehl-Sisca (Ed.), *The science and art of self care*. Norwalk, Conn.: Appleton-Century-Crofts, 1985, pp. 171–180.

45. Branch, M. Self-care: Black perspectives. In J. Riehl-Sisca (Ed.), *The Science and art of self care*. Norwalk, Conn.: Appleton-Century-Crofts, 1985, pp. 181–188.

46. Futrell, M., Brovender, S. , McKinnon-Mullett, E., & Brower, H. T. *Primary health care of the older adult*. North Scituate, Mass.: Duxbury Press, 1980.

47. Green, L. W. How to evaluate health promotion. *Hospitals*, October 1, 1979, *53*, 106–108.

48. Green, L. W. Evaluation and measurement: Some dilemmas for health education. *American Journal of Public Health*, February, 1977, *67*, 155–161.

49. Breslow, L., & Somers, A. R. Life-time health monitoring program. *New England Journal of Medicine*, 177, *296*, 601–608.

50. Sechrist, W. Causal attribution and personal responsibility for health and disease. *Health Education*, March–April, 1983, *14* (2), 51–54.

51. Ibid., p. 53.

52. Ibid., p. 54.

CHAPTER *9*

Developing a Health
Protection–Promotion Plan

The major focus of this chapter is on the development of holistic plans for health protection and health promotion of clients, both individuals and families. To maximize positive outcomes from health planning, the client must be an active participant in the planning process. Relying on clients to make decisions concerning desirable health goals and means to attain them promotes positive perceptions of worth and affirms the ability of individuals and families to improve health status.

Genuine dialogue between the provider and client is a prerequisite to sound health planning and maintenance of behavior change. The role of the nurse is to *assist* clients with health planning rather than to *control* the process. During assessment, the nurse and client develop a mutual understanding of (1) values, beliefs, and perceptions that affect health and health-related behaviors of the client; (2) expectations of important referent groups; (3) behavioral options potentially available to the client; (4) the interaction of social–ethnical–cultural background with health practices; (5) potential or actual barriers to self-care; and (6) existing support systems for health-promoting behaviors. Developing a systematic plan for behavior change provides an opportunity for the client to express stabilizing and actualizing tendencies in purposeful ways directed toward increasing wellness and enhancing life satisfaction.

The Health Protection–Promotion Plan should be reasonable in terms of demands on the client and the time frame allocated for accomplishment of desired health or health-related goals. Knowledge and skills already possessed by the client should be optimally used in the planning process. Capitalizing on positive health practices currently a part of personal or family life style prevents overloading the client with a barrage of self-imposed or implied demands for major life changes.[1]

Health planning is a dynamic process in which flexibility to meet the changing needs of individuals and families is critical. The plan systematically lends direction but does not dictate goals that must be attained or behaviors that must be learned. It is possible at any point to revise the plan or return to a former step in order to create a more positive growth experience for the client.[2] A viable Health Protection–Promotion Plan should assist the client in developing a realistic sense of direction and control over life, particularly in the area of health. Programs for change must be personalized for a specific individual or family in terms of the plan of action and approaches to measuring or monitoring progress.[3] The ultimate goal of health planning and implementation is to make health protection and health promotion a way of life that individuals and families enjoy.

THE HEALTH-PLANNING PROCESS

The process for developing a Health Protection–Promotion Plan will be outlined below. Each step in the process will be discussed separately, and materials for actual use with clients will be presented. Tailoring the process and materials to meet the needs of specific individuals or families is the responsibility of each professional nurse providing educative–supportive care. The following nine steps actively involve both the client and the nurse in the health-planning process:

1. Review and summarize data from assessment
2. Identify strengths and competencies of the client
3. Identify health goals and related areas for improvement
4. List possible behavior changes
5. Prioritize behavior changes based on client's perception of desirability and difficulty
6. Make a commitment to behavior change
7. Identify effective reinforcements or rewards
8. Determine barriers to behavior change
9. Develop time frame for implementation of plan

Specific approaches that can be used to initiate and sustain behavioral change will be discussed in Chapter 10.

Review and Summarize Assessment Data

During assessment, a wealth of information is shared between nurse and client. The reduction of this information to manageable proportions is an important step in developing the Health Protection–Promotion Plan. Through the summary process, the individual or family can gain new insights concerning positive qualities and resources that may previously have been un-recognized. In addition, the client gains increased awareness of the range of behaviors that can be acquired or learned.

Summary statements in response to each of the questions identified below can organize assessment data in concise and meaningful form. Both the nurse and the client should retain a copy of the assessment summary for continuing reference during the health planning process.

1. What are the client's most salient values?
2. To what extent are values and actions consistent?
3. Are there preexisting problems that need to be considered in developing a Health Protection–Promotion Plan?
4. To what extent does the client wish to assume responsibility for personal–family health?
5. What positive health practices does the client already engage in?
6. What is the client's overall life-style pattern?
7. For what chronic illnesses is the client at risk?
8. What is the level of fitness of the client?
9. What is the nutritional status of the client?
10. What sources of stress does the client experience?
11. How does the client handle stress?
12. Who are the significant others that serve as a support system for the client?
13. How does the client meet spiritual needs?
14. What is the client's current level of knowledge related to prevention and health promotion?
15. What additional motivation, knowledge, or skills does the client need to acquire to enhance present self-care skills?
16. What does the client perceive as the benefits of life-style change?
17. What potential or actual barriers to change exist?

Clients can be guided through the review and summary process by the nurse during clinic appointments or home visits.

Identify Strengths and Competencies of the Client

Every client brings unique strengths to the health-planning task. These assets should be identified, acknowledged, and reinforced by the nurse. Strengths may be in any of the following areas: consistency between values and actions, physical fitness, weight management, ability to cope with stress, spiritual solidarity, family patterns of health behavior, or extent of health knowledge. Each individual or family seen by the nurse already has a system of health care practices in place that includes conscious behaviors and unconscious habits. The nurse and client should achieve consensus on areas in which the client is already taking informed and responsible health or health-related action.

For self-care directed toward health protection and promotion to be effective, it must be compatible with the client's cultural and experiential background.[4] Clients will carry out health behaviors in ways that fit their cultural beliefs and current levels of knowledge and skill. The client's sense of cultural or ethnic pride and esteem can be reinforced during the health-planning process. Cultural practices supportive of health should be integrated into the overall health plan.

Through teaching, guidance, and support, the nurse nurtures and enhances existing competencies to meet health needs. Self-care demands of individuals may vary according to age, sex, developmental maturity, and health status. The self-care demands of families may vary by family composition, developmental stage, and role demands. While clients will differ in their requirements for self-care and in their competencies for self-management, it is important that the nurse emphasize to all clients their own importance as "primary self-care agent."

The format for developing a Health Protection–Promotion Plan for an individual client is presented in Figure 9–1. The format for designing a Health Protection–Promotion Plan for a family appears in Figure 9–2. In both planning tools, a section is provided in which individual and family health care strengths can be identified.

Identify Health Goals and Areas for Improvement

The next step in the planning process is to identify personal or family health goals and related areas for improvement. The client may not be motivated to make all the changes in current life style that the nurse considers desirable. Systematically reviewing areas for potential change can assist clients in making informed choices concerning the behavioral changes on which they will focus in the initial Health Protection–Promotion Plan.

The nurse should communicate to the client the excitement of change and continuing growth during health counseling sessions. The nurse should avoid making clients feel guilty or inadequate in regard to current health practices. Health goals and related areas for improvement should be listed on the Health Protection–Promotion Plan. After the list has been made, the individual or family can prioritize the areas for improvement in terms of importance. Letting the client determine priorities and supporting efforts to make changes in the areas selected is part of the educative–supportive role of the nurse.

Many clients will initially place high priority on areas of health protection where the threat of illness is tangible and easily understood. Decreasing risk for specific chronic health problems fits the medical orientation of the vast majority of Americans. Measures for risk reduction are often conceptualized by clients as being more concrete than measures for health promotion. Health-hazard appraisal–health-risk appraisal has been widely used as a framework for presenting health information to adult populations and for providing personalized feedback regarding the potential impact of lifestyle changes recommended.[5] A high level of client familiarity or interest in risk reduction would indicate to the nurse that health protection may be the most meaningful area for emphasis in early health planning. Mastery of

Designed for: _____

Home Address: _____

Home Telephone Number: _____

Occupation (if employed): _____ _____

Work Telephone Number: _____

Birth Date: _____ Date of Initial Plan: _____

Current Health Problems (if any): _____

_____

Chronic Illness for Which at "Moderate or High Risk": _____

_____

List Major Risk Factors: _____

_____

_____

_____

_____

Physical Fitness Status: Height _____ Weight _____

Percent Body Fat _____

Recovery Index _____

Current Dietary Patterns: Protein Intake (%) _____

Carbohydrate Intake (%) _____

Fat Intake (%) _____

Stress Status: Life-Stress Score _____

Major Sources of Stress _____

_____

_____

_____

Usual Signs of Distress _____

_____

_____

STAI Scores: State _____

Trait _____

Figure 9–1. Format for an individual health promotion–protection plan. (continued)

Perceptions of Control:

MHLC Scores: Internal _____

Chance _____

Powerful Others _____

Rank Order of "Health" in Health-Values Scale _____

Top-Ranked Five Priorities Health-Values Scale

_____

_____

Purpose in Life (Spiritual Status) _____

_____

Self-Care Strengths of the Client

Self-Care Measures

Nutritional Practices

Physical or Recreational Activity

Sleep Patterns

Stress Management

Figure 9–1. (continued)

Self-Actualization

Sense of Purpose

Relationships with Others

Environmental Control

Use of Health Care System

Others

Personal Health Goals	
GOALS	CLIENT PRIORITY (1 = MOST IMPORTANT)

Figure 9–1. (continued)

Areas for Improvement in Self-Care			
Target Health Goal:			
HEALTH PROTECTION/ PROMOTION AREAS TO BE STRENGTHENED (MAY USE CATEGORIES UNDER SELF-CARE STRENGTHS OR ADD OTHER RELEVANT CATEGORIES)	CLIENT PRIORITY (1 = MOST IMPORTANT)	SPECIFIC BEHAVIOR CHANGES	CLIENT PRIORITY (1 = MOST DESIRABLE)
List below the top-priority areas for change as designated by client.			
List below the two most desirable behavior changes in each area as designated by the client.			

Figure 9–1. (continued)

Designed for (Family Name): _____

Family Form: _____

Family Members:

NAME	SEX	POSITION IN FAMILY	BIRTH DATE	OCCUPATION (IF EMPLOYED)
_____	__	_____	____	_____
_____	__	_____	____	_____
_____	__	_____	____	_____
_____	__	_____	____	_____
_____	__	_____	____	_____
_____	__	_____	____	_____

Home Address: _____

Home Telephone: _____

Work Telephone Number: _____

Cultural Background: _____

Spiritual–Religious Orientation: _____

Type of Housing: _____

Major Formal Roles of Family Members: _____

_____

_____

Community Affiliations of Family: _____

_____

_____

_____

_____

_____

Communication Patterns (Verbal and nonverbal, including expression of caring/affection):

Figure 9–2. Format for a Family Health Promotion–Protection Plan (continued on next page).

Family Decision-Making Patterns:

Family Values with Highest Rank:

1. _____

2. _____

3. _____

4. _____

5. _____

Rank Order of Health as a Value (if not listed above):

_____

Value Conflicts in Family (if any):

Goals Important to Family:

MUTUAL GOAL OR SPECIFIC
TO DYAD (D) OR TRIAD (T)

_____   _____

_____   _____

_____   _____

_____   _____

Family Strengths:

Figure 9–2. (continued)

Major Sources of Stress for Family and Perceived Ability to Deal with Stressors:

Current or Recent Family Developmental or Situational Transitions:

Family Concerns or Challenges:

Family Self-Care Patterns

Current Health Protecting or Preventive Behaviors (e.g., immunization, self-examination, periodic screening/examination by health professionals, avoidance of toxic exposure, use of seat belts):

Current Health-Promoting Behaviors (Life Style Review):
    Nutritional Practices:

    Physical–Recreational Activities:

    Sleep–Relaxation Patterns:

    Stress Management:

Figure 9–2. (continued)

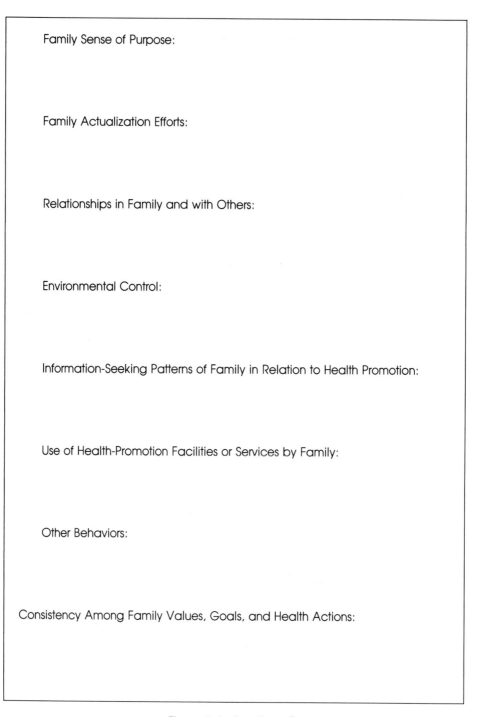

Family Sense of Purpose:

Family Actualization Efforts:

Relationships in Family and with Others:

Environmental Control:

Information-Seeking Patterns of Family in Relation to Health Promotion:

Use of Health-Promotion Facilities or Services by Family:

Other Behaviors:

Consistency Among Family Values, Goals, and Health Actions:

Figure 9–2. (continued)

Family Health Goals	
GOALS	FAMILY PRIORITY (1 = MOST IMPORTANT)

Figure 9–2. (continued)

Areas for Improvement in Family Health			
Target Health Goal:			
AREA OF CHANGE (SEE CATEGORIES UNDER FAMILY SELF-CARE PATTERNS)	SPECIFIC BEHAVIOR CHANGE	FAMILY PRIORITY (1 = MOST DESIRABLE)	APPROACHES SELECTED TO FACILITATE FAMILY CHANGE

Figure 9–2. (continued)

Evaluation of Progress Toward Change in Family Life Style

Two weeks:

One month:

Three months:

Six months:

One year:

Figure 9–2. (continued)

health-protection measures will often motivate clients to consider making additional life-style changes directed toward health promotion. It appears that once clients make changes to decrease specific threats to health, they gain new awareness of the many possibilities for enhancing health and well-being.

List Possible Behavior Changes

People evaluate their own behavior using internal subjective criteria or external standards established by others. Often people are aware that "something is wrong" or that their current behavior is not as desirable as it might be, but they are unable to identify specific changes that can be made to improve health status. Clients may give emotional cues concerning the behavior that they wish to change. Examples of such cues include:

"I don't like the way that I look!"

"I'm so fat that I hate myself!"

"I get mad at myself for being so uptight!"

Emotions are legitimate feelings on the part of clients to which the nurse should be sensitive in order to recognize areas of concern. A constructive program of change can only begin after specific behavioral or emotional difficulties or dilemmas have been concretely identified.[6]

At this point, the client should be encouraged to look at each area in which improvement is desired and determine what behaviors currently practiced are supportive or nonsupportive of the desired change. For instance, if the client values a slim, healthy figure and has the goal of losing weight, eating "junk foods" is inconsistent with both values and goal. The client should be assisted in examining major value–behavior inconsistencies that exist. Alternative actions that are both healthful and enjoyable to the client need to be substituted for the inconsistent behaviors. It is unfortunate that what individuals and families have learned to prefer within the American life style is often detrimental to health. While our bodies thrive on adequate intake of complex carbohydrates, proteins, and unsaturated fats, the American culture encourages consumption of simple carbohydrates and large amounts of saturated fats. Body needs and socially acquired preferences are frequently at odds with one another.

In identifying possible behavior changes, no territory of behavior should be off limits for exploration. The more open the individual or family is in discussing health concerns with the nurse, the higher the probability of developing an exciting and challenging health-promotion plan. Often, areas that the client is reluctant to discuss, such as marital relationships, human sexuality, spirituality, and family cohesiveness, are the most crucial in which to make changes in order to enhance well-being.

Prioritize Behavior Changes

Prioritizing possible behavior changes in terms of desirability to the client is a critical step in the development of a Health Protection–Promotion Plan. It is at this point that clients select from all the behavioral options available those behaviors that are appealing and that they are willing to try. This brings the client full circle from assessing current health status and life style, through considering areas of desired improvement and reviewing behavioral options, to actually identifying those behaviors to be changed in order to accomplish desired goals. At this point in the health-planning process, a cohesive plan of action begins to emerge.

The client's priorities for behavior change will reflect values; activity preferences; estimates of cognitive, affective, and psychomotor skills; subjective probabilities for success in learning; and ease with which target behaviors can be integrated into life style. No one is in a better position than the client to know what changes are feasible given current health status, life style, support systems, and environment.

Make a Commitment to Behavior Change

Through identification of new behaviors that the client is willing to try, a verbal commitment is made to change. However, the client may be more motivated to follow through with selected actions if the personal commitment is formalized through a written contract. While contracts or written agreements between two or more parties have been used in business transactions for many years, use of a *behavioral contract* in helping relationships is relatively new. In a behavioral contract, individuals or families negotiate a realistic behavior change with themselves or significant others. The contract contains specific information about (1) the change to be made, (2) the way the change is to be accomplished, (3) the individual or family members who are to engage in the change, (4) the time frame in which behavior is to be accomplished, and (5) the consequences of meeting or not meeting the terms of the agreement. Behavioral contracts used by the nurse are generally of two types: nurse–client contracts and self-contracts. Each type will be discussed separately, and illustrations of sample contracts will be provided.

Nurse–Client Contract. This type of contract can be defined as any working agreement continuously renegotiated between nurse and client.[7] A contract provides direction for the helping relationship through identification of mutual objectives and responsibilities of each party to the contract. Contracts allow clients to participate actively in their own care by choosing goals that can be realistically accomplished.

Sloan and Schommer identify components of the nurse–client contracting process as follows:

1. Mutual exploration of health problems, concerns and goals between nurse and individual or family
2. Establishment of mutually agreeable health goals
3. Mutual exploration of resources available to accomplish goals
4. Development of a plan specifying steps and methods for achieving goals
5. Negotiation of division of responsibilities between client and nurse

6. Mutual agreement on time limit to accomplish goals
7. Mutual evaluation of progress toward accomplishment of goals in designated time frame
8. Modification, renegotiation, or termination of contract to meet needs of the client[8]

Through nurse–client contracting, both parties to the contract are clear on who will be responsible for what. Generally, the client is responsible for carrying out certain behaviors, while the nurse is responsible for providing information, training, counseling, or specific reinforcement–rewards. The nurse, as the health care professional involved in the contract, bears the additional responsibility of providing helpful input and continuing feedback to the client concerning the adequacy of performance of activities identified in the contract. It is also critical that the nurse be consistent and conscientious in managing the reinforcement–reward contingencies of the contract. Failure in fulfilling this commitment will destroy the trust and confidence placed in the nurse by the client.

Herje has identified the following characteristics as important for nurse–client contracts:

1. Goals contracted for should be realistic
2. Behavior related to achievement of goals should be measurable
3. Goals should be stated in positive terms
4. Behavior indicative of goal attainment must be rewardable[9]

The nurse–client contract provides incentives for behavior change rather than relying solely on individual persistence or will power. Rewards selected should be immediate as often as possible and reinforcing to the client. The client should understand that rewards will be withheld when the terms of the agreement are not met. However, penalties should not be imposed on the client by the nurse for failure to reach performance goals, as this may create resentment and hostility and threaten the integrity of the nurse–client relationship.

A nurse–client contract may be made with an individual or a family unit. A sample format for a nurse–client contract made with an individual is presented in Figure 9–3. A sample format for a nurse–client contract negotiated with a family appears in Figure 9–4. When contracting with a family, all members are party to the contract, actively participating through fulfillment of specific responsibilities. As an example, a family may agree to brisk walk, jog, or bicycle together 2 to 3 times each week. A family may agree to make specific modifications in their nutritional practices, such as increasing vegetables in their diet to two servings per day. Contracting can be fun for the entire family. Children especially enjoy contracting and are excellent in following through with the commitments that they make and in supporting and encouraging others to follow through also. Family members, because of their continuing contact and emotional connectedness, can serve as important sources of encouragement, reinforcement, and reward for one another. The role of the nurse is to assist families to stay well; to value physical, psychological, spiritual, so-

---

Nurse–Client Contract and Agreement

Statement of Health Goal: _____ *Decreased feelings of stress and tension* _____

I _____ *Jim Johnson* _____ promise to _____ *use progressive relaxation* _____
　　　　　(client)

_____ *techniques (four-muscle groups) upon arriving home from work each day* _____
(Client Responsibility)

for a period of _____ *one week* _____ , whereupon,

_____ *Kathy Turner* _____ will provide _____ *a copy of* _____
　　　　　(nurse)

_____ *Herbert Benson's book, Relaxation Response* _____
(Nurse Responsibility)

on _____ *Saturday, March 7th* _____ to me.
(date)

If I do not fulfill the terms of this contract in total, I understand that the designated reward will be withheld.

Signed: _____
　　　　　　　　　　　　　　　(client)

　　　　　　_____
　　　　　　　　　　　　　　　(date)

　　　　　　_____
　　　　　　　　　　　　　　　(nurse)

　　　　　　_____
　　　　　　　　　　　　　　　(date)

Figure 9–3. Sample nurse–client contract for an individual client.

cial, and environmental well-being; and to establish and maintain healthy and fulfilling family life styles.[10] Family contracting is one nursing strategy useful for accomplishing the above goals.

The extent to which the contract has worked must be evaluated. Did the client accomplish the goal fully, partially, or not at all? If failure occurred, what were the reasons? How could the contract be reorganized so that the probability of successful completion is high? Does the contract need to be

---

Nurse–Client Contract and Agreement

Statement of Health Goal: _____ *Improve eating habits* _____

We _____ *The Nichols* _____ promise to *eat two servings of*
                              (family)

_____ *vegetables and two servings of fruit daily* _____
                              (family responsibility)

for a period of _____ *one week* _____ whereupon,

_____ *Lana Buxton* _____ will provide _____ *four movie theater* _____
                              (nurse)

_____ *tickets at the Strand Theater* _____
                              (nurse responsibility)

on _____ *Friday, April 10th* _____ to us.
                              (date)

If we do not fulfill the terms of this contract in total, We understand that the designated reward will be withheld.

Signed: _____
                              (family representative)

               _____
                              (date)

               _____
                              (nurse)

               _____
                              (date)

Figure 9–4. Sample nurse–client contract for a family.

renegotiated? Should the contract be terminated? Careful analysis of the contracting process and evaluation of subsequent outcomes will permit the nurse and client to design contracts that successfully move clients toward desired health goals. Success in fulfilling the agreements in the contract enhances the client's self-esteem and problem-solving abilities. The client gains increased confidence in meeting future health needs.

Self-Contract. A self-contract is a commitment of individuals or families to themselves to perform specific behaviors for a previously identified reinforcement that is attractive and motivating.[11] Since the client is responsible for both the behavioral commitment and for conveying the reward, immediate reinforcement is possible. Self-contracting is an effective approach for enhancing the client's control over behavior, thus creating a sense of independence, competence, and autonomy. The client does not become overly dependent on the nurse for reinforcement but instead serves as the source of rewards for positive health behaviors.

Ultimately the client must learn to manage a reward system that is supportive of emerging positive health practices. The sooner the client can participate in self-contracting as an adjunct to nurse–client contracting, the more confident the client will become in the ability to initiate and sustain behavior change. An example of a self-contract for an individual is presented in Figure 9–5. A family self-contract appears in Figure 9–6.

A word of caution is in order regarding self-contracting. In many instances, individuals or families with a low self-concept or little perceived control over health may not feel compelled to meet their own expectations or demands. The motto "to thine own self be true" is not taken seriously. Without the external expectations of the nurse, there is little follow-through on specific activities to meet contract terms. When this occurs, the nurse should discuss with the individual or family their feelings about independence in self-care. In addition, emphasizing clients' strengths and their ability to accept responsibility in nurse–client contracts can enhance self-esteem and increase the probability of successful self-contracting in the future.

Identify Effective Reinforcements

Identifying effective sources of reinforcement or reward for engaging in new health-protecting or health-promoting behaviors is an important step in planning for implementation of the Health Protection–Promotion Plan. It is important to distinguish between external and internal reinforcement. External rewards generally refer to tangible objects or experiences that are reinforcing for the client. Objects that can be used for reinforcement include books, personal care products, educational pamphlets, self-care materials, or passes to exercise gyms or health spas. Cash value is not necessarily a good index of reinforcement value. Experiential rewards may be 15 minutes with the nurse to talk about anything that the client wishes, an opportunity to meet with a physical fitness consultant free of charge, or the opportunity to borrow a program of audiocassettes on some health topic of importance to the client. Pleasurable family activities such as trips, sports, or picnics also can have strong reinforcement value. Family activities should frequently be used as rewards, since they can increase family communication, cohesiveness, and sense of purpose.

The reinforcement value of any external reward depends on the client's perception of its desirability or utility and the probability with which the client believes that the target activity will actually be followed by the reward.

Self-Contract

Personal Health Goal: _____ *Change Dietary Habits* _____

I _____ *Doris Downs* _____ promise myself that I will _ *follow* _

_ *the sample menus for a 1200 calorie diet for breakfast, lunch, and* _

_ *dinner* _ for a period of _____ *two days* _____ ,

whereupon I will _____ *buy myself a new pair of earrings* _____

on _____ *Wednesday, June 8th* _____ .

Signed _____

Date _____

Figure 9–5. Sample individual self-contract.

Self-Contract

Family Health Goal: _____ *Get more exercise* _____

We _____ *The Stones* _____ promise each other that we will _____ *go* _____

_____ *swimming at the "Y" once a week* _____ for a period of _ *three weeks* _

whereupon we will _____ *buy the newest version of Trivial Pursuit* _____

on _____ *Friday, February 10th* _____ .

Signed: _____

_____

_____

Date _____

Figure 9–6. Sample family self-contract.

If the client highly values the reinforcement offered and is certain that the appropriate behavior will be reinforced, the probability of the client taking action is high. If the reward is of little value to the client, and the probability of attaining it is viewed as minimal, little motivation will exist to engage in the target behavior.

Internal rewards are intangible but can be highly reinforcing to indi-

Developed by: _____   (name)
External Rewards (list below and rank according to desirability, 1 = most desirable)
Objects: Available   Potentially Available
Experiences: Require Advanced Planning   Do Not Require Advanced Planning
Internal Rewards (list below)

Figure 9–7. Reward-and-reinforcement list.

Behavior: Learn to Use Progressive Relaxation as One Approach to Handling Stress	
Component of Behavior	**Reward or Reinforcement**
Attend first class session at 9 A.M. Saturday at the county health department	Watch the football game in the afternoon on TV
Use relaxation audiotape at home for 20 minutes of practice	
Sunday	Call John and visit for a while
Monday	Spend an hour at the driving range
Tuesday	Buy a new paperback novel
Wednesday	Praise myself for having practiced relaxation each day thus far
Thursday	Invite Harry and Jim over to play pool
Friday	Take my family to a movie
Attend second class session at 9 A.M. Saturday at the County Health Department	Take an orange juice break afterwards with Bret, a class member
Practice relaxation techniques for 20 minutes providing my own cues rather than using the tape	
Sunday	Go for a short drive and enjoy the scenery
Monday	Spend 30 minutes reading my new novel
Tuesday	Buy myself a new bottle of aftershave lotion
Wednesday	Praise myself for persistence and successful practice
Thursday	Allow myself to linger in a warm shower longer than usual
Friday	Go to stock car races with the family
Keep my weekly record of relaxation practice	The nurse will provide a copy of *Relaxation Response* by Herbert Benson

Figure 9–8. Reward/reinforcement plan.

viduals and families. Internal reinforcement can be defined as self-praise, increased satisfaction, enhanced self-image, or feelings of self-esteem as a result of completing a designated behavior. The important advantages of internal reinforcement include (1) the client is in control of reward contingencies and (2) reinforcement can be administered immediately in any situation.

Reinforcements, to be optimally effective in rewarding positive health behaviors, cannot be left to happenstance. Planning a reward system ahead of time ensures that reinforcements will be available as they are needed and that they will be objects, experiences, or internal states that are highly valued by clients. In Figure 9–7, a sample reward-and-reinforcement list is presented. An outline of a reward–reinforcement plan is presented in Figure 9–8. The plan provides a course of action with reinforcement points carefully identified for shaping the specific behavior selected. Use of rewards for behavior and life style change will be discussed in more detail in Chapter 10.

Determine Barriers to Change

All individuals and families experience barriers to making changes in behavior. While some obstacles cannot be anticipated, others can be planned for and overcome or their potential for impact considerably weakened before initiating the change process. If the client is aware of possible barriers and has formulated plans for dealing with them should they arise, successful behavior change is more likely to occur.

Barriers to effective health behavior can arise from inside clients themselves, from significant others, or from the environment. Internal barriers to change may be lack of motivation, fatigue, boredom, giving up, lack of appropriate skills, or disbelief that behavior can be successfully changed. Family members can impose considerable barriers if they encourage continuation of health-damaging behaviors or if they actively discourage attempts at behavior change. Environmental barriers that may inhibit positive change include lack of space or appropriate setting in which to carry out the selected activity; dangers within the immediate environment, such as heavy traffic or high crime rate; and inclement weather or inappropriate climate. The client should be assisted by the nurse in dealing with these environmental barriers or in locating another setting appropriate for health activities.

Develop a Time Frame for Implementation

Changes toward more positive health practices need to be made over a period of time in order to allow new behaviors to be learned well, integrated into one's life style, and stabilized. Attempting to change or initiate a number of new behaviors all at once may result in confusion, discouragement, and abandonment of the Health Protection–Promotion Plan by the client. Whether the client is attempting to reduce risk for chronic diseases or to enhance health status, gradual rather than abrupt change is desirable. Just as health education for self-care must proceed at the pace of the learner rather than at that of the nurse, changes in behavior must be sequenced in reasonable steps appropriate for the client.

Developing a time plan for implementation allows appropriate knowledge and skills to be mastered before a new behavior is implemented. For example, it is difficult to warm up before brisk walking or jogging if the client has no idea of what appropriate warm-up exercises are. The time frame for developing a given behavior may be several weeks or several months. If the client is rewarded for accomplishing short-term goals, this provides encouragement for continuing pursuit of long-term objectives. A meaningful plan requires that deadlines be set for accomplishing specific goals. Adher-

Designed for:	*Jim Thorpe*
Home Address:	*486 N. Walden*
Home Telephone Number:	*(303) 875-3111*
Occupation (if employed):	*Chemical engineer*
Work Telephone Number:	*(303) 872-1334*
Birth Date: *8/3/41*	Date of Initial Plan: *4/2/80*
Current Health Problems (if any):	*Transient elevations in blood pressure*
Chronic Illness for Which at "Moderate or High Risk":	*Cardiovascular disease*
List Major Risk Factors:	*(1) Father died from heart attack at*
	58 years of age, (2) 25% overweight,
	(3) 41–50% fat in diet, (4) sedentary
	occupation, (5) moderate to high stress,
	(6) periodic BP readings as high as 150/90.
Physical Fitness Status:	Height *6'0"* Weight *218 lbs.*
	Percent Body Fat *23%*
	Recovery Index *162*
Current Dietary Patterns:	Protein Intake (%) *13%*
	Carbohydrate Intake (%) *43%*
	Fat Intake (%) *44%*

Figure 9–9. Sample individual health protection–promotion plan.

Stress Status:			
	Life-Stress Score		*154*
	Major Sources of Stress		*Work*
			Finances
	Usual Signs of Distress		*Difficulty sleeping;*
		muscles tense and stiff	
	STAI Scores:	State	*40*
		Trait	*38*
Perceptions of Control:	MHLC Scores:	Internal	*56*
		Chance	*28*
		Powerful Others	*38*

Rank Order "Health" in Health-Values Scale   *4*

Top Ranked Five Priorities Health-Values Scale   *Happiness*

         Inner harmony

         A sense of accomplishment

         Health

         Self-respect

Purpose in Life (Spirituality):   *Believes in a supreme being and in life after death. Attends church regularly.*

Self-Care Strengths of the Client

Self-Care Measures

  Drinks 6–8 glasses of water/day
  Does not smoke
  Does not take laxatives
  Knows what blood pressure and pulse readings should be
  Uses soft toothbrush and dental floss regularly

Figure 9–9. (continued)

Self-Care Strengths of the Client

Nutritional Practices
 	
   Eats breakfast daily
   Eats three meals/day
   Adds little or no salt to food
 	
Physical or Recreational Activity
 	
   Plays golf 1–2 times per week
   Maintains good posture
   Walks up stairs rather than riding elevator
 	
Sleep Patterns
 	
   Gets 7 hours of sleep/night
   Sleeps on a firm mattress
 	
Stress Management
 	
   Can laugh at self
   Understands the relationship between stress and illness
   Enjoys spending time in unstructured activities
 	
Self-Actualization
 	
   Maintains an enthusiastic and optimistic outlook on life
   Is a member of two community-service groups
   Is aware of personal strengths and weaknesses
   Respects own accomplishments
 	
Sense of Purpose
 	
   Believes that life has purpose
 	
Relationships with Others
 	
   Is close to family and enjoys spending time with them in camping and recreational activities
   Communicates easily with others
   Perceives self as well-accepted by co-workers
 	
Environmental Control
 	
   Does not permit smoking in house and car
   Provides resources to meet personal needs
   Maintains safe living area
 	
Use of Health Care System
 	
   Reports unusual signs or symptoms to a physician

Figure 9–9. (continued)

Personal Health Goals	
GOALS	CLIENT PRIORITY (1 = MOST IMPORTANT)
Decrease risk for hypertension	1
Learn to relax	2
Maintain desired weight	3
Achieve consistency between personal priorities and allocation of time	4

Areas for Improvement in Self-Care

Target Health Goal: *Decrease risk for hypertension*

Health Protection–Promotion Areas to Be Strengthened (may use categories under self-care strengths or add other relevant categories)	Client Priority (1 = most important)	Specific Behavior Changes	Client Priority (1 = most desirable)
Increased physical activity	1	Brisk walk 4 times/week for 45 minutes	1
		Begin jog-walk exercise	4
		Swim at the "Y" 4 times/ week	2
		Play tennis at the "Y" 2 times/week	3
Monitor blood pressure	2	Have blood pressure checked at health department once a month	2
		Have physician check blood pressure every 3 months	3
		Buy blood pressure cuff and learn to take own pressure	1

Figure 9–9. (continued)

Areas for Improvement in Self-Care			
Target Health Goal: *Learn to relax*			
Health Protection–Promotion Areas to Be Strengthened (may use categories under self-care strengths or add other relevant categories)	Client Priority (1 = most important)	Specific Behavior Changes	Client Priority (1 = most desirable)
Understand my body's response to stress	3	*Observe my own reactions in tense situations*	2
		Review my responses on "signs of distress"	1
		Ask people close to me how I act when tense	3
Identify areas of stress in my life	2	*Discuss my life-stress review with the nurse*	1
		Make a list of personally stressful situations as they occur	2
		Talk to my wife about sources of stress in the home	3
		Talk to my boss about sources of stress on the job	4
Learn specific relaxation skills	1	*Read* Relaxation Response *by Herbert Benson*	2
		Attend series of classes on relaxation techniques	1
		Attend classes in yoga	3
		Purchase a set of audiotapes on relaxation skills	4

Figure 9–9. (continued)

Areas for Improvement in Self-Care			
Target Health Goal: *Maintain desired weight*			
Health Protection–Promotion Areas to Be strengthened (may use categories under self-care strengths or add other relevant categories)	Client Priority (1 = most important)	Specific Behavior Changes	Client Priority (1 = most desirable)
Change eating habits	*1*	*Decrease number and sodium content of between-meal snacks*	*1*
		Become familiar with basic food groups	*3*
		Avoid eating anything after 7 P.M. at night except low-calorie snacks	*2*
		Plan an 1800 calorie low-sodium diet to follow	*4*
		Go on a crash diet	*undesirable*
Target Health Goal: *Achieve consistency between personal priorities and allocation of time (family first priority)*			
Health Protection/Promotion Areas to Be Strengthened (may use categories under self-care strengths or add other relevant categories)	Client Priority (1 = most important)	Specific Behavior Changes	Client Priority (1 = most desirable)
Learn to use time at work more efficiently	*3*	*Develop time-management plan*	*2*
		Arrive at work a half hour earlier	*3*
		Learn to say "no" when asked to complete additional tasks outside my area of responsibility	*1*

Figure 9–9. (continued)

Areas for Improvement in Self-Care			
Target Health Goal: *Achieve consistency between personal priorities and allocation of time (family first priority)*			
Health Protection– Promotion Areas to Be Strengthened (may use categories under self-care strengths or add other relevant categories)	Client Priority (1 = most important)	Specific Behavior Changes	Client Priority (1 = most desirable)
Improve relationship with my wife	*1*	*Arrange to take my wife out for lunch*	*1*
		Buy flowers or a special gift for my wife	*3*
		Express appreciation to my wife for meal preparation	*2*
Improve relationships with my son and daughter	*2*	*Set aside a specific time each week to go bike riding with my son and daughter*	*2*
		Arrange to take my son and daughter (wife, too) to a baseball game	*3*
		Spend time one evening each week visiting with my son and daughter and listening to what they have to say	*1*
		Take my son, daughter, and their friends roller skating	*4*
List below the top-priority areas for change as designated by client.			
Increase physical activity *Learn specific relaxation skills* *Change eating habits* *Improve relationship with my wife*			

Figure 9–9. (continued)

List below the two most desirable behavior changes in each area as designated by the client.

Increase physical activity
  Brisk walk 4 times/week for 45 minutes
  Swim at the "Y" 4 times/week

Learn specific relaxation skills
  Attend relaxation classes
  Read Relaxation Response *by Herbert Benson*

Change eating habits
  Decrease number and sodium content of between-meal snacks
  Avoid eating after 7 P.M. at night

Improve relationship with my wife
  Arrange to take my wife to lunch
  Express appreciation to my wife for preparing meals

Figure 9–9. (continued)

ence to deadlines should be encouraged, with changes made only when the time frame must be shortened or lengthened to make it more conducive to permanent behavior change.

REVISIONS OF THE HEALTH PROTECTION–PROMOTION PLAN

A schedule for periodic review of the Health Protection–Promotion Plan should be established. Revisions should be carried out during counseling sessions, with both the client and the nurse contributing to the process. Impetus for changes in the plan may result from mastery of target behaviors, changes in client's values and priorities, or awareness of new options available to the client. Outdated plans fail to provide impetus or direction for change and thus become uninteresting and meaningless to the client. Periodic revision and updating of the health plan provides a systematic approach for movement of the client toward higher levels of health.

SUMMARY

The Health Protection–Promotion Plans presented in this chapter provide individuals and families with a systematic approach to improving health practices and life style. Sample plans are presented in Figures 9–9 and 9–10 to assist the reader in further understanding how the Health Protection–Promotion Plan can be used as the basis for wellness care. All clients should be provided with a health portfolio that contains their Health Protection–Promotion Plan and other relevant health records.

246

Designed for (Family Name): *The Thompsons*

Family Form: *Blended Family*

Family Members:

NAME	SEX	POSITION IN FAMILY	BIRTH DATE	OCCUPATION (IF EMPLOYED)
Bill	M	Father	9/39	Truck driver
Janet	F	Mother	8/41	Receptionist
Allison	F	Daughter (B.T.)	7/69	Student
John	M	Son (J.T.)	6/71	Student
Dana	F	Daughter (J.T.)	9/72	Student

Home Address: *518 S. Greenwood*

Home Telephone Number: *736–1846*

Work Telephone Number: *736–9476*

Cultural/Background: *German ancestry*

Spiritual–Religious Orientation: *Christian Faith, Methodist*

Type of Housing: *Two-story house in established area of town with older homes*

Major Formal Roles of Family Members: *Bill: father, husband, employee; Janet: mother, wife, employee, hospital volunteer; Allison: daughter, sibling, cheerleader; John: student, basketball player, tennis player; Dana: student, Girl Scout; all: church members*

Community Affiliations of Family: *Grace Methodist Church, Kiwanis Club, Pep Club*

Figure 9–10. Sample family Health Protection–Promotion Plan. (continued)

Communication Patterns (Verbal and nonverbal, including expressions of caring/affection):
Bill and Janet (open)
Parents and children (generally open, sometimes guarded)
Affection expressed primarily through facial expressions and gestures

Family Decision-Making Patterns:
Generally democratic
Janet tends to make health care decisions; Bill dominates decisions concerning large expenditures. All members contribute to decisions about family vacations and activities.

Family Values with Highest Rank:

    1. *A comfortable life*

    2. *Health*

    3. *Happiness*

    4. *Self-respect*

    5. *An exciting life*

Rank Order of Health as a Value (if not listed above):

    _____

Value Conflicts in Family (if any):
Parents are more traditional in their orientation than children. Janet and Bill concerned about saving money, children interested in spending money.

Goals Important to Family:

	MUTUAL GOAL (M) OR SPECIFIC TO DYAD (D) OR TRIAD (T)
Achieving financial security	*D Bill and Janet*
Maintaining an attractive appearance	*M*
Staying healthy	*M*
Good grades in school	*T Allison, John, Dana*

Family Strengths:
    Bill and Janet married for 3 years and seem to get along well; children enjoy school and sports; Janet interested in planning nutritious meals for the family; family has been able to handle stressful situations arising from adults and children with different family life styles now being blended; no major health problems evident.

Figure 9–10. (continued)

Major Sources of Stress for Family (if any) and Perceived Ability to Deal with Stressors:
Allison and Dana share a room, which sometimes creates problems.
Bill occasionally accused of giving preferential treatment to Allison. In general, have been able to handle stressful situations well.

Current or Recent Family Developmental or Situational Transitions:
John—going to high school
Janet—death of mother
Allison—planning for separation and college attendance

Family Concerns or Challenges:
Staying healthy and attractive
Spending more time together as a family, especially with Allison going to college next year

Family Self-Care Patterns

Current Health-Protecting or Preventive Behaviors (e.g., immunization, self-examination, periodic screening/examination by health professionals, avoidance of toxic exposure, use of seat belts):
Regular dental check-ups—Allison, John, Dana
Pap smear every two years—Janet
Use seat belts
Sporadic breast self-examination—Janet

Current Health-Promoting Behaviors (Life-style Review):

Nutritional Practices:
Eat fast foods frequently
Eat junk foods—Bill, John, and Dana
Evening meals usually at home, nutritional quality varies

Physical/Recreational Activities:
Sedentary, little exercise—Bill, Janet, Allison, Dana
Plays basketball and tennis 2–3 times per week—John

Sleep/Relaxation Patterns:
Sleep 8 hours per night—children
Sleep 6 hours per night—Bill and Janet
Watch TV for relaxation

Stress Management:
Family members have trouble managing their time to get things done
Bill procrastinates on "home projects"
No formal training in relaxation skills

Figure 9–10. (continued)

Family Sense of Purpose:
> *Life purpose centers around helping children to "make something of themselves" and around church activities. Believe in life after death.*

Family Actualization Efforts:
> *Janet attends cooking classes and has taken some courses at the local junior college.*
> *Bill is enrolled in a mechanics class.*
> *Dana takes modern dance.*

Relationships in Family and with Others:
> *The Thompsons have several families at church with whom they are close friends. Cordial to neighbors but spend very little time visiting with them as are too busy with own activities. Family activities are few as family members have differing demands on their time*

Environmental Control:
> *Seem to be in control of home environment. No readily apparent health hazards.*

Information-Seeking Patterns of Family in Relation to Health Promotion:
> *Janet and Bill listen to the health cable TV network. Family subscribes to* Prevention *magazine*

Use of Health Promotion Facilities or Services by Family:
> *Bill used to play handball 2 to 3 times per week 2 years ago.*
> *Janet and Allison have attended aerobics classes together.*

Other Behaviors:
> *Bill and Janet have participated in the National Cancer Society Fund Drive for the past 3 years.*

Consistency among Family Values, Goals, and Health Actions:
> *Major inconsistencies appear to be (1) value placed on good nutrition but "junk food" consumed frequently, (2) value placed on health and appearance but sedentary life style for four out of five family members. John maintains a high level of physical activity.*

Family Health Goals

GOALS	FAMILY PRIORITY (1 = MOST IMPORTANT)
Get more exercise (all members)	2
Lose weight (Bill and Janet)	5
Spend more time in family activities (all members)	1
Express affection more openly with one another (all members)	4
Eat fast food and refined sugars less frequently (Janet, Bill, Allison, Dana)	3

Figure 9–10. (continued)

Areas for Improvement in Family Health			
Target Health Goal: Spend more time in family activities; get more exercise (combined two goals)			
AREA OF CHANGE (SEE CATEGORIES UNDER FAMILY SELF-CARE PATTERNS)	SPECIFIC BEHAVIOR CHANGE	FAMILY PRIORITY (1 = MOST DESIRABLE)	APPROACHES SELECTED TO FACILITATE FAMILY CHANGE
Physical-recreational activities and relationships in family	*Plan a weekly family bike trip*	*2*	*Weekly plan for specific rewards/ reinforcements*
	Play tennis together at the "Y" weekly	*3*	*Associative learning by exercising together in same place repeatedly*
	Go to a movie together at least every other week	*4*	
	Work out at the "Y" Personal Fitness Center two times per week together	*1*	

Figure 9–10. (continued)

Evaluation of Progress Toward Change in Family Life Style

Two weeks:
  First week—Exercised together twice.
  Second week—Exercised together twice.

One month:
  During previous 2 weeks, exercised together at "Y" 2 times each week.

Three months:
  No exercise sessions at "Y" during previous week.

Six months:
  Exercising together at the "Y" on the average of 1 time per week.

One year:
  Exercise frequency at "Y" per week varies between 1 to 2 times. Bill, Janet, and Allison exercise together more than with John and Dana, whose interests in exercising fluctuate from week to week. Family members need assistance in increasing frequency of exercise to 3 times per week. Re-evaluate family goals.

Figure 9–10. (continued)

REFERENCES

1. Litwack, L., Litwack, J. M., & Ballou, M. B. *Health counseling.* New York: Appleton-Century-Crofts, 1980.
2. Hames, C. C., & Joseph, D. H. *Basic concepts of helping: A holistic approach.* New York: Appleton-Century-Crofts, 1980.
3. Allen, R. The importance of cultural variables in program design. In M. P. O'Donnell & T. H. Ainsworth (Eds.), *Health promotion in the workplace.* New York: Wiley, 1984, pp. 69–95.
4. Caley, J. M., Dirksen, M., Engalla, M., & Hennrich, M. L. The Orem self-care nursing model. In Riehl, J. P., & Roy, C. (Eds.), *Conceptual models for nursing practice* (2nd ed.). New York: Appleton-Century-Crofts, 1980, p. 304.
5. Weiss, S. M. Health hazard–health risk appraisals. In J. D. Matarazzo, S. M. Weiss, J. A. Herd, & N. E. Miller (Eds.), *Behavioral health: A handbook of health enhancement and disease prevention.* New York: Wiley, 1984, pp. 275–294.
6. Martin, R. A., & Poland, E. Y. *Learning to change: A self-management approach to adjustment.* New York: McGraw-Hill, 1980.
7. Sloan, M. R., & Schommer, B. T. The process of contracting in community nursing. In B. W. Spradley (Ed.), *Contemporary community nursing.* Boston: Little, Brown, 1975, pp. 221–229.
8. Ibid., pp. 224–225.

9. Herje, P. A. Hows and whys of patient contracting. *Nurse Educator*, January–February 1980, *5*, 30–34.

10. Johnson, R. Promoting the health of families in the community. In M. Stanhope & J. Lancaster, *Community health nursing: Process and practice for promoting health*. St. Louis: C. V. Mosby, 1984, pp. 330–360.

11. DeRisi, W. J., & Butz, G., *Writing behavioral contracts*. Champaign, Ill.: Research Press, 1975.

PART IV

Strategies for Prevention and Health Promotion:
The Action Phase

While the stategies in the preceding section have been focused on facilitating informed decision making by the client about health behaviors, this section will present specific actions that the client can take to protect and enhance personal health status. The strategies presented in each chapter can be used by the client in implementing the Health Protection–Promotion Plan. Since the dynamics of behavior change are important for both client and nurse to understand, strategies for change will be presented and the roles of both nurse and client in the change process discussed. Approaches to exercise and physical fitness, nutrition and weight control, stress management, and building and strengthening social support systems will be presented. It is the intent of this section to provide the nurse with specific information and counseling strategies to be used in facilitating and supporting the client in efforts to attain better health and increased life satisfaction.

CHAPTER *10*

Modification of Life Style

Every human being has the potential for becoming more purposeful in life, more competent in managing health, and more self-actualized through developing unique personal resources. Realization of human potential is achieved primarily through progressive change, a natural part of the life process.[1] Lifton has described change as a formative process that consists of "creating, maintaining, breaking down and recreating viable form."[2] According to Lewinian theory, change is a process characterized by three critical stages: unfreezing, changing, and refreezing.[3,4] During unfreezing, there is a developing awareness of the need to change and an increasing desire for change. During changing, the client considers alternative behaviors and makes a commitment to engage in specific health actions. The third stage of the change process is refreezing. The purpose of refreezing is to maintain new health behaviors over time and incorporate supporting attitudes and values related to the new health behaviors into the self-system.[5]

Because of man's creative and problem-solving abilities, self-directed change is possible. Acknowledgment of the potential of clients for self-modification recognizes their human dignity, autonomy, and right to choose how they will live.[6] Self-change can be defined as new behaviors that clients willingly undertake to achieve self-selected goals or desired outcomes. In order to engage in self-change effectively, certain behavior modification skills must be acquired. These skills include: self-observation (self-monitoring), self-instruction, self-reinforcement, and self-evaluation.[7] Self-modification has the following characteristics:

- It applies the laws of learning
- It concentrates on specific actions, thoughts, or emotions
- It places heavy emphasis on positive reinforcement
- It allows individuals to design and carry out their own learning program based on self-selected goals[8]

In order for individuals and families to gain increased control over their own health status, the right set of internal and external conditions must be created to support desired behaviors.

Behavior modification and life-style change represent the action phase of health behavior. Behavior change is preceded by preparatory adjustments for action such as learning, thinking, and deliberation.[9] These preparatory adjustments have been dealt with in the preceding chapters as the decision-making phase of health behavior. Nursing strategies during the action phase include: (1) assisting clients in the identification and use of relevant cues to elicit desired behaviors, (2) providing instruction and assistance to clients in using self-change strategies, (3) reducing barriers to illness-prevention and health-promotion activities, (4) supporting and reinforcing efforts of clients to make changes in behavior, and (5) assisting clients in evaluating the impact of new behaviors on feelings of well-being and health status. During the action phase, the nurse serves as a catalyst for behavior change, suggests alternative solutions to the client, assists the client with various steps of the change process, and links the client with appropriate community resources to facilitate behavior change and maintenance efforts.[10]

The action phase of health behavior is depicted in Figure 10–1. Level of readiness to act is largely a consequence of the decision-making phase. Cues of varying intensity, depending on the level of readiness that exists, are essential to activate behavior. On the other hand, barriers can impede constructive health actions on the part of clients. Following initial action, the client may continue the new behavior without reservation, look for additional information to support the new behavior, or reconsider other action alternatives. Long-term change consists of initiation and continuation of positive health practices. Research to date has dealt primarily with interventions for initiating behavior change. Strategies to facilitate long-term maintenance of health-promoting behaviors and integration of such behaviors as a permanent component of life style need to be developed and empirically tested.

Factors that need to be considered in facilitating client change toward a healthier life style include the following:

- Reasons for change
- Available knowledge and skills to initiate and sustain change
- Ratio of payoffs for present behavior in relation to anticipated payoffs for change or new behaviors
- Extent of support for changed behavior within the social and physical environment[11]

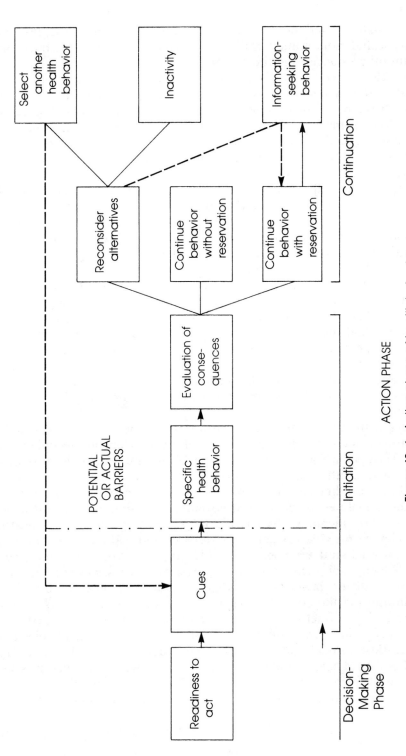

Figure 10–1. Action phase of health behavior.

257

The climate created for change is extremely important. Throughout the action phase, individuals and families need to have input from the nurse and significant others concerning their strengths (strength bombardment) in order to increase perceptions of effectiveness. Feelings of efficacy determine how hard persons will strive to adopt a new behavior and how long they will persist with the behavior despite difficulties.[12] Expectations of efficacy are based on four primary sources of information: personal performance, observing others' accomplishments, verbal persuasion or other types of influence, and states of physiological arousal from which individuals judge their inner resources and competence.[13]

The nurse as a helping professional must have an accurate, empathetic understanding of the life situation of the client and provide support and positive regard in order to facilitate change.[14] A client can best recognize and accept both strengths and limitations if an interpersonal environment exists between the nurse and client that is characterized by caring, personal authenticity, and open communication.[15]

As an example of client services focused on behavior modification, nurses at the Nursing Consultation Center, Pennsylvania State University, provide individual and family counseling as well as group programs to assist clients in evaluating and modifying life style patterns to enhance individual and family health-generating potential. In addition, the center also provides assistance to clients with chronic illness to enable them to develop a life style that supports healthful and productive living. The services of the center are available to residents of the community as well as students, faculty, and staff of the university.

Nurses at the UCLA Center for Health Enhancement Education and Research provide another excellent example of involvement in life-style interventions. The Center is an outreach arm to the community, providing disease prevention and health promotion services. From their experiences with clients, Jordan-Marsh and her colleagues have developed a conceptual framework to: provide guidelines for persons to initiate and maintain health-behavior changes, develop meaningful curricula for supporting life-style or health-behavior change, provide a structure for research and evaluation, and provide for continuity as staff members are added or replaced.[16] The conceptual framework focuses on the impact of support structures, styles of living, and change processes on health status. Health status, the outcome by which success in altering life style is measured, is viewed by the Center staff as consisting of three dimensions: functional status, or the ability to carry out tasks of daily living and to fulfill the challenges of one's social roles and responsibilities; clinical status, which encompasses the physical and biochemical aspects of health; and psychological status, which involves the sense of well-being, mental and emotional state, perception of the quality of life, and integration of strengths and resources toward maximizing personal potential.

Eight internal processes that are viewed as facilitating change in the individual are: readiness appraisal, goal decisions, resource consultation, strategy decisions, commitment check, stress inoculation, experimentation, and self-evaluation.[17] While a complete description of the work of the Center and the supporting conceptual framework is beyond the scope of this chapter, efforts of nurses in this setting provide an example of the valuable contributions that nurses can make to developing effective behavior change programs.

STRATEGIES FOR CHANGE

Specific approaches for initiating self-modification to be discussed in this chapter include: (1) self-confrontation, (2) cognitive restructuring, (3) modeling, (4) operant conditioning, (5) counterconditioning, and (6) stimulus control. Strategies presented for maintaining new health behaviors include: (1) publicizing commitment, (2) associative learning, (3) recording progress, and (4) intermittent reinforcement. When working with an individual or with a family, one particular technique may be chosen or several different techniques may be combined in a more complex behavior change program. It is critical that both nurse and client be involved in decisions concerning approaches to be used for the change of behavior.

Self-Confrontation

At the core of every individual's value system is the self-concept. Self-concept represents beliefs about personal competence and worth. Personal values and beliefs and the values and beliefs of others provide standards of conduct by which the self-concept is evaluated. Threats to self-concept directly affect feelings of self-esteem. When a contradiction exists between values and self-concept or behaviors and self-concept, it can be resolved with the least effort by changing values that are less central or by changing behaviors to be consistent with self-concept.[18]

Self-confrontation as a counseling approach is based on the premise that change results from the arousal of an affective state of dissatisfaction within the client due to recognition of chronic inconsistencies in his or her values, beliefs and behavior system or between the personal system and that of individuals whom the client admires and wishes to emulate. The extent to which dissatisfaction is aroused depends on the client's recognition of inconsistencies.[19] Once significant dissatisfaction is experienced, it is assumed that the person will *change* values, attitudes, and behaviors to make them more integrated with one another—and, more important, to make them more consistent with self-concept.[20]

Self-confrontation → Self-dissatisfaction → Cognitive or
(recognition of   behavioral
(inconsistencies)   change

Contradictions or inconsistencies that are of most concern to the client are the focus for intervention.

Self-confrontation has been shown to be effective in facilitating both values and behavior change. In reviewing a large number of studies in which self-confrontation techniques were used, it was found that value rankings changed in 21 of 22 studies, attitudes changed in 7 of 9 studies, and behavioral changes occurred in 6 out of 13 studies. Behavioral changes have been noted in some studies for as long as 13 to 90 weeks following a "single-dose" intervention.[21]

The Rokeach Value Survey presented in Chapter 7 is the instrument most frequently used in self-confrontation. However, the author suggests that "health" be added to the list of terminal values if the nurse intends to use the instrument for this purpose. The nurse may also wish to consider using the Health-Values Scale discussed in Chapter 7 for self-confrontation counseling.

Administration of the Rokeach Value Survey or Health Values Scale provides the basis for discussing values–values or self-concept–values inconsistencies. For instance, valuing *family security* but not *mature love* or *true friendship* represents a value–value conflict, while thinking of oneself as a robust and energetic person yet placing low value on *health* represents a self-concept–value inconsistency. Clients who consider themselves robust and healthy but find that they begin to breathe heavily and perspire when climbing stairs are experiencing a contradiction between self-concept and behavior. Recognition of this inconsistency may cause some clients to begin brisk walking or jogging to enhance physical fitness, thus meeting specific standards that are part of the self-concept.

The client may also use self-confrontation by contrasting the behavioral consequences of continuing a health-damaging behavior with the consequences of discontinuing the behavior. For example, the nurse can ask the client to list several activities that would be possible if smoking were discontinued, then predict events or restrictions on behavior that would be likely to occur if smoking behavior were not changed. This approach to the analysis of the consequences of two opposing behaviors creates a sense of disequilibrium in the client by contrasting "what is or will be" with "what could be." With the perception of a threat to the self-system from potential loss of old behaviors and the necessity to develop new behaviors, the client may respond with denial of the need to change or with anxiety.[22] In using this strategy, the nurse must evaluate the extent to which the client can tolerate disequilibrium and also provide support and encouragement to lessen resultant anxiety.

Another approach to self-confrontation is to have the client examine personal value rankings compared to referent groups that the client admires or wishes to emulate.[23] For instance, clients might look at their value hierarchy in comparison to normative rankings of individuals who are in excellent health or who are avid health-promotion enthusiasts (joggers, bicyclists, or people who meditate regularly). Seeing differences between personal values and those of important reference groups, clients may rethink their own values and reorganize the value hierarchy to approximate more closely that of the group that they wish to be like.[24]

While much of the clinical work that has been done with self-confrontation techniques has been in the area of racism and prejudice, the approach has excellent potential as a health-protection–promotion intervention. It is highly possible that for some individuals, a fundamental shift in personal values may be required before there is acceptance of responsibility for health; that shift might be prerequisite to a significant health-related behavior change.

In an interesting study conducted by Conroy,[25] self-confrontation techniques were used as an approach to smoking cessation. He asked his experimental group to view two charts showing the instrumental value ranking of smokers and the instrumental value rankings for quitters (nonsmokers). The values of *self-discipline* and *broadmindedness* were outlined in red. These values were selected because previous research has shown that smokers and quitters differed significantly on their ranking of these two values. Smokers ranked *broadmindedness* third and *self-discipline* eighth, whereas quitters ranked *broadmindedness* eighth and *self-discipline* first. The difference in ranking was discussed with the clients, and they were asked to indicate their extent of admiration for people who had been able to quit smoking. They were then encouraged to compare their own value rankings with those of smokers and quitters.

After completion of the smoking clinic, values were again surveyed; the rank order of *self-discipline* in the experimental group had increased significantly, while no significant changes had occurred in raking of *broadmindedness* or other values. Increase in rankings of *self-discipline* were closely correlated with amount of dissatisfaction expressed by clients with their own preclinic value rankings. In reviewing the behavioral effects at the conclusion of the clinic period, the experimental group had reduced its smoking rate to 5 percent of its preclinic rate, whereas the control group still reported 28 percent of its preclinic rate.

A significant difference was apparent for a period of 2 months following termination of the experiment. This difference eventually became dissipated in a high rate of recidivism.[26] However, it is important to note that the self-confrontation treatment produced significantly greater short-term effects than a variety of other more typical smoking-clinic treatments. It is widely recognized that smoking represents an addictive behavior, like drinking, overeating, and misuse of drugs, that is highly resistant to change. Attempts to change addictive behaviors result in symptoms of withdrawal and psychological difficulties because of the pervasive role that such behaviors play in life style. Thus, successful use of self-confrontation in decreasing addictive behaviors portends even greater effectiveness for self-confrontation techniques in promoting positive health practices.

Several explanations have been proposed to explain the impact of self-confrontation as a counseling technique. One explanation is the value-mediation hypothesis, which states that since the individual functions holistically, a change in values will result in subsequent changes in behavior. A change in one part of the system results in a modification of the whole. Another explanation is that behavior change occurs directly from recognized inconsistencies between self-concept and behavior rather than indirectly through value change. The specific mechanisms whereby self-confrontation works still need to be identified.

Research to determine normative attitudes and values of individuals who routinely practice health-protecting and health-promoting behaviors would provide meaningful information on which to base nursing interventions. From this information, materials could be developed for use with clients to increase the incidence of protective–promotive behaviors and decrease the incidence of health-damaging behaviors. Conroy has suggested that in order for health professionals to change the American life style significantly through individual and group interventions, the following steps must be taken.

1. Educate the public as to its role and responsibility for health maintenance.
2. Identify through research the attitudes and values that support health-protection and health-promotion behaviors and sustain health-damaging behaviors.
3. Provide effective methods for altering not only attitudes and values but specific health-related behaviors.[27]

The professional nurse is encouraged to use self-confrontation techniques in health counseling, carefully evaluating their impact on different client groups and with a variety of differing health values, attitudes, and behaviors. For further information on the clinical use of self-confrontation techniques, the reader is referred to additional sources.[28–30]

Cognitive Restructuring

Attention to clients' thinking, imagery, and attitudes toward self are relatively new areas for exploration in the change process. Cognitive restructuring as an intervention technique was developed by Ellis and Grieger to assist counselors in dealing with these phenomena. The approach is frequently referred to as rational–emotive therapy.[31] Not only a therapeutic technique, it also represents an interesting approach to increasing clients' beliefs in personal control of their environment. The basic assumption behind the approach is that the way that individuals label or evaluate a specific situation determines their emotional reaction to the situation. Individuals as a result of experience develop generalized sets of beliefs about various situations or social interactions in their own lives, and these expectancies (self-generated) mediate or determine their emotional and behavioral reactions in any specific situation.[32] The critical factor in determining an individual's response is not the actual situation as much as what the person says internally (e.g., appraisals, attributions, and evaluations in the form of self-statements or self-generated images) before or during the target event.[33]

The self-statement is an important concept in cognitive restructuring. It can be defined as a covert verbalization that elicits emotional reactions. Since self-statements represent covert behavior, their impact is only indirectly observable through the client's self-reports and the overt actions for which the self-statements are assumed to be the mediating link between internal or external stimulus and behavioral response. The task of the nurse is to help clients recognize the messages they give themselves about their health and health-related behaviors and to help them correct problematic patterns of thinking and dysfunctional beliefs.[34]

The process of self-statements and self-evaluation begins early in life. The child develops a self-directing and self-reacting verbal repertoire from observation of the self-administered praise and criticism of adults.[35] Self-administered praise can facilitate performance and feelings of esteem. Invariably self-criticism inhibits behavior. The nurse should be aware of the fact that what sometimes appears to be a skill deficit in self-care may be self-inhibition of the appropriate response. This inhibition is the result of inappropriate self-statements.

Maladaptive emotions are often mediated by irrational self-statements that the client generates in specific situations. If negative emotions are aroused because individuals unthinkingly accept certain illogical premises or irrational ideas, then there is good reason to believe that clients can be taught to think more logically and rationally and thereby create positive emotional states rather than negative ones that in return change behavior and life experiences in positive directions.

Velten[36] found that the reported moods of clients varied as a function of the self-referenced statements that they read. When individuals were given positive statements to read, such as "I feel great," and "My life is wonderful," positive moods prevailed. When individuals were given negative statements to read, such as "I have too many bad things in my life," or "I feel like my life is falling apart," negative moods were dominant. These data and those of other researchers support the ABC framework proposed by Ellis and Grieger[37] for explaining the impact of self-generated thoughts or ideas on responses to specific environmental events:

- A → Activating experience or event
- B → One's beliefs about A (rational or irrational)
- C → Emotional–behavioral consequences

While the A and C components are quite easy to identify, analyzing self-generated thoughts and emotions at the time of the event is more difficult. However, for effective cognitive restructuring to take place, self-generated thoughts (self-statements) must be accurately recalled and carefully analyzed.

Irrational self-statements are often brought about by overgeneralization from past unpleasant experiences ("I'll never lose weight"), self-blame ("I don't have any will power"), and negative self-attributions ("I'm weak and no good"). Irrational self-statements result in decreased self-esteem, depression, and lack of success in attempts at behavior change.[38] Distortion of reality through overgeneralizations is a major source of irrational beliefs. Compare the following:

- Irrational belief (derived from   "I'll never be thin again!"
  overgeneralization)
- Rational belief   "I have difficulty losing weight."

Ellis has suggested that irrational beliefs frequently can be identified by looking at the "shoulds" or "musts" in clients' lives or at their beliefs concerning powerlessness or lack of control. There are five common irrational beliefs:[39]

1. I must be loved by everyone (Social rejection implies personal inadequacy)
2. I should do everything that I do exceptionally well (One must be thoroughly competent in all aspects of life)
3. I am powerless to determine whether I experience health and happiness or misery
4. It is better to avoid life's difficulties rather than face them
5. I cannot change myself or my surroundings[39]

To the extent that clients hold expectations that are inconsistent with reality (irrational self-statements), they are likely to experience failure in making the health-related changes in their lives that they wish to make. Self-statements constitute internal cues to behavior. If internal cues are irrational, desired behaviors will not occur. A number of studies have shown positive relationships among interpersonal anxiety, text anxiety, speech anxiety, and the extent of irrational beliefs.[40–42] Further research is needed to determine the impact of irrational beliefs on health behaviors.

Goldfried and Sobocinski[43] have outlined the steps for applying the psychological principles of cognitive restructuring to clinical intervention with clients. The goal of the intervention is to teach clients to think more rationally, increase the incidence of positive emotions and positive self-appraisal, and thus gain greater control over their own lives and health. The specific steps of cognitive restructuring are the following:

1. *Help clients accept the fact that self-statements mediate emotional arousal.*
   Self-statements and emotional arousal to specific situations may occur automatically and without deliberate effort or conscious thought. Self-statements and associated emotions must be brought into conscious thought in order to deal constructively with their impact on health practices.

2. *Assist clients in recognizing the irrationality in certain beliefs.* Encourage the client to observe and challenge personal self-statements. The client should explore how he or she may be misinterpreting life events. The nurse should support the client in challenging irrational health-related beliefs, particularly those that are most troublesome. The client might ask the following questions:

- What evidence supports my belief?
- What parts of my beliefs are true? What parts are false?
- Am I sticking close to reality (actual facts) in my self-statements, or am I overreacting and distorting events?

    The client should be encouraged by the nurse to offer arguments for the irrationality of self-defeating beliefs.

3. *Help clients understand that the inability to initiate or sustain desirable behaviors frequently results from irrational self-statements.* Negative emotional responses can be maintained by self-generated thoughts indefinitely and to the point where they automatically inhibit behavior without client awareness. Clients need to stop thinking irrationally in order to facilitate constructive behavior change.

4. *Help clients modify their irrational self-statements.* Have the client write down rational self-statements that represent responses to troublesome situations. Keep statements short so that they can be rehearsed in the target situation. Rehearsal of rational self-statements decreases the incidence of irrational self-statements. Clients can learn with practice to talk to themselves rationally and to give cues that support positive emotional states. Examples of rational self-statements are "Calm down," "Relax," "Concentrate on the present," "This isn't so bad," "This situation is challenging," and "I'll conquer this one, given a little time."

Imagery can be used to assist the client in practicing rational self-statements.[44] Imaginary presentations of troublesome situations can be described to the client by the nurse and overt or covert rehearsal of rational self-statements carried out. The client should be encouraged to take at least 10 minutes each day for imagery and rehearsal of positive self-statements. Practice is essential to achieve cognitive restructuring. The ultimate goal for clients is to think about themselves and others more sensibly in the future. Through modifying internal thoughts and imagery, overt behavior can be changed.[45,46]

Modeling

Another approach to assisting clients in changing toward more positive health practices is that of modeling. Modeling consists of observing the behavior of others who have successfully achieved the goal that clients have set for themselves. Modeling is especially helpful when clients are aware of their specific goal but are uncertain about the exact behaviors that should be developed in order to move toward the goal.[47] In early life, children learn a great deal through modeling. This form of learning is continued into adulthood. Individuals acquire social skills and learn how to relate with others through observing the interactions of persons whom they respect and admire.

The nurse can serve as an important role model for health-protecting and health-promoting behaviors. Inherent in the nurse's professional role is the responsibility to provide a model of healthful living that is attractive to clients and consequently emulated by individuals to whom care is provided. Health practitioners' personal physical fitness can have a great impact on their credibility when they are recommending life-style changes to clients. If health professionals smoke, are overweight, or do not exercise regularly, their credibility in the eyes of clients is diminished. A "do as I say, not as I do" approach to behavior change by health practitioners is detrimental to the success of any disease prevention–health promotion program. Those professionals involved in health fields must look closely at their own behavior before recommending life-style changes to others.[48]

The following considerations are important in the effective use of modeling to facilitate behavior change:

- There must be models available with whom the client can identify
- The client must take an active role in the selection of appropriate models
- The learner must have an opportunity to actually observe the desired behaviors and must attend to important aspects of the behavior
- The client must have the requisite knowledge and skills to reproduce the behavior
- The client must perceive incentives or rewards for imitating the target behaviors
- The learner must have the opportunity for overt or covert rehearsal of the target behaviors

By carefully choosing models that have achieved goals the client desires, opportunities can be provided to observe the model in events that contain the behaviors the client wishes to adopt. For example, how does an individual who is slim and trim eat? How much? Which foods? How long does eating take? What other behaviors does he or she engage in while eating? The client can acquire many useful ideas from models for modifying personal health behaviors.

Some clients may feel that it is undesirable to imitate others, that it results in artificial behaviors or that it is not genuine. However, the use of models does not imply that kind of imitation. Actually, the most economical kind of human learning is by imitation. By observing good models, complicated behavior sequences can often be repeated accurately on the first performance. This kind of imitation occurs throughout life and is a very natural process. Observing models gives ideas for behavior rather than a rigid sequence of actions that the client is expected to perform.[49] Observation of others also enriches the client's thinking regarding the range of behavioral options available.

It is important that the nurse and client mutually participate in the selection of appropriate models with whom the client can identify. This is particularly important when the cultural and ethnic backgrounds of the nurse and client differ. Models should be individuals who are frequently available during the initial learning stage and ones whom the client respects. The success of many self-help groups can be partially explained through modeling techniques that generate new ideas for behavior or coping strategies for specific problems. The fact that health professionals are generally held in very high esteem by clients places the nurse in an important position as a potential role model.

Actual observation of target behaviors is important to successful imitation. It is even more important that the client attend to key aspects of the behavior so as to benefit from the example. For instance, if verbal behavior rather than nonverbal behavior is the important point of observation, the client should be aware of this fact. If the nurse serves as the model, attention can be called to important aspects of behavior. If this is not the case, the client may have to be primed or assisted ahead of time to organize observations around the key points to be observed. Once attention has been directed to the critical aspects of a behavior sequence, learning from role models will be more efficient and effective.

It should be apparent to the nurse before model observation whether the client has the requisite knowledge and skills to reproduce the desired behavior. While it is optimum to develop the required skills prior to the modeling sequence, skills can be learned as part of the modeling process. The nurse as a model should not only demonstrate skills (e.g., warm-up exercises) that the client desires to learn, but also explain, provide needed information, and express personal feelings about the target behavior. This helps the client to think more holistically about and rehearse the behavioral sequence.

The client must perceive some incentive or reward for imitating the model's behavior. The incentive may be increased social effectiveness in relationships with others, improved eating patterns, or enhanced physical fitness. Verbal rewards by the nurse, such as praise and recognition, are often potent in promoting efforts to learn new behaviors. Self-praise and self-satisfaction are covert rewards that the client can administer for successfully performing modeled behaviors.

As a final note, opportunities for rehearsal of observed behaviors is critical to allow the client to internalize the verbal and nonverbal cues to behavior, such as limb position or muscle tension. Overt rehearsal is much more effective than covert rehearsal and should be encouraged immediately after observation whenever possible. Overt rehearsal allows the nurse to determine the efficacy of learning and provide feedback through suggestions for refining the client's performance of the target behaviors.

Operant Conditioning

One of the most effective self-modification techniques available to clients is operant conditioning. It is based on the premise that all behaviors are determined by their consequences. If positive consequences result, the probability is high that the behavior will occur again. If negative consequences occur, the probability is low for the behavior's being repeated. A commonly repeated fallacy is that operant conditioning represents manipulation of the client by the nurse. This is not true: When self-modification is the focus of nursing intervention, clients control the selection of behaviors to be changed and reinforcement contingencies to be used; that is, clients select what they will change, how they will change, and the rewards that they will receive for change. Self-modification through operant conditioning gives the client the means of achieving personal health goals.

The client must be in complete control of the change process if new health behaviors are to be initiated and sustained. Positive reinforcement (reward) rather than negative reinforcement (removal of an aversive condition) or punishment (aversive experience) provide the motivation for behavior change. Behaviors that are to be reinforced must be clearly delineated in the Health Protection–Promotion Plan described in Chapter 9. Clients must be aware of what marks the beginning and end of the target behavior and how the behavior that they wish to reinforce is different from other related behaviors. A behavior such as "eats slowly" is too general and cannot be accurately observed. What is "slowly"? When does the specific behavior begin and end? "Pauses between bites during the meal and lays fork on plate" is a concrete behavior that can be clearly observed. Behaviors to be reinforced must be countable so that reinforcement can be appropriately used.

Collecting Baseline Data. If a client wishes to increase the incidence of a specific health-promoting behavior or decrease the incidence of a health-damaging behavior, it is important that an initial frequency count of the target behavior (baseline data) be obtained so that extent of progress toward the desired change can be accurately assessed. Counts of occurrence of the behavior may be made in total or in situation-specific or time-specific categories. The instrument or form on which behavior is to be recorded must be portable so that it is always available when the target behavior occurs. Total counts may be made on a small manual counter or calculator. Categorical counts are usually recorded with paper and pencil. A 3 × 5 index card is a convenient size for the client to carry.[50]

An example of a daily record of smoking behavior is presented in Figure 10–2. For many behaviors, times and situations are important because they represent the configuration of cues in which the behavior occurs. The period of baseline data collection can end when (1) the client has a good estimation

Behavior to Be Observed:	Smoking	
Observation Categories:	Morning Afternoon Evening	
Method of Coding Behavior:		E = Smoking after or during eating and drinking S = Smoking while nervous in a social situation D = Smoking while driving the car O = Smoking at other times
Smoking Record		

Date: Tuesday, August 26		
Morning	Afternoon	Evening
E E D O S S S E	O S S D S E E E	E O

Date: Wednesday, August 27		
Morning	Afternoon	Evening
E E E D D S S E E	S S S S D D E E E E	S E O

Figure 10–2. Self-observation sheet. *(From Self-Directed Behavior: Self-Modification for Personal Adjustment, by D. L. Watson and R. G. Tharp. Copyright © 1972 by Wadsworth, Inc. Reprinted by permission of the publisher, Brooks/Cole Publishing Company, Monterey, California.)*

of how often the target behavior occurs, or when (2) the client is confident that he or she understands the patterns of occurrence of the target behavior.[51] Data from daily records can be compiled and graphed as illustrated in Figure 10–3.

Self-observation or monitoring can increase the client's awareness of the frequency of health-protecting, health-promoting, and health-damaging behaviors. Common reactions include "I didn't know that I smoked that much" or "I didn't realize that I smoke as much in the afternoon as I do in the morning." Self-observation before initiating a program to support behavior change provides a means of assessing client progress.[52]

It must be noted that while self-observation can be used to collect baseline data about the frequency with which health-related behaviors occur, studies of smoking cessation and other behavioral changes have failed to show sustained effects from self-observation or self-monitoring alone without use of other self-modification techniques.

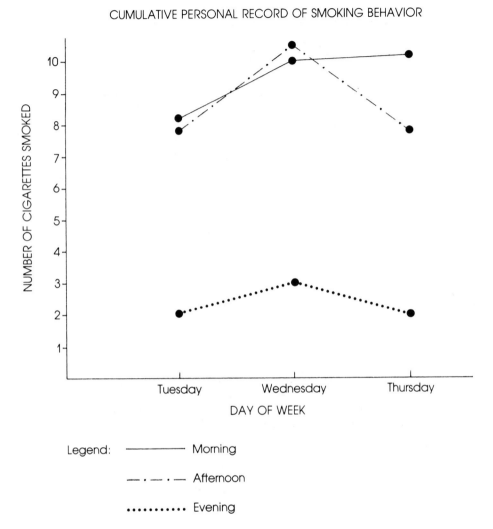

Figure 10–3. Sample cumulative graph of health-damaging behavior.

Using Reinforcement Contingencies. Appropriate use of reinforcement is extremely important in operant conditioning for self-directed behavior change. The reinforcements used in modifying health behaviors should be carefully selected, as described in Chapter 9. They should be important to the client, accessible for immediate use, and potent enough to motivate behavior.

Tangible or social reinforcers serve as effective sources of motivation. Activities as well as objects can be tangible reinforcers according to the Premack Principle.[53] This principle states that if Event A is more probable than Event B when the individual has both options available, Event A can function as a reinforcer if access to A is contingent on first performing B. For example, going to the movie (A) may be made contingent on brisk walking for 2 miles (B). When tangible and social reinforcers (praise, attention, approval) are paired, they become synergistic, each enhancing the potency of the other.[54] A combination of both may be needed initially to facilitate the acquisition and practice of new health behaviors. As health practices become stabilized, less tangible sources of reinforcement are needed to sustain actions.

As soon as possible the client should be encouraged to use self-generated reinforcers such as complimentary thoughts or images. Covert self-reinforcement is the most versatile source of reward. The client has complete control over administration of self-praise and self-compliments. Once a new behavior is occurring regularly, the results of the behavior itself may provide adequate reinforcement. Losing weight, feeling more relaxed, or feeling more energetic all are consequences of health behaviors that have reinforcing properties.

The time frame for application of reinforcement is critical. Immediate reinforcement is highly desirable, particularly in the early phases of self-change. Immediate reinforcement that is self-administered provides clients with moment-by-moment control over their own behavior. Initially, continuous reinforcement is also advisable. Continuous reinforcement promotes rapid learning of the desired behaviors. Intermittent reinforcement applied later stabilizes the behavior and makes it resistant to extinction. Over time, the nurse should decrease active participation in the reinforcement system of the client. Fading can occur in a number of ways. The nurse may move from tangible reinforcers to social reinforcers or from continuous reinforcement to intermittent reinforcement and then to complete fading.[55] Reinforcement may also be increasingly delayed as a form of fading.

Using an organized approach for reinforcement of positive health behaviors generally promotes extinction of undesirable behaviors as a result of lack of reinforcement. Health-promoting and health-damaging behaviors are frequently incompatible. Increasing one automatically decreases the occurrence of the other. In fact, one of the reasons for infrequent occurrence of desired behaviors may be that an undesirable behavior competes with the desired behavior and interferes with its performance. Questions that the client can ask in order to identify a positive health behavior that is incompatible with a negative one include the following:[56]

- Is there some directly opposite behavior that I would like to increase?
- What behaviors would make it impossible to perform the undesired behavior?
- If an incompatible positive behavior cannot be identified, is there a basically meaningless act that can be substituted for the undesirable behavior, e.g., folding hands in lap to prevent nail biting?

This approach, which emphasizes substitution or replacement as opposed to denial, can maintain a positive climate for behavioral change even when health-damaging behaviors that have become a habit for the client are being extinguished.

Shaping Behavior. Many behaviors are too complex to be acquired all at once. Gradually shaping desired behaviors is an effective approach to making permanent changes in life style. Shaping occurs when closer and closer approximations of the final behavior are rewarded. Reinforcement through the shaping process is contingent on increasingly higher levels of performance by the client. An example of shaping is the following:

- Brisk walk for 15 minutes 2 days of first week
- Brisk walk for 20 minutes 3 days of second and third week
- Brisk walk for 30 minutes 3 days of fourth and fifth week
- Brisk walk for 45 minutes 4 days of sixth and seventh week
- Brisk walk for 60 minutes 4 days of eighth and ninth week

Each step toward the final behavior should be mastered before the next step is attempted. The client can control the size of incremental steps to be rewarded and the rate at which the desired behavior is acquired.

Problems that clients are likely to experience in the process of shaping behaviors include plateaus when progress seems impossible, cheating by reinforcing inadequate levels of performance, and problems in persistence (sometimes referred to as will power). These problems should be anticipated and dealt with constructively, either through increased use of tangible reinforcers or through potent social reinforcers during plateau periods when persistence is waning.

The nurse responsible for guiding the client in self-modification should be skilled with shaping techniques. Two books have been written especially for nurses on the subject: *Behavior Modification: A Significant Method in Nursing Practice*, by LeBow,[57] and *Behavior Modification and the Nursing Process*, by Berni and Fordyce.[58]

Coverant Conditioning. Efforts at conditioning within psychology have stretched beyond operant conditioning of overt behavior to operant conditioning of covert processes that precede behavior. Covert processes are self-generated thoughts or images that are only indirectly observable through self-report of clients or observation of subsequent actions. A covert operant (coverant) is an idea that initiates behavior. It can serve as an internal cue for subsequent action. For example, the statement, "I'd really enjoy having a cigarette; it would make me feel relaxed and calm," can be the first step to actual overt behavior (in this case, health-damaging behavior). If occurrence of the thought or coverant can be decreased, the behavior that generally follows will be less likely to occur. One approach to conditioning coverants is the positive reinforcement of coverants that will result in positive behaviors. One example is saying "stop" when the undesirable coverant occurs and substituting a desirable coverant, such as "If I don't smoke, my breath will smell sweet and I will be more desirable to be around." Reinforcements for coverants may be overt or covert. Overt reinforcement consists of using objects, experiences, or interactions with others as rewards for appropriate coverants, while covert reinforcement includes use of self-praise or self-encouragement.

Conditioning covert behaviors is an emerging area of exploration; more research needs to be conducted before the parameters for clinical use of covert conditioning are clearly identified. For further information on this technique, a number of sources can be consulted.[59-62]

Counterconditioning

Counterconditioning is a classical conditioning procedure that is frequently referred to as systematic desensitization. The aim of this approach to behavior change is to break an undesirable bond between a stimulus (conditioned stimulus) and a response (conditioned response). A conditioned response often represents an irrational or maladaptive response to one or more specific situations that has become automatic.

The goal of counterconditioning is to replace the undesirable stimulus–response bond with a more desirable one. For instance, anxiety may be replaced by relaxation in stressful situations, preventing the occurrence of the negative emotional response. Relaxation is actually incompatible with the previously conditioned response (anxiety). Stress management, to be discussed in Chapter 13, is an excellent illustration of this clinical technique.

Counterconditioning can be carried out by use of imagery or in real-life situations. For example, when clients are being desensitized to stressful situations, they can be asked to imagine increasingly stressful events while they remain in a protected environment. Relaxation rather than tension represents the stimulus–response bond that the client is attempting to achieve. Once the client can relax during stressful imagery, relaxation techniques can be applied to stressful situations in real life. It is interesting to note that symptom substitution or displacement of anxiety seldom occur when counterconditioning is used to decrease the occurrence of negative emotions in specific situations.[63]

Stimulus Control

By changing the antecedents of behavior, that is, the events that precede behavior, it is possible to decrease or eliminate undesired behavior and increase desired outcomes. The locus of attention in stimulus control is on the antecedents of behavior, rather than on its consequences as in operant conditioning. In order to use stimulus control effectively, the client must have accurate information about when and where desirable behaviors could occur more frequently and under what conditions undesirable behaviors occur. The client must arrange for environmental cues to be encountered such as promote only desired behaviors. As indicated in the Health Belief Model and the proposed Health Promotion Model, cues are critical elements during the action phase.

During the decision-making phase, the client determines which health actions will be taken and achieves a certain level of readiness to act. This mobilized energy must be activated by an instigating event that can be either external or internal. The level of cue intensity needed to initiate behavior is directly related to the level of readiness of the client following the decision-making phase. People in a state of readiness to take a specific action appear to have a lowering of perception if not of sensory thresholds to specific stimulation relevant to their goal. Generally, the higher the level of readiness, the lower the intensity of the cue needed to activate appropriate behavior. Figure 10–4 illustrates this relationship. Cues that surpass optimum intensity usually inhibit behavior rather than facilitate it.[64]

Multiple cues potentiate each other. Internal cues can be coupled with external cues, for example, "feeling good after brisk walking" coupled with "the invitation from spouse to take a walk." Table 10–1 presents an overview of possible cues to taking health-protecting and -promoting action.

Individuals define for themselves the cues that are relevant based on past knowledge and experience. For some clients, a postcard reminding them of an exercise class may be an adequate prompting for attendance, while for

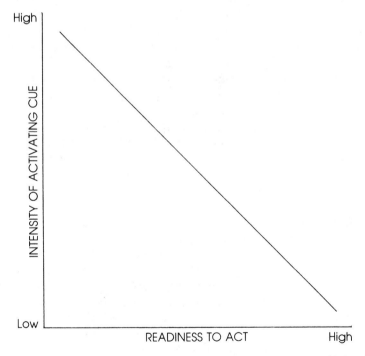

Figure 10–4. Relationship of readiness to take health actions and intensity of cues needed to activate behavior. *(From Rosenstock, I.M. Why people use health services. Milbank Memorial Fund Quarterly, July 1966. 44, 94–127. With permission.)*

TABLE 10-1. POSSIBLE CUES FOR HEALTH-PROTECTING AND HEALTH-PROMOTING ACTIONS

Internal Cues
Bodily states, e.g., feeling good, feeling energetic, recognizing aging, fatigue, cyclical discomfort

Affective states, e.g., enthusiasm, motivation for self-preservation, high level of self-esteem, happiness, concern

External Cues
Interactions with significant others, i.e., family, friends, colleagues, nurse, and physician

Impact of communication media, e.g., motivational messages from television, radio, newspapers, advertisements, and special mailings

Visual stimuli from the environment, e.g., passing a diabetic screening clinic, billboards, attendance at a health fair, passing a gym or exercise center, or viewing others participating in target activity

---

other clients a personal call from the nurse and several reminders from spouse may be needed to initiate action. The nurse must be aware of effective cues for specific clients in order to prompt positive health behaviors with success. Dimensions of cues to be considered include relevance, strength (intensity), number, duration, and synergistic potential.

Some cues are successful in prompting a given behavior much of the time, while others vary in effectiveness from one time to another or one situation to another. Cues may also be action specific. A configuration of cues that triggers relaxation may not be the cues that trigger exercise or appropriate eating behavior.

The nurse, family, environment, or client may serve as the source of behavioral cues. Since the extent to which nurses can provide cues to action is limited, an important part of their professional role is to assist clients in (1) developing sensitivity to appropriate cues, (2) increasing chances for encountering appropriate cues and, (3) developing a system of internal cues that consistently trigger desired actions. It is important to remember that verbal and nonverbal cues, regardless of their source, must be consistent with each other. Any incongruity between cues can confuse and frustrate the client and inhibit action.

Antecedents of behavior need to be carefully analyzed in order to create a configuration of cues that will prompt specific health protecting–promoting behaviors. The client should describe the setting(s) in which the health-related behavior has occurred previously or could occur:

- *Physical setting*—Describe the setting(s) in which the behavior occurs. Describe when, where, and what is present.
- *Social setting*—Describe who is present when the behavior occurs and what they are doing.
- *Intrapersonal setting*—Describe what the client is thinking, feeling, or doing. What did the client say or think to him- or herself just before the behavior occurred?

Through controlling cues or antecedents, the incidence of target behaviors can be modified. The nurse can assist the client in learning how to change cue configurations to elicit desired behaviors. Specific approaches to stimulus control will be presented below.

Cue Restriction or Elimination. Situational cues for undesired behaviors can sometimes be eliminated. When such cues cannot be totally eliminated, they can often be reduced. For instance, the cues to eating may be reduced to one room in the house, the kitchen or dining room. This is called stimulus narrowing or cue restriction. A setting can also be selected that is incompatible with an undesirable response (cue elimination). Examples include sitting in "no-smoking" areas of restaurants or eating meals only with nonsmokers if cessation of smoking is the goal. Through stimulus narrowing or reduction, the target behavior comes under the influence of only a few cues. By localizing the cues that activate behavior, arrangements can be made for limited encounter with these cues. In successful cue elimination, extinction of the behavior should result.

Cue Expansion. In cue expansion, the number of stimuli that prompt desired behavior is increased. For instance, while personal preparation of food at home in one's own kitchen may prompt small servings of meats, fruits, and vegetables, the environment of a restaurant may prompt selection of rich entrees and desserts. An expanded configuration of cues can prompt health-promoting behavior in a variety of different settings. For instance, being given a menu at a restaurant can provide cues for looking at salad and vegetable options as opposed to less nutritious and higher caloric offerings. By expanding the range of cues that elicit specific responses, desirable behaviors can occur more frequently and with greater regularity. Gaining conscious control over behavior rather than responding automatically will assist the client in acting more rationally and more in line with personal health goals.

Controlling antecedents of behavior through the restriction, elimination, or expansion of cues can assist clients in creating internal and external cue configurations supportive of positive health practices. Stimulus control is an important approach to successfully modifying behavior and life style.

Barriers to Change

Interference with action can arise from external barriers within the environment, such as lack of facilities, materials, or social support, or from internal barriers, such as lack of knowledge, skills, or appropriate affective or motivational orientation on the part of the client. The professional nurse facilitates the action phase by assisting clients in minimizing or eliminating barriers to action. It is futile to encourage clients to take actions that are highly likely to be blocked or frustrated.

Internal barriers to self-modification toward more positive health practices can result from a variety of sources:

- Unclear short-term and long-term goals
- Insufficient skill to follow through with self-modification approach
- Perceptions of lack of control over environmental contingencies (cues, reinforcements, time) related to the target behavior
- Lack of motivation to pursue selected health actions

Barriers such as these often reflect insufficient planning or preparation for action during the decision-making phase.

Clients who find their course of action thwarted may reevaluate the decisions made regarding practice of specific health behaviors. They may seek more information to support change in behavior, discard the selected action in favor of another, rationalize the behavior as unnecessary, or deny the relevance of the selected health goal.

The interaction of level of readiness and barriers to action is depicted in Table 10–2. Consequences for the client and appropriate nursing actions are also presented. Action, conflict, or inactivity can result from differing levels of readiness and blocks to action. When clients evidence a high level

TABLE 10-2. INTERRELATIONSHIPS AMONG LEVEL OF READINESS TO TAKE HEALTH ACTIONS, BARRIERS, CONSEQUENCES FOR CLIENTS, AND NURSING INTERVENTIONS

Level of Readiness	Barriers to Action	Consequences for Client	Nursing Interventions
High	Low	Action	Support and encouragement; provide low-intensity cue
High	High	Conflict	Assist client in lowering barriers to action
Low	Low	Conflict	Provide high-intensity cue
Low	High	No action	Assist client in lowering barriers to action and then provide high-intensity cue

of readiness to engage in health-protecting–promoting behaviors and barriers are low, only a low-intensity cue is needed to activate behavior. A high-intensity cue under these conditions may actually be aversive. When readiness is high and barriers to action are also formidable, barriers need to be reduced or eliminated. When both readiness and barriers are low, readiness to act should be increased in order to initiate action. When readiness is low and barriers high, both factors should be addressed in order to allow constructive behaviors to occur.

Significant others can serve as barriers to health actions. One of the most important sources of information about the appropriateness of our own beliefs and actions are the attitudes and behaviors of others. When family members or other persons or groups disagree or are neutral or apathetic toward health behaviors, the extent of inhibition created for the client depends on the following factors:

- The relevance of disagreeing persons or groups
- Attractiveness to the client of disagreeing persons or groups
- Extent of disagreement of relevant persons or groups
- Number of persons relevant to the client who are in disagreement with behavior
- Extent to which client is self-directed rather than other-dependent

As the nurse listens to the client's account of efforts at implementation of health practices, he or she may well be able to provide insights concerning blocks to desired behavior. By analysis of the environment in which the behavior is to occur and preparation of the client with the appropriate knowledge and skills to deal constructively with potential or actual barriers to implementation, the nurse can facilitate accomplishment of personal health goals meaningful to the client.

Maintaining Behavior Change

Changes in behavior that are transient accomplish little in enhancing client health status. Not only must behavior be sustained in the environment in which it is learned, but the behavior must be generalized to other situations. Factors that affect continuation of positive health behaviors include:

- Number of personal beliefs and attitudes that support the target behavior
- Extent of affective and cognitive commitment to target behavior
- Ease of incorporating behavior into life style
- Extent to which behavior is intermittently reinforced or rewarded
- Degree of future orientation of the client
- Amount of activity involved in making the decision to take action
- Personal attractiveness of incompatible actions
- Centrality of health as a value
- Extent to which decision to take action has been communicated to others

The maintenance phase is indeterminate in length, extending from beginning stabilization of the new behavior throughout the client's life span. Three approaches for maintaining new behaviors will be discussed briefly.

Publicizing Commitment. A commitment to a specific course of action to improve health should have the following properties: it should be an active decision on the part of the client, it should be made public or communicated to as many persons as possible, it should involve deliberate effort, and it should be internally motivated and uncoerced.[65] Commitment to a course of action can be formalized through nurse–client, family–client, or self–contracts, as discussed in Chapter 9. Making commitment to change behavior a matter of public knowledge will often provide support, validation, and social pressures from others to maintain the target behavior over an extended period of time. In fact, individuals who also believe that they should take similar actions may join the client in a collegial endeavor that provides continuing support and camaraderie.

Associative Learning. The repeated pairing of stimulus and response results in associative learning. Such learning results in behaviors that become automatic and are maintained on a stimulus–response level with little conscious effort. Many habits of daily living that individuals engage in, such as brushing teeth, showering, and dressing, are formed through associative learning.[66] Habit formation results in stable patterns of behavior that are partially independent of reinforcement contingencies. When a behavior is stabilized to the point that it no longer needs reinforcement or requires only intermittent reinforcement, a habit has been developed.

The nurse can assist clients in associative learning by helping them plan for certain health-promoting behaviors to occur repeatedly in the same setting or context. For example, a client can exercise each noon in the company fitness center, 3 to 5 days a week. The client should head to the fitness center promptly at noon, allowing absolutely nothing else to interfere with the scheduled exercise activity. The decision to exercise or not exercise should not even be considered each day. The client should avoid any opportunity for choice once the initial commitment to exercise has been made. When the client arrives at the fitness center, the stimuli of the locker room, exercise equipment, and co-workers jogging or bicycling will prompt the client to get into proper attire, warm up, and start to exercise. After a period of time, if associative learning has occurred, exercising at noon should become a habit just like brushing teeth or showering.[67]

Recording Progress. Clients can be encouraged to keep a graph that depicts their progress over time in developing and continuing positive health practices. The frequency, intensity, or duration of the behavior may be graphed to illustrate vividly the accomplishments of the client. Self-appraisal of successes and the extent to which behavior has actually changed provides a source of reward and reinforcement for continuing health-promoting actions.

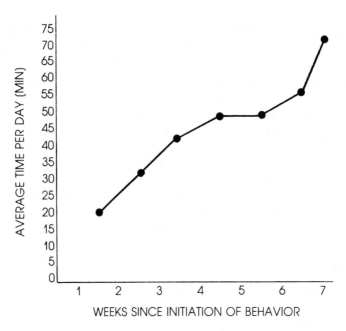

Figure 10–5. Progress chart for brisk walking.

A sample of a progress chart for brisk walking is presented in Figure 10–5. In some corporate fitness centers, computerized records of employee progress are maintained. Employees can track their progress in miles run during a month or total calories expended in exercise activities. These records can become part of the employee's comprehensive health portfolio.

Intermittent Reinforcement. Intermittent reinforcement has been shown to be more effective than continuous reinforcement in sustaining behaviors. Intermittent reinforcement is carried out by requiring greater frequency, intensity, or duration of the target behavior before reward is given, as compared to continuous reinforcement. The amount of reinforcement may be varied, and the latency of reinforcement may be varied as well. These reward contingencies can be manipulated by the client, family, or nurse.

Intermittent reinforcement maintains the novelty of rewards and the interest of clients while avoiding saturation and decreased effectiveness of reinforcement contingencies. Without certainty of reward but with some probability of attaining it, positive behaviors have been shown to persist over long periods of time.

Ethics of Behavior Change
Within the nursing profession, the right of autonomy and self-determinism of the client is a major tenet of professional practice in situations where autonomous behavior is not a threat to the health and welfare of other human

beings. Thus, individuals and families should be allowed to select their behavioral patterns and life style based on sound information from health professionals or other credible information sources. Not all members of society will choose the most healthful behaviors, and this is their right when their actions do not affect others.[68] As the nurse assists clients who have sought help in adopting health-promoting life styles, authoritarian and coercive strategies should be avoided. Allowing clients to assume leadership in self-modification is an ethical, nonmanipulative approach to improving the health of individuals and families.

SUMMARY

A number of behavior-change strategies have been presented in this chapter. The reader is referred to other sources for additional discussion of varying approaches to behavior modification and for specific structured exercises that can be used with clients to assist them in adopting healthier life styles.[69,70] The nurse in assisting individuals and families to modify health behaviors not only promotes desired changes but provides clients with skills for continuing self-change and self-actualization.

REFERENCES

1. Schwitzgebel, R. K., & Kolb, D. A. *Changing human behavior: Principles of planned intervention.* New York: McGraw-Hill, 1974.
2. Lifton. R. J. *The life of the self.* New York: Simon & Schuster, 1976.
3. Lewin, K. *Field theory in social science.* New York: Harper, 1951.
4. Schein, E. H., & Bennis, W. G. *Personal and organizational changes through group methods: The laboratory approach.* New York: Wiley, 1965.
5. Williams, D. D., & Davis, J. H. Change and persistence: A paradox in promoting health behaviors. *Journal of Community Health Nursing,* 1984, *1* (1), 21–26.
6. Kanfer, F. H. The many faces of self-control, or behavior modification changes its focus. In R. B. Stuart (Ed.), *Behavioral self-management: Strategies, techniques and outcomes.* New York: Brunner/Mazel, 1977, p. 5.
7. Kazdin, A. E. *Behavior modification in applied settings* (2nd ed.). Homewood, Ill.: The Dorsey Press, 1980.
8. Watson, D. L., & Tharp, R. G. *Self-directed behavior: Self-modification for personal adjustment.* Monterey, Calif.: Brooks/Cole, 1972.
9. Shibutani, T. A cybernetic approach to motivation. In Buckley, W. (Ed.), *Modern systems research for the behavioral scientist.* Chicago: Aldine, 1968.
10. Cobb-McMahon, B. A., Williams, D. D., & Davis, J. H. Changing health behavior of community health clients. *Journal of Community Health Nursing,* 1984, *1* (1), 27–31.
11. Kanfer, F. H., & Karoly, P. Self-control: A behavioristic excursion into the lion's den. *Behavior Therapy,* 1972, *3,* 398–416.
12. Chesney, M. A. Behavior modification and health enhancement. In J. D. Matarazzo, S. M. Weiss, J. A. Herd, et al. (Eds.), *Behavioral health: A handbook of health enhancement and disease prevention.* New York: Wiley, 1984, pp. 338–350.

13. Ibid.
14. Sauber, S. R. *Preventive educational intervention for mental health.* Cambridge, Mass.: Ballinger, 1973, p. 74.
15. Otto, H. *Group methods to actualize human potential.* Beverly Hills, Calif.: Holistic Press, 1970.
16. Jordan-Marsh, M., Gilbert, J., Ford, J. D., Kleeman, C. Life-style intervention: A conceptual framework. *Patient Education and Counseling,* 1984, *6* (1), 29–38.
17. Ibid.
18. Rokeach, M. *The nature of human values.* New York: Free Press, 1973.
19. Ibid.
20. Lockwood, A. L. Notes on research associated with values clarification and value therapy. *The Personnel and Guidance Journal,* May 1980, 606–608.
21. Ibid., p. 608.
22. Williams & Davis, op. cit., p. 22.
23. Lockwood, op. cit., p. 608.
24. Rokeach, M., & McLellan, D. D. Feedback of information about the values and attitudes of self and others as determinants of long-term cognitive and behavioral change. *Journal of Applied Social Psychology,* 1972, *2,* 236–251.
25. Conroy, W. J. Human values, smoking behavior, and public health programs. In Rokeach, M. (Ed.), *Understanding human values: Individual and societal.* New York: Free Press, 1979.
26. Ibid., p. 200.
27. Ibid., pp. 202–207.
28. Rokeach, M., & Cochrane, R. Self-confrontation and confrontation with another as determinants of long-term value change. *Journal of Applied Social Psychology,* 1972, *2,* 283–292.
29. Greenstein, T. Behavior change through value self-confrontation: A field experiment. *Journal of Personality and Social Psychology,* 1976, *34,* 254–262.
30. Grube, J., Greenstein, T. N., Rankir, W. L., & Kearney, K. Behavior change following self-confrontation: A test of the value-mediation hypothesis. *Journal of Personality and Social Psychology,* 1977, *35,* 212–216.
31. Ellis, A., & Grieger, R. *Handbook of rational-emotive therapy.* New York: Springer, 1977.
32. Goldfried, M. R. The use of relaxation and cognitive relabeling as coping skills. In Stuart, R. B. (Ed.), *Behavioral self management: Strategies, techniques and outcomes.* New York: Brunner/Mazel, 1977, pp. 82–116.
33. Meichenbaum, D. H., & Turk, D. The cognitive, behavioral management of anxiety, anger and pain. In Davidson, P. (Ed.), *Behavioral management of anxiety, depression and pain.* New York: Brunner/Mazel, 1976.
34. Kendall, P. C., & Turk, D. C. Cognitive-behavioral strategies and health enhancement. In J. D. Matarazzo, S. M. Weiss, J. A. Herd, et al. (Eds.), *Behavioral health: A handbook of health enhancement and disease prevention.* New York: Wiley, 1984, pp. 393–405.
35. Kazdin, op. cit., p. 259.
36. Velten, E., Jr. A laboratory task for induction of mood states. *Behavior Research and Therapy,* 1968, *6,* 473–482.
37. Ellis & Grieger, op. cit. pp. 8–9.
38. Martin, R. A., & Poland, E. Y. *Learning to change: A self-management approach to adjustment.* New York: McGraw-Hill, 1980, pp. 159–160.

39. Ellis, A. *Reason and emotion in psychotherapy.* New York: Lyle Stuart, 1962.
40. Meichenbaum, D. H., Gilmore, J. B., & Fedoravicious, A. Group insight versus group desensitization in treating speech anxiety. *Journal of Consulting and Clinical Psychology*, 1971, *36*, 410–421.
41. Trexler, L. D., & Karst, T. O. Rational–emotive therapy: Placebo and no treatment effects on public speaking anxiety. *Journal of Abnormal Psychology*, 1972, *79*, 60–67.
42. Osarchuk, M. *A comparison of a cognitive, a behavioral therapy and a cognitive plus behavioral therapy treatment of test anxiety in college students.* Unpublished doctoral dissertation. Adelphi University, 1974.
43. Goldfried, M. R., & Sobocinski, D. The effect of irrational beliefs on emotional arousal. *Journal of Consulting and Clinical Psychology*, 1975, *43*, 504–510.
44. Goldfried, M. R., op. cit., pp. 97–99.
45. Redd, W. H., & Sleator, W. *Take charge: A personal guide to behavior modification.* New York: Random House, 1976.
46. Blittner, M., Goldberg, J., & Merbaum, M. Cognitive self-control factors in the reduction of smoking behavior. *Behavior Therapy*, 1978, *9*, 553–561.
47. Watson & Tharp, op. cit., p. 134.
48. Sensenig, P. E., & Cialdini, R. B. Social-psychological influences on the compliance process: Implications for behavioral health. In J. D. Matarazzo, S. M. Weiss, J. A. Herd, et al. (Eds.), *Behavioral health: A handbook of health enhancement and disease prevention.* New York: Wiley, 1984, pp. 384–392.
49. Watson & Tharp, op. cit., pp. 74–75.
50. Ibid., p. 84.
51. Ibid., p. 97.
52. Ibid., p. 108.
53. Martin & Poland, op. cit., p. 21.
54. Deibert, A. N., & Harmon, A. J. *New tools for changing behavior.* Champaign, Ill.: Research Press, 1978, pp. 18–25.
55. Berni, R., & Fordyce, W. E. *Behavior modification and the nursing process.* St. Louis: C. V. Mosby, 1977, p. 68.
56. Watson & Tharp, op. cit., p. 137.
57. LeBow, M. D. *Behavior modification: A significant method in nursing practice.* Englewood Cliffs, N.J.: Prentice-Hall, 1973.
58. Berni & Fordyce, op. cit.
59. Daniels, L. K. An extension of thought-stopping in the treatment of obsessional thinking. *Behavior Therapy*, 1976, *7*, 131.
60. Wolpe, J., & Lazarus, A. A. *Behavior therapy techniques.* New York: Pergamon, 1966.
61. Girdano, D. A., & Everly, G. S. *Controlling stress and tension: A holistic approach.* Englewood Cliffs, N.J.: Prentice-Hall, 1979, pp. 153–154.
62. Hays, V., & Waddell, K. J. A self-reinforcing procedure for thought stopping. *Behavior Therapy*, 1976, *7*, 559.
63. Agras, W. S. *Behavior modification: Principles and clinical applications.* Boston: Little, Brown, 1972.
64. Edgell, S. E., & Castellan, N. J. Configural effect in multiple cue probability learning. *Journal of Experimental Psychology*, 1973, *100*, 310–314.
65. Sensenig & Cialdini, op. cit., p. 386.
66. Hunt, W. A., Matarazzo, J. D., Weiss, S. M., & Gentry, W. D. Associative learning, habit, and health behavior. *Journal of Behavioral Medicine*, 1979, *2*, 111–124.

67. Pender, N. J. Self-modification. In Bulechek, G. M., & McCloskey, J. C., (Eds.), *Nursing interventions: Treatments for nursing diagnoses.* Philadelphia: Saunders, 1985, pp. 80–91.

68. O'Connell, J. K., & Price, J. H. Ethical theories for promoting health through behavioral change. *Journal of School Health,* October 1983, *53* (8), 476–479.

69. Mahoney, M. J. *Self-change: Strategies for solving personal problems.* New York: Norton, 1979.

70. Tubesing, N. L., & Tubesing, D. A. *Structured exercises in wellness promotion: A wholeperson handbook for trainers, educators, and group leaders.* Duluth, Minn.: Whole Person Press, 1984.

CHAPTER 11

Exercise and
Physical Fitness

Today, many Americans are older physically than their chronological age because of long-term neglect of bodily needs and sedentary life style. Most urban dwellers are underactive but highly stressed, leading to lack of energy, low productivity, and limited enjoyment of daily life. These individuals have been labeled "physically disadvantaged" by Cantu.[1] While this term is often considered to apply only to persons with chronic health problems or physical disabilities, individuals who are overweight, sedentary, or both should also be included in this classification regardless of chronological age.

Modern life style fosters unfitness. During childhood and adolescent years, most individuals focus on the competitive aspects of sports in school athletic programs and do not develop a commitment to systematic exercise as an important lifetime activity.[2] In a study of the fitness level of children, Godin and Shephard[3] found that adolescent boys were more active physically than girls. The girls showed a marked decline in strenuous exercise from grades seven to nine. Thus, for many individuals, particularly females, sedentary life styles may emerge early in life and be highly resistant to change. While some individuals are genetically endowed with stronger physical constitutions than others, most Americans cheat themselves out of months, years, or even decades of good health by inappropriate physical activity habits.[4] Years of inactivity are a major causative or contributing factor to degenerative changes that occur with aging or chronic illness.

Physical fitness is critical for dynamic, fulfilling, and productive living. It is an important expression of both the stabilizing and actualizing tendencies in human beings. No Health Protection–Promotion Plan is complete without an individualized exercise program that takes into consideration the present level of fitness of the client and any existing health problems.

Fortunately, over the past few years, regular exercise has been increasingly recognized by Americans as contributing to personal health. In the Surgeon General's Report, *Healthy People,* national goals call for participation in regular and vigorous physical activity by 90 percent of youth and 60 percent of adults by 1990. Present estimates indicate that 41 to 51 percent of adults are sedentary, while only one-third of all adults participate in exercise on a weekly basis. Just 15 percent are believed to expend an energy equivalent (1500 kcal per week) that is of epidemiological or physiological significance.[5] Given the prevalence of sedentary life styles in the American population, a major challenge for health care professionals is to assist clients of all ages in increasing physical fitness through systematic, habitual exercise.

BENEFITS OF EXERCISE

Many studies have indicated that frequent strenuous exercise associated with a continuous and significant elevation of pulse for 20 to 30 minutes helps protect individuals against the threat of heart attacks, improves physical well-being, and increases feelings of vitality. Paffenbarger et al.,[6] in a 16-year study of 16,936 Harvard alumni, found that for individuals who exercised vigorously expending 2000 or more calories per week, mortality rates were one-quarter to one-third lower than among less active men. With or without consideration of hypertension, cigarette smoking, obesity, or history of early parental death, mortality rates were significantly lower among the physically active. Evidence also suggests that there is a relationship between regular exercise, productivity, and improved psychological states.[7-9] Sidney and Shephard[10] found that adults who participated vigorously in a physical training program showed decreased anxiety and improved body image. The major positive effects of systematic exercise are summarized in Table 11–1. While a detailed discussion of the many benefits of exercise is beyond the scope of this chapter, the reader is referred to a number of sources in which an in-depth analysis of the benefits of exercise is presented.[11-16]

Decline in physical fitness often occurs with age. For example, by age 70, some women may lose up to 70 percent of their bone mineral mass. There is also a significant decrease in lean body mass and basal metabolism rate. However, these degenerative processes and many others can be markedly slowed by a systematic physical activity program. The basic components of fitness include the following:[17]

- Cardiorespiratory endurance—capability of heart, blood vessels, and lungs to function at optimum efficiency in delivering nutrients and oxygen to tissues and removing wastes

TABLE 11–1. POSITIVE INFLUENCES OF CHRONIC ENDURANCE PHYSICAL EXERCISE

Blood Vessels and Chemistry
  Increase blood oxygen content
  Increase blood cell mass and blood volume
  Increase fibrinolytic capability
  Increase efficiency of peripheral blood distribution and return
  Increase blood supply to muscles and more efficient exchange of oxygen and carbon
    dioxide
  Reduce serum triglycerides and cholesterol levels
  Reduce platelet cohesion or stickiness
  Reduce systolic and diastolic blood pressure, especially when elevated
  Reduce glucose intolerance

Heart
  Increase strength of cardiac contraction (myocardial efficiency)
  Increase blood supply (collateral) to heart
  Increase size of coronary arteries
  Increase size of heart muscle
  Increase blood volume (stroke volume) per heart beat
  Increase heart rate recovery after exercise
  Reduce heart rate at rest
  Reduce heart rate with exertion
  Reduce vulnerability to cardiac arrythmias

Lungs
  Increase blood supply
  Increase diffusion of O_2 and CO_2
  Increase functional capacity during exercise
  Reduce nonfunctional volume of lung

Endocrine (Glandular) and Metabolic Function
  Increase tolerance to stress
  Increase glucose tolerance
  Increase thyroid function
  Increase growth hormone production
  Increase lean muscle mass
  Increase enzymatic function in muscle cells
  Increase functional capacity during exercise (muscle oxygen uptake capacity)
  Reduce body fat content
  Reduce chronic catecholamine production
  Reduce neurohumeral overreaction

Neural and Psychic
  Reduce strain and nervous tension resulting from psychologic stress
  Reduce tendency for depression
  Euphoria or "joie de vivre" experienced by many
  Improved body image

Reprinted from Cantu, R.C. Toward fitness: Guided exercise for those with health problems. New York: Human Sciences Press, 1980. With permission.

- Muscular strength—capacity of muscles to exert maximal force against a resistance
- Muscular endurance—capacity of muscles to exert force repeatedly over a period of time
- Flexibility—ability to use muscles and joints through maximum range of motion
- Motor skill performance—ability of nerves to receive messages that result in smooth, coordinated muscle movement

A physically fit person generally has a lower heart rate and more rapid recovery (return to resting rate) for any given exercise work load than does a person

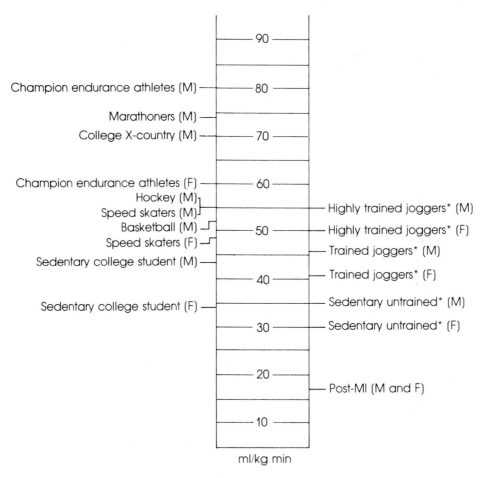

Figure 11–1. Maximal oxygen uptake values for selected activity groups. F: female; M: male. An asterisk indicates that values are for middle-aged adults. [*Reprinted from Getchell, B. Physical fitness: A way of life (2nd ed.). New York: Wiley, 1979. With permission*).

who is unfit. Maximal oxygen uptake (aerobic capacity) is an important measure of fitness. During treadmill stress test or bicycle ergometer test, use of special equipment that analyzes oxygen and carbon dioxide content of expired air allows determination of maximal or submaximal oxygen uptake.[18] Maximal uptake can be used for young adults, while submaximal uptake (50 and 75 percent of the age-computed maximal rate) is a safer procedure for older or sedentary individuals. Maximal oxygen uptake is expressed in milliliters of oxygen consumed per kilogram of body weight in a minute. Figure 11–1 depicts maximum oxygen uptake values for selected activity groups.

A well-planned physical activity program can increase aerobic capacity by 20 to 30 percent, improve cardiorespiratory endurance, enhance muscle strength, and improve flexibility. A significant change in level of physical fitness can be achieved. The rest of this chapter will be devoted to discussion of various types of exercise and fitness programs. The reader is referred back to Chapter 6 for information concerning physical fitness evaluation.

THE ROLE OF THE NURSE

Nurses are familiar with the importance of exercise such as passive or active range of motion for the bedridden patient or ambulation during hospitalization to prevent the undesirable and hazardous effects of immobility. The nurse's role in preventing deterioration of fitness for the patient is a well-defined one. In contrast, the concept of promoting physical fitness for purposes of health protection and promotion among individuals and families has been largely ignored in nursing curricula. As a result, most nurses know little about this aspect of health promotion, even though it is one of the most important factors in preventing disability and increasing health and wellness.[19]

The nurse should be able to evaluate physical fitness of clients independently or in collaboration with an exercise physiologist and incorporate knowledge of physiology, chemistry, and anatomy (Krebs cycle, cell physiology, cardiovascular dynamics) into practical approaches to exercise. Blair[20] presents an excellent overview of various approaches for assessing exercise habits and physical fitness of clients. The nurse should not only instruct, support, and evaluate clients during physical fitness activities but should serve as a role model of the physically fit adult. Personal experience with exercise and fitness activities increases the enthusiasm of the nurse for such programs and promotes understanding and empathy for clients during the early experiences of muscle soreness, fatigue, and slow progress.

Many nurses are actively involved in providing nutrition and weight-control programs for adults in the community and children in school settings. Nurses who provide services to families have the responsibility for assisting family members to plan group or individual physical fitness activities. Wellness programs in many hospitals are coordinated by nurses and place major emphasis on physical training programs. Nurses functioning in these settings should be familiar with the basic principles of exercise prescription. Guidelines for developing exercise prescriptions are provided by Ribisl.[21]

PRE-EXERCISE CONSIDERATIONS

All individuals who have a family or personal history of cardiovascular disorders, present previous signs or symptoms of cardiovascular disease, or are over 35 years of age should obtain a complete physical examination before beginning an exercise program. The physical examination should include a family history, blood lipid profile, resting blood pressure, resting 12-lead electrocardiogram, and exercise 12-lead electrocardiogram.[22] A treadmill stress test or bicycle ergometer test is also recommended. If the client's personal physician is not familiar with these physical fitness tests or does not have the proper equipment to administer them, the client should request the name of a physician qualified to conduct such an evaluation.

The aerobic capacity of the client as well as heart rate and rhythm patterns during testing are important considerations in structuring an appropriate exercise program. The nurse should work closely with clients and their physicians in implementing individualized physical activity programs. Exercise programs should be re-evaluated at regular intervals to determine client adherence and appropriateness.

PROPER BREATHING

Learning to breathe is the first thing that newborn infants do, but many children, adolescents, and adults develop inefficient and improper breathing patterns. When breathing is inappropriate or inadequate, all parts of the body, including muscles and brain, are affected by a shortage of oxygen. Proper breathing is not just a matter of the inhalation and exhalation of air; it includes the expansion of all parts of the lungs as well as correct posture to make this expansion possible. The proper movement of the diaphragm is critical for effective breathing. It should lower (contract) during inhalation and curve up into the thorax (relax) during exhalation. This type of breathing, referred to as diaphragmatic or abdominal breathing, is important throughout each day, but it is particularly important during exercise, when cells of the heart and muscles need increased oxygen.

Because of limited space, the physiology of breathing will not be discussed here. Instead, several breathing exercises will be described that the nurse can teach clients in order to promote maximum expansion of lungs and increased benefits from exercise.

Nickolaus Breathing Technique[23]
This exercise increases the client's awareness of breathing patterns, helps gain control of breathing, increases lung capacity, and relaxes the total body

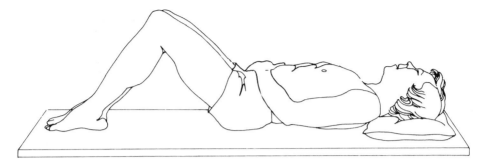

Figure 11–2. Body position and alignment for Nickolaus breathing technique.

in preparation for exercise. It can be incorporated as part of the warm-up routine.

The client should be instructed to lie on the floor (rug or mat is preferred, but a blanket may be used), with knees bent to keep lower back against the floor and knees and feet 6 to 8 inches apart. The body should be aligned as illustrated in Figure 11–2, with feet on the floor, toes turned slightly inward so that the arches are lifted. Chin should be toward chest, with mouth slightly open. The client should imagine lying in bed, relaxed, letting everything go, just before drifting off to sleep. The hands should be placed on the stomach, with middle fingers meeting at the navel so that the client can feel the up-and-down movement of abdominal muscles. The client should inhale slowly through the nose to the count of 4, letting the diaphragm descend and abdomen rise. The breath should flow upward into the chest, expanding the upper part of the torso. The air should then be allowed to flow out through the nose and mouth, gently contracting muscles of the chest then those of the abdomen. With abdominal contraction, the lower part of the back should make solid contact with the floor. This exercise should be repeated six times.

It is important to maintain an even flow in breathing with inhalation and exhalation performed in a steady and continuous fashion. The only tension that should be felt during exhalation is in the abdomen.

Diaphragmatic Breathing (Sitting Position)[24]
If the client prefers, diaphragmatic breathing can be performed while sitting in a straight-backed chair. The client should assume a comfortable position, with feet resting flat on the floor and hands placed one over the other at the navel as illustrated in Figure 11–3. Eyes should remain open. The client should imagine a giant balloon, in the abdomen below the hands, which he or she is attempting to fill with air. The hands will raise as the imaginary balloon is filled. The client should continue inhalation through the nose until the balloon is "filled to the top." Total length of inhalation should be 5 to 7 seconds. The client should inhale through the nose, since this allows the air to be warmed and moistened, and aids in the removal of impurities. Air inhaled through the mouth may be too cold for comfortable deep breathing.

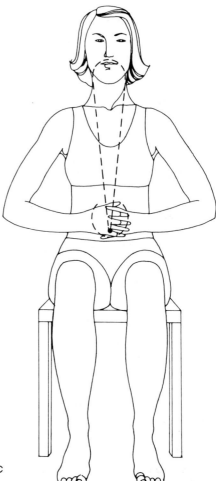

Figure 11–3. Sitting position for diaphragmatic breathing.

The breath should be held momentarily while the phrase "I feel calm" is repeated slowly. The air can then be exhaled to "empty the balloon." During exhalation the raised abdomen and chest recede. This breathing exercise should be repeated 4 to 5 times in succession at least 8 or 10 times per day. If lightheadedness occurs, decrease length of inhalation or number of repetitions.

Complete Breathing[25]

This technique is taken from yoga and is a combination of coordinated postural movements and breathing. The starting position for complete breathing is illustrated in Figure 11–4A. Knees should be together, with hips resting on heels and frontal part of head resting on the floor. This position is assumed after complete exhalation. The body should be raised as in Figure 11–4B

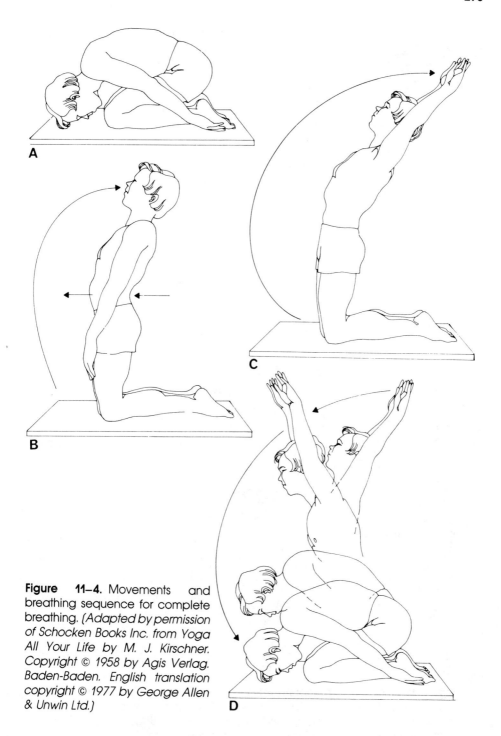

Figure 11-4. Movements and breathing sequence for complete breathing. *(Adapted by permission of Schocken Books Inc. from Yoga All Your Life by M. J. Kirschner. Copyright © 1958 by Agis Verlag. Baden-Baden. English translation copyright © 1977 by George Allen & Unwin Ltd.)*

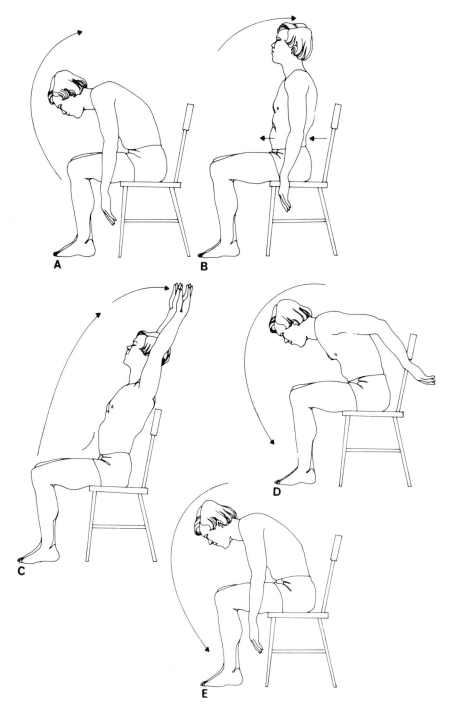

Figure 11–5. Modified complete breathing technique for the elderly or disabled. *(Adapted by permission of Schocken Books Inc. from* Yoga All Your Life *by M. J. Kirschner. Copyright © 1958 by Agis Verlag, Baden-Bagen. English translation copyright © 1977 by George Allen & Unwin Ltd.)*

when air is inhaled; abdomen should move out, and the hollow in the back should be prominent. The client should raise arms above his or her head while holding his or her breath for 1 to 2 seconds (Fig. 11–4C). During exhalation, the starting position is slowly assumed again (Fig. 11–4D) in preparation for the next sequence. This exercise should be practiced 6 to 8 times in succession 3 to 4 times per day; it can be modified for the elderly or disabled as illustrated in Figure 11–5.

Summary

Correct breathing is essential for good cardiopulmonary function. As with any skill, practice is important in mastering appropriate breathing techniques. Use of appropriate diaphragmatic breathing will greatly enhance vitality and facilitate endurance during active exercise.

CHARACTERISTICS OF GOOD EXERCISE

A program of exercise that promotes physical fitness should have the following characteristics from the client's perspective.[26]

- It should be enjoyable
- It should be vigorous enough to make use of a minimum of 400 calories

TABLE 11-2. TARGET HEART RATE AND HEART-RATE RANGE BY AGE GROUP

Age	Your maximum heart rate* (beats/min)	Your target heart rate (75% of the maximum in beats/min)	Your target heart-rate range (between 70 and 85% of the maximum in beats/min)
20	200	150	140 to 170
25	195	146	137 to 166
30	190	142	133 to 162
35	185	139	130 to 157
40	180	135	126 to 153
45	175	131	123 to 149
50	170	127	119 to 145
55	165	124	116 to 140
60	160	120	112 to 136
65	155	116	109 to 132
70	150	112	105 to 123

*Maximum heart rate is the greatest number of beats per minute that your heart is capable of. During exercise, your heart rate should be approximately 70 to 85 percent of this maximum.
Reprinted from Kuntzleman, C.T. The complete book of walking. New York: Simon & Schuster, 1979, p. 96. With permission.

- It should sustain the heart rate at 70 to 85 percent of maximum potential for 20 to 30 minutes (approximately 120 to 150 beats)
- It should produce rhythmical movements, with muscles alternatively contracting and relaxing
- It should be repeated for 30 to 60 minutes, 4 to 5 days per week
- It should be systematically integrated into the client's life style

Recreational activities that achieve target heart rate and thus develop cardiopulmonary and muscular endurance include running, swimming, cross-country skiing, cycling, rowing, handball, basketball (if played vigorously), and squash.[27] Brisk walking can also be used, since it is continuous, rhythmical movement. However, walking takes a longer period of time than the above recreational activities to achieve target heart rate. Table 11–2 presents target heart rate and heart-rate range by age. Sports not recommended as beneficial in conditioning include golf, bowling, baseball, softball, and volleyball, as they do not provide continuous, rhythmic activity.

WARMING UP FOR EXERCISE

A warm-up period before extended exercise is important in order to increase blood flow to heart and skeletal muscles, enhance oxygenation of tissues, and loosen (decrease tension) and strengthen muscles. The warm-up period need take no longer than 10 to 15 minutes and should be immediately followed by endurance exercise. Some exercise specialists differentiate between warm-up and stretching exercises and believe that there is less likelihood of injury from stretching exercises if they are carried out after the endurance regimen but prior to cool-down. The following is a suggested warm-up sequence of exercises:

1. Walk briskly for 1 minute
2. Jog for 45 seconds
3. Walk briskly for 30 seconds
4. Arm circles
5. Jumping jacks
6. Lateral bend
7. Head rotation
8. Side leg raises
9. Single leg raise and knee hug
10. Push-ups (floor or wall)

Each of the warm-up exercises except jogging and walking will be described below. Jogging and walking will be dealt with at length later in this chapter under Endurance Exercises. The reader is referred to the references at the end of the chapter for other activities that can be used in warm-up routines.

Arm Circles

This warm-up exercise increases the flexibility of muscles in the arm and shoulder region. The client should stand with feet shoulder-width apart and arms at sides. Arms should make large sweeping circles, with elbows straight, swinging arms from the shoulders.[28] The inward cross-body and outward cross-body arm circles and forward (swimming crawl motion) and backward (backward swimming crawl) arm circles are illustrated in Figure 11–6. Ten repetitions of each type of arm circles are recommended.

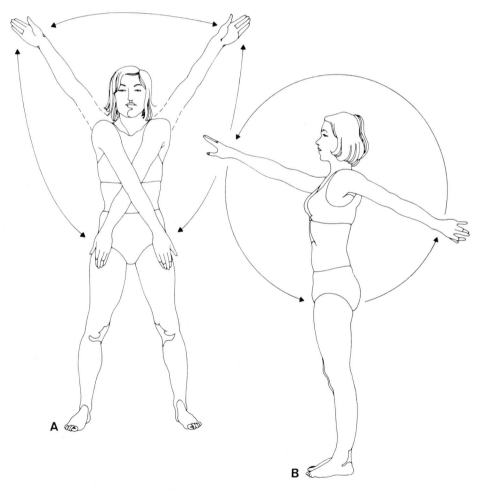

Figure 11–6. Arm circles.

Jumping Jacks

This exercise is frequently used as part of the warm-up routine. It stretches and loosens major muscle groups within the arms and legs. The client should start with feet together and hands at sides. When jumping to the position with feet apart, arms should be kept straight and swung up over head. Ten to 20 jumping jacks should be repeated at a comfortable tempo. Figure 11–7 illustrates the jumping jack exercise.

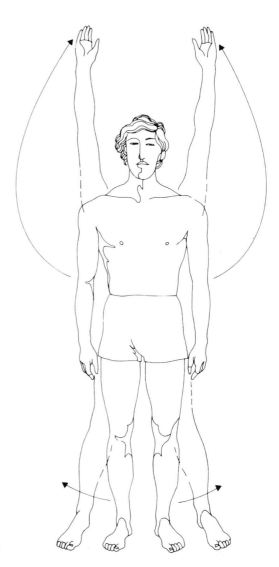

Figure 11–7. Jumping jacks.

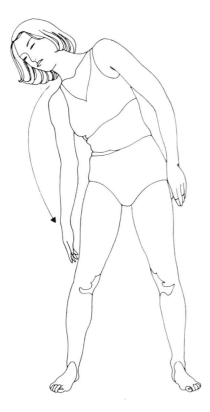

Figure 11–8. The lateral bend.

Lateral Bend

This warm-up exercise is intended to loosen and stretch the lateral muscles of the trunk and back. Feet should be about shoulder-width apart, arms at sides. By bending laterally, the client should reach down the right leg with the right hand until he or she feels a pulling sensation in the back. At this point, the client should straighten to upright position and repeat the same stretching movement on the left side. Ten repetitions are recommended. The lateral bend is illustrated in Figure 11–8.

Head Rotation

The client should assume a sitting position, with arms comfortably resting at sides. While the client breathes in, the chin should be dropped forward to the chest. The client should roll the head to the left, then to the back, stretching the chin toward the ceiling. As the head is rolled to the right and forward again, the client should exhale. This is an excellent exercise for increasing the flexibility of neck muscles and is particularly recommended for individuals who spend a great deal of time at desk work. Figure 11–9 illustrates

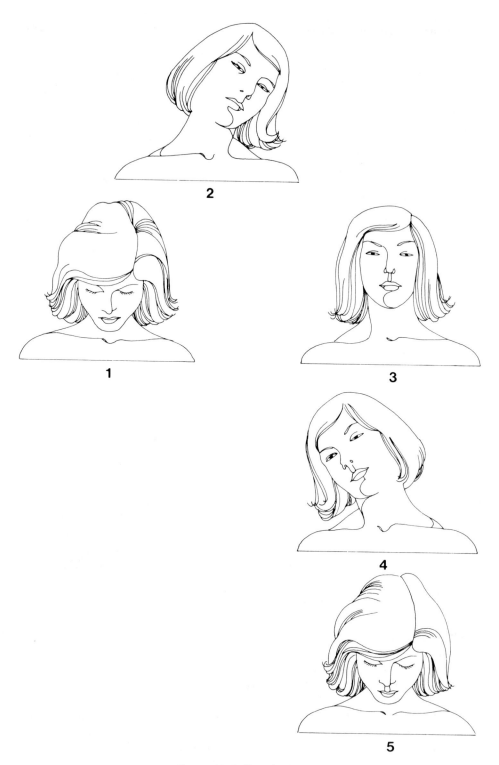

Figure 11–9. Head rotation.

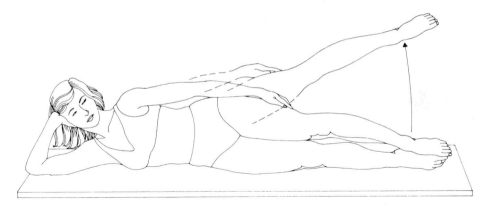

Figure 11–10. Side leg raises.

head rotation. Repetitions should be increased from 5 to 15, as tolerated. The client should be informed that initially some dizziness may occur; therefore, this exercise should never be performed in a standing position.

Side Leg Raises

This exercise stretches and strengthens the lateral hip muscles and is a good conditioning exercise. The client should lie on his or her right side in extended position, with head resting on right hand as shown in Figure 11–10. The client raises the left leg as high as possible above the horizontal position and then returns to starting position. After completing repetitions for one side, the client repeats the exercise on the other side. Fifteen to 25 repetitions are recommended.

Single Leg Raise and Knee Hug

This exercise is intended to strengthen low back and abdominal muscles while increasing the flexibility of hip and knee joints. The client assumes a reclining position as illustrated in Figure 11–11 and raises extended left leg about 12 inches off the floor, slowly bending the knee and moving it toward the chest. The client then places both hands around the knee and pulls it gently toward his or her chest as far as possible. The leg is then slowly extended to the starting position. This exercise is repeated 3 to 5 times with each leg.

Wall Push-Ups

This exercise is intended to strengthen arm, shoulder, and upper back muscles while stretching chest and posterior thigh muscles. The client should stand erect facing the wall with feet about 6 inches apart, arms extended, and palms of hands against the wall. The client slowly bends the arms and lowers body toward the wall, until cheek almost touches the wall. The body is then slowly pushed away from the wall, extending arms and returning to original

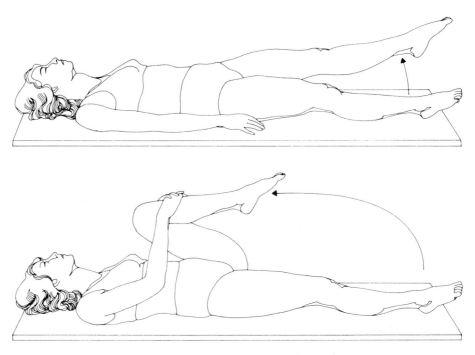

Figure 11–11. Single leg raise and knee hug.

position. This exercise should be repeated 5 to 10 times as illustrated in Figure 11–12. Traditional floor push-ups can also be used if the level of fitness of the client permits more exertion than required by wall push-ups.

The client who is just beginning a physical exercise program will need to select three or four warm-up exercises initially, completing 5 to 10 repetitions of each. As endurance exercise is continued, repetitions can be increased, different warm-up exercises can be selected for variety, or others can be added to extend the time spent in warm-up. Cool weather usually requires a longer warm-up period than does warm weather.

STRETCHING EXERCISES

Loss of joint and muscle flexibility often occurs with aging. Flexibility is defined as the extent to which the client is able to move joints and muscles through full range of motion. Since walking and running do little for flexibility, stretching exercises are extremely important in the maintenance of physical fitness. Stretching exercises can:[29]

- Reduce muscle tension and increase feelings of relaxation
- Promote circulation

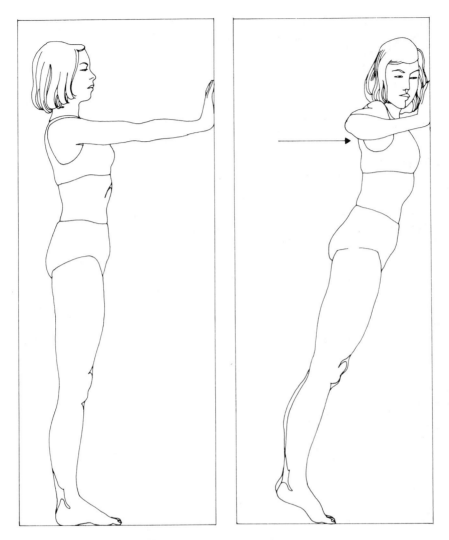

Figure 11–12. Wall push-ups.

- Lengthen muscles after exercise
- Increase range of motion of joints and increase flexibility
- Prevent injuries such as muscle strain
- Help coordination by allowing for freer and easier movement
- Possibly inhibit the onset of chronic inflammatory conditions such as arthritis, bursitis, and tendonitis

Stretching exercises put more strain on muscles than do warm-up exercises. Excessive stretching, just like excessive jogging, can produce injuries. After the body is warmed up or after the endurance phase of exercise, stretching can be carried out with much less discomfort and concern for injury. Stretching exercises should be done slowly and the stretched position held for 15 to 30 seconds. The client should avoid stretching too far. As the client becomes more flexible, stretching positions can be held longer and the muscle can be stretched a bit further.[30]

Because of limited space, only a few stretching exercises will be presented here. The reader is referred to the references at the end of the chapter for more detailed information on stretching routines.

Back-Stretch

The back is extremely vulnerable to injury, and many Americans suffer from chronic back problems. This exercise stretches the back and neck muscles and promotes greater strength and flexibility. The client should stand erect with feet shoulder-width apart and bend forward at the waist, letting arms, shoulders, and neck relax. The client should go to the point where a slight stretch is felt in the back of the legs. If the client cannot reach the floor, the hands can be placed on the legs to provide support. When straightening back up, the knees should be slightly bent to avoid pressure in the lower back. Figure 11–13 illustrates the back-stretch exercise. Five to 7 repetitions are recommended initially. If the client is elderly or disabled, back-stretch exercise can also be done sitting in a chair. Knees are placed apart, feet flat

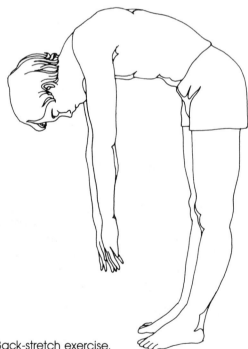

Figure 11–13. Back-stretch exercise.

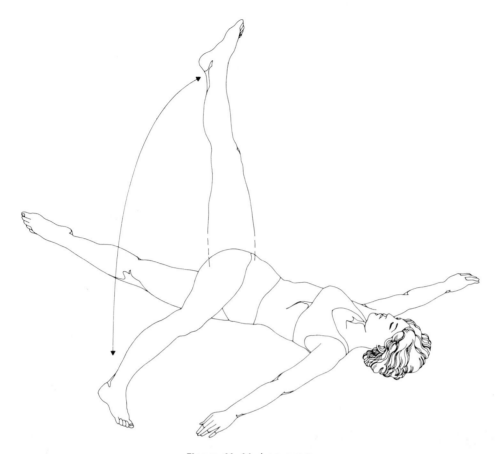

Figure 11–14. Leg overs.

on the floor, with the body gently lowered between the knees. The fingers and palms of the hands should touch the floor. This exercise is particularly effective in dealing with postural strain following typing, driving, sewing, or other forms of sedentary work.[31]

Leg Overs

The purpose of this exercise is to stretch the rotator muscles of the lower back and pelvic region. The client should lie on back with legs extended and arms extended at shoulder level with the palms up. The leg should be kept straight as it is raised to the vertical position (toes pointed). The opposite leg should remain on the floor in extended position. The vertically extended leg should reach across the body to the opposite hand and then be returned to the vertical position as shown in Figure 11–14. The exercise should be repeated with each leg for 4 to 10 repetitions.

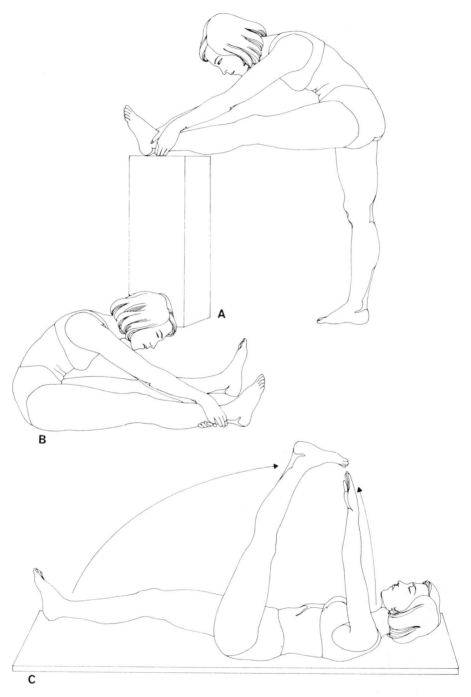

Figure 11–15. Hamstring-stretching exercises. **A.** Standing hamstring stretcher. **B.** Sitting hamstring stretcher. **C.** Lying-down hamstring stretcher.

Hamstring Stretcher

This exercise can be done in three different positions as illustrated in Figure 11–15.

In the standing position (Fig. 11–15A), one leg is raised and the heel of the foot rests on a table or chair. The client should lean toward the raised foot until stretching is felt in the thigh. This position should be held for several seconds, with care being taken not to overstretch.

In the sitting position (Fig. 11–15B), knees should be extended with legs spread apart at a 45-degree angle. The client should bend forward at the waist, grasping one ankle with both hands and trying to touch the head to the knee until stretching is felt in the back of the leg. This position should be held for 5 to 7 seconds.

In the lying-down position (Fig. 11–15C), the client is on his or her back on the floor or bed. Arms are raised perpendicular at right angles to the body. Each leg should be kept straight but swung up gently toward the fingers. Five to 10 repetitions with each leg are recommended.[32] The lying-down position may be easier for elderly individuals to use. The purpose of the exercise is to stretch the lower-back muscles and hamstring muscles, which shorten considerably with age or in women from wearing high-heeled shoes.

Trunk Rotator

This exercise is performed to stretch the muscles of the lower back, buttocks, and waist. The client should begin by standing with feet shoulder-width apart and hands with fingers interlaced behind head. First the client should lean to the right and continue moving in a clockwise direction, down and up to the left and back to the original position, in a circular motion. The circular motion should be repeated in a counterclockwise direction.[33] Six to 8 repetitions in each direction are recommended. The body motion for the trunk rotator is depicted in Figure 11–16.

Cat's Arch

This exercise is intended to stretch the muscles of the lower back, waist, and stomach. The client should begin by getting down on hands and knees, keeping elbows straight and knees bent at a 90-degree angle. The stomach should be pushed toward floor and the back bent downward. This will cause extension of the back muscles. Then the client should arch his or her back like an angry cat. In attempting to do this, the client should pull in the stomach muscles as much as possible and push the lower back towards the ceiling. This exercise is excellent for increasing the flexibility of the lower back, particularly after sitting behind a desk for long periods of time.[34] Figure 11–17 depicts the two different positions to be assumed during this stretching exercise. Six repetitions are recommended initially, increasing to 15 to 20 as tolerated.

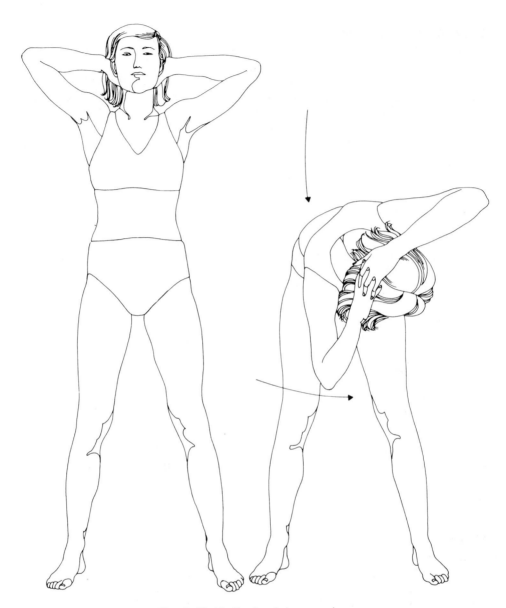

Figure 11-16. Trunk-rotator exercise.

Stretching Exercises for Feet and Ankles

The feet and ankles are extremely important in most endurance activities and thus should be given careful attention in stretching and flexibility exercises. Lying in the position shown in Figure 11–18, with the knee flexed, the foot can be circled clockwise until the toe is pointed away and then flexed back to its starting position. This exercise should be repeated only five times with each foot, since cramping may occasionally occur. If cramping does occur, the foot should be relaxed until cramping subsides, and then the exercise can be continued.

Foot flexion is also illustrated in Figure 11–18. In this exercise, the foot is arched by extending the metatarsal but keeping the toes flexed. The toes are then pointed and flexed again, and then the entire foot is flexed. This exercise should also be repeated five times with each foot. These exercises

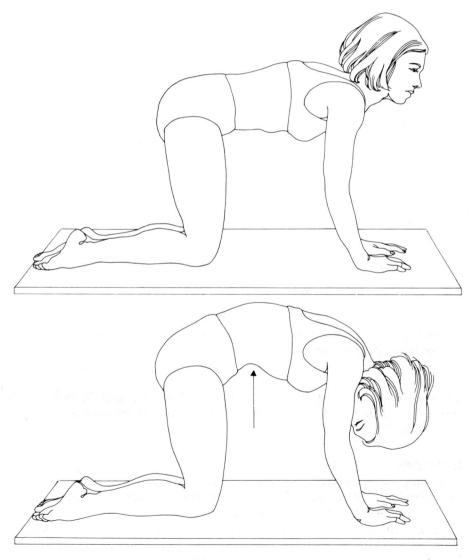

Figure 11–17. The cat's arch.

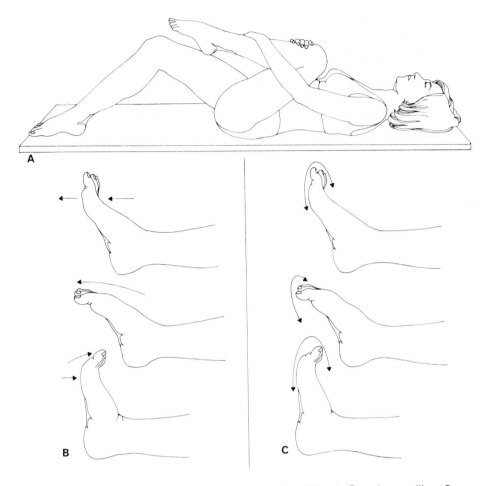

Figure 11-18. Stretching exercises for feet and ankles. **A.** Exercise position. **B.** Foot flexion. **C.** Foot/ankle circles.

can be carried out while sitting in a chair with the leg slightly raised if the physical condition of the client makes this position more feasible.

Summary

Stretching exercises strengthen muscles, ligaments, and tendons and develop flexibility in the body's muscles and joints. This increases physical readiness to engage in endurance exercise as well as greater ease and comfort in carrying out the activities of daily living. The number and type of stretching exercises appropriate for each individual must be determined through mutual discussion and planning between the nurse and the client.

ENDURANCE EXERCISES

A systematic program of endurance exercise can result in cardiopulmonary and muscular conditioning. Endurance exercises should be integrated into life style, since continued practice is essential for long-term health-protection and health-promotion benefits. Maintaining physical fitness is a lifelong process that can be enjoyable, rewarding, and challenging to the client. Endurance exercises to be discussed in this chapter include walk-jog, jogging, and walking. These are the least expensive and usually the most convenient endurance exercises for clients to perform.

Critical aspects of self-care important for all individuals engaged in a physical fitness program include the following:

1. The feet should be well cared for, since they are subjected to increased stress and friction during endurance exercise
2. A good pair of running shoes should be worn for all endurance exercises. Characteristics of good shoes include:[35]
   - Cushioned soles
   - Ample toe room
   - Heel elevation from $\frac{1}{2}$ to $\frac{3}{4}$ inches above sole
   - Good support
   - Oxford type
   - Leather, allowing feet to breathe
   - Sole that flexes at the ball of foot but not at the midpoint
3. Clean, snug-fitting socks should be worn during exercise to prevent the development of pressure points and blisters
4. Endurance exercises should not be carried out during the hottest or most humid hours of the day in warm weather
5. Endurance exercise should not be carried out immediately following a meal. The client should exercise before eating or wait $1\frac{1}{2}$ to $2\frac{1}{2}$ hours after eating a full meal
6. Workout should be preceded by drinking an increased amount of clear liquids (e.g., water, juice). Water loss from the body is markedly increased during endurance exercise
7. From $1\frac{1}{2}$ to $2\frac{1}{2}$ hours before exercise, ingestion of small to moderate amounts of high-carbohydrate foods can increase glucose reserves
8. Maintenance of an adequate intake of salt and potassium prevents muscle cramps
9. Excessive stretching during warm-ups should be avoided
10. Shin splints can be prevented by running or walking on soft or semisoft rather than hard surfaces. The surface should also be relatively flat rather than hilly to prevent excessive fatigue
11. If injury to achilles tendon (inflammation, partial rupture, or complete rupture) occurs, ice should be applied immediately, and activity should be reduced

TABLE 11-3. COMPETENCY-BASED OBJECTIVES FOR A TEACHING PLAN ON EXERCISE

The consumer of health should be able to:
Express personal concept of health.

Examine personal views in regard to health and physical fitness.

Relate his or her general health and illness history.

Relate his or her specific (if available) health–illness information (e.g., blood pressure, weight, diet, smoking habits, electrocardiogram results, specific blood chemistry results such as cholesterol and triglyceride levels, personality characteristics, etc.).

Express personal likes and dislikes of physical activity.

Recognize that exercise is a part of but not the sole factor of health maintenance.

Locate exercise resources in the community.

Plan a time schedule when exercises could be included without altering the client's life style.

Conjointly plan an exercise program with his or her doctor and nurse/teacher.

Recognize aerobic exercises that either are or are not appropriate for the client.

Describe suitable clothing to wear during exercising.

Explain the importance of a warm-up period.

Describe the symptoms of angina and muscle strain that would indicate cessation of activity.

Demonstrate how to monitor a pulse before, during, and after exercise.

Compare vital signs and physical changes during and after exercise to resting vital signs.

Demonstrate emergency actions (CPR) that may be necessary during group exercising activities.

Question exercise fads and nonprofessional literature on exercise.

Compare his or her progress over a period of time.

Plan for medical and nursing/teaching follow-up.

Value his or her progress and perseverence in habit formation and health maintenance.

Choose by virtue of his or her individual right to terminate the program.

Adapted from Borgman, M.F. Exercise and health maintenance. *Journal of Nursing Education,* January 1979, *16,* 6–10. With permission.

The nurse is responsible for assisting the client in developing specific competencies related to efficient and effective use of endurance exercise for physical conditioning. Borgman[36] has identified competency-based objectives for a teaching plan on exercise as an aspect of health maintenance. These objectives are presented in Table 11–3. Review of the competencies required indicates the complexity of physical endurance activities. The client must be able to plan adequately for exercise, prepare for exercise, monitor physical status during exercise, take appropriate actions if problems arise, and appraise personal progress.

Walk-Jog

This endurance exercise is appropriate for clients of all ages. Interspersing walking and jogging provides variation and distributes periods of physical stress over a span of time. Following warm-up exercises, the client should begin a period of jogging that lengthens throughout the conditioning program. In the beginning, jogging for 30 seconds followed by walking for an equal amount of time allows the client to adjust to increased physical activity. The client should jog erect, with the spine extended to maximize comfort. As the amount of time spent in jogging increases, the client will develop greater concentration on the smoothness and rhythm of body movement. Increased awareness of breathing, muscular contractions, relaxation, sensations of lightness, and enjoyment will characterize the activity.

Clients should be able to take their radial or carotid pulse for 10 seconds and multiply by 6 during both jogging and walking segments of the walk-jog. The heart rate should be within the target heart rate range during jogging (see Table 11–2), dropping somewhat during walking segments. If heart rate is not initially at target level, it will increase as the jogging periods are lengthened. If heart rate is above this level during jogging, changing to brisk walking and shortening the next segment is suggested. A plan for developing a walk-jog program is presented in Table 11–4. Clients should continue at each level until they have mastered that walk-jog combination and then move on to the next. If problems are encountered in moving to the next step, such as excessive fatigue, marked breathlessness, or faintness, the client should return to the previous level for a period of 3 to 5 days before attempting the next level of conditioning the second time.

Clients should be cautioned to proceed judiciously. If they are over 50 years of age and have been sedentary, it is wise to have them brisk walk on a progressive schedule for 10 to 12 weeks before beginning the walk-jog routines.

Jogging

Through jogging, the client reaches target heart rate (70 to 85 percent maximum) more rapidly than in a walk-jog routine. However, continuous jogging is more physically demanding than walk-jog and should never be attempted as the initial endurance exercise. It is recommended that the client com-

TABLE 11–4. PROGRESSIVE WALK-JOG PROGRAM

Level	Jog	Walk	Repeats
1	30 sec	30 sec	4 sets (work up to 12 sets for 3 consecutive days)
2	1 min	30 sec	6 sets (work up to 12 sets for 3 consecutive days)
3	1½ min	30 sec	6 sets (work up to 12 sets for 2 consecutive days)
4	2 min	30 sec	6 sets (work up to 10 sets for 2 consecutive days)
5	4 min	1 min	4 sets (work up to 6 sets for 2 consecutive days)
6	8 min	2 min	2 sets (work up to 4 sets on 2 consecutive days)
7	12 min	2 min	2 sets
8	15 min	3 min	2 sets
9	20 min	3 min	2 sets

plete the previously described walk-jog routine before attempting continuous jogging.

Jogging or running are the forms of endurance exercise that result in the highest caloric expenditure per minute. Females expend 9.1 kcal/min^{-1} at 81.9 percent VO$_2$ maximum, as compared to males, who expend 15.5 kcal/min^{-1} at 81.1 percent VO$_2$ maximum. Weight makes a difference in the amount of calories burned, particularly for jogging, although similar patterns are found for walk-jog and walking.[37] The higher the weight, the more calories that are burned.

Following completion of the walk-jog routine, continuous jogging should be carried out initially for a period of time no longer than 20 minutes. Clients should carefully evaluate their tolerance of continuous endurance activity by checking their pulse every 5 minutes during jogging and by noting any unusual physical symptoms. After 10 to 14 days of jogging continuously for 20 minutes, clients can increase jogging time to 30 minutes. If this is tolerated well for a period of 2 weeks, the jogging period can be increased to 35 or 40 minutes. This is an adequate length of time to allow heart rate to rise and to sustain target heart rate at conditioning level for 30 minutes.

Individuals who jog continuously have reported altered psychological states, such as euphoria, heightened inner awareness, or increased feelings of control during jogging. Some report decreased attention to environmental surroundings or that jogging results in a "natural high."[38] Because of increased internal focus and decreased attention to surroundings during jogging, the client should take precautions to minimize chances of injury. The client should never jog at night when unseen obstacles may cause serious trauma or jog in an area of heavy traffic.

Discussion of jogging as an endurance exercise in this chapter has been brief. For additional information, the reader is referred to the references at the end of the chapter and to several excellent books.[39-41]

Walking

This endurance exercise is safe for people of all ages. It can be tailored to individual differences and a wide range of fitness levels. Since fewer calories are expended in walking when compared to jogging, the client must walk briskly twice as long to achieve comparable levels of conditioning. Kuntzleman[42] has stated that an adult male burns the number of calories equivalent to one pound of fat (approximately 3500 calories) in 12 hours of brisk walking. The number of calories expended depends on walking rate (mph) and body weight. For comparable amounts of walking, individuals who weigh more expend greater energy than do individuals who weigh less. Brisk walking is extremely important during periods of attempted weight loss as it prevents the loss of lean body tissue and bone minerals.

The positive outcomes from a systematic walking program are many and varied. Walking can result in the following:

- Decreased percentage body fat
- Improved circulation
- Increased muscle tone in legs
- Decreased problems of constipation
- Improved mental state, with decreased depression and anxiety
- Improved recovery index following exercise
- Lowered blood pressure
- Improved physical fitness
- Decreased risk of coronary heart disease
- Decreased bone demineralization

Walking at 70 to 85 percent of maximum heart rate for at least 20 minutes three times per week will improve physical fitness. Walking at 70 to 85 percent of maximum heart rate for 30 minutes or longer four times per week can decrease the risk of coronary heart disease. If at the rate of walking selected by the client, pulse does not reach target level, rate of walking or length of walk must be increased to achieve a training effect. The barometer for how much walking the client can tolerate early in the walking program is the level of fatigue, breathlessness, or uncomfortable symptoms experienced. If after walking, the client seems excessively tired for more than an hour, the walk may be too strenuous. The client can walk more slowly or for a shorter period of time until tolerance is increased for more sustained efforts.

Regarding the psychological effects of walking, a study of a group of men over 50 years of age indicated that after several weeks of walking for 15 minutes per day, neuromuscular tension was decreased more effectively than it was from using standard dosages of tranquilizers over the same period of time.[43] Walking can promote feelings of serenity and relaxation. Consequently, it is an important adjunct to other stress-management techniques that the client may choose to use.

In order to maximize the benefits from a walking program, a number of suggestions can be made to the client:

- Walk naturally
- Wear good shoes with adequate support
- Let arms hang loosely at sides
- Hands, hips, knees, and ankles should be relaxed
- Feet should strike the ground at the heel
- Push off with toes when walking
- Use heel-to-toe rolling motion
- Breathe naturally
- Walk for fun as well as for fitness

Several ways that the client can make walking more enjoyable include inviting someone to walk along and visit, varying the route taken for the walk to provide the aesthetics of different environments, and "getting into the walk" by appreciating the pleasurable body sensations of smooth, coordinated movement.

Other endurance exercises that are beyond the scope of this book include swimming, running, bicycling, and rope skipping. The reader is referred to references at the end of this chapter for further information on these activities.

Summary

In summary, all clients engaged in endurance exercise should have well-developed self-monitoring skills. Clients participating in endurance exercises should not only understand how and when to check their own pulse but should also know what symptoms to look for as an indication of a possible problem. The nurse should counsel the client concerning the following symptoms and emphasize the need for the client to seek medical attention if they occur.[44]

- Chest or arm pain
- Marked increase in shortness of breath
- Irregular heart beat
- Light-headedness, fainting
- Nausea and vomiting with exercise
- Unexplained weight changes

- Muscle or joint problems
- Prolonged fatigue
- Muscle weakness
- Unexplained changes in exercise tolerance

COOLING DOWN

Following endurance exercise, cooling down is important. This phase of the workout provides a 5- to 10-minute recovery period following strenuous activity to allow circulation to gradually return to normal, preventing pooling of blood in muscles and possible fainting. Cooling down is important since in endurance exercise, blood pressure, body temperature, heart rate, and lactic acid within the muscles are all increased. Cooling down appropriately promates elimination of waste products from the muscles, maintains blood flow to and from the muscles, and allows body temperature and heart rate to decrease slowly. Inappropriate cooling down can make the client feel sore and nauseated. At the end of the cooling-down period, the heart rate of the client should be below 100.

Several exercises can be used during the cooling-down period. Five will be presented in this chapter for the client to consider. Exercises selected for cooling down should not allow a rapid drop in heart rate; there should be a gradual decrease in heart rate over a period of 5 to 10 minutes.

Walking and Deep Breathing

An excellent exercise for cooling down is walking briskly for 5 minutes, breathing deeply. Diaphragmatic breathing fully aerates the lungs and facilitates continuing oxygenation of blood following endurance exercise. As the client walks, he or she can also shake head and arms in a relaxed manner (shakedown). The shakedown further loosens tight muscles.[45]

Straight Arm and Leg Stretch

This exercise strengthens abdominal muscles while stretching the muscles of the arms. The client should lie flat on the floor with legs together and arms at the sides. The buttocks and abdomen are tensed so that the back is flat against the floor. The client should slowly move arms and legs outward along the floor as far as possible, hold for 5 seconds, and return to a starting position. Five to 10 repetitions of this exercise are recommended. The two positions to be assumed during the exercise are shown in Figure 11–19.

Achilles Stretcher

This exercise is helpful in stretching the heel cord on the lower part of the calf muscle (Achilles tendon). The client should face the wall, an arm's distance away, with knees straight, toes slightly inward, and heels flat on floor.

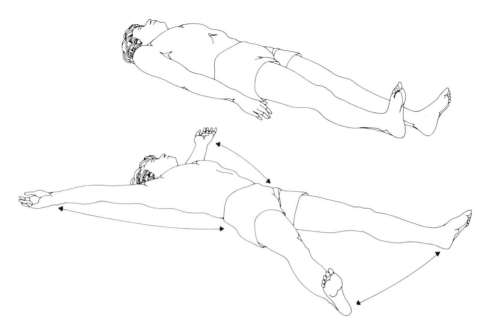

Figure 11–19. Straight arm and leg stretch.

With hands resting on the wall, the client should lean his or her body forward by bending elbows slowly. It is important that legs and body be kept straight and heels be on the floor. Five to 10 repetitions of this exercise are recommended. See Figure 11–20 for illustration of this exercise.

Half Knee Bend

This exercise is helpful in toning the hips, thighs, and buttocks, as well as in allowing gradual cooling down following endurance exercise. The client should assume a starting position with hands on hips and feet separated about shoulder width. As the exercise begins, the arms should be swung forward up to shoulder height and the knees bent about half-way, with heels kept on the floor. From this position, the client should return to the starting position. Figure 11–21 depicts the action sequence. Six to 8 repetitions are recommended initially, with frequency gradually increased to 12 to 15. The client can also progress to full knee bends as personal tolerance allows.[46]

Bent-Knee Half-Curl[47]

This exercise strengthens abdominal muscles and maintains activity during cooling down. The client should assume a lying-down position, with knees bent at a 45- to 90-degree angle and feet flat on the floor. Hands should be interlaced behind head. Tucking chin into chest, the client should curl forward until shoulders are about 10 to 14 inches off the floor. This position should be held for 2 to 4 seconds. The client should slowly return to the starting position. Three to 4 repetitions are recommended initially, with frequency increased to 6 to 8 as conditioning progresses. The sequence to be followed in completing this exercise is depicted in Figure 11–22.

Conclusion

Any of the activities described in the section on Stretching Exercises can also be used for cooling down. Clients should vary their routine to maintain personal interest and also to determine those exercises that are most effective in facilitating a slow decrease in heart rate.

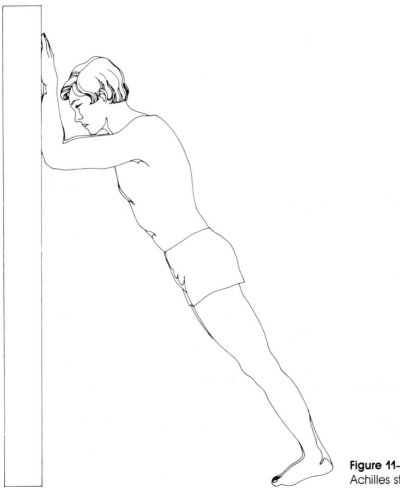

Figure 11–20.
Achilles stretcher.

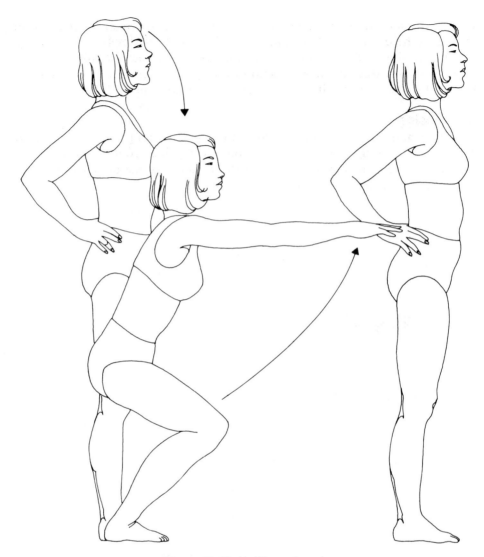

Figure 11–21. Half knee bend.

CONTINUATION OF EXERCISE PROGRAM

To maintain physical fitness, it is critical that clients continue their exercise program as an integral part of their personal life style. Drop-out rates as small as 11 percent and as large as 70 percent have been reported for physical-activity programs within the first 6 weeks. What can the nurse do to promote consistent practice of behaviors directed toward improving and maintaining

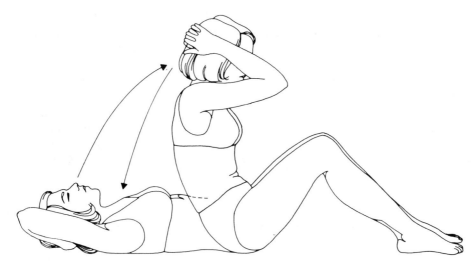

Figure 11–22. Bent-knee half-curl.

physical fitness? Some suggestions for assisting the client in maintaining behavioral consistency include the following:

- Setting both short-term and long-term goals
- Letting others know of intention to exercise regularly
- Recording progress
- Making a time commitment
- Choosing the best time of the day and establishing a pattern (habit of regular physical activity)
- Selecting a specific place in which to exercise
- Dressing the part in clothing appropriate for exercise
- Thinking the part by concentrating on enjoyment and feelings of well-being during exercise
- Varying warm-up and cool-down exercises
- Walking or running with others, particularly family members with similar fitness goals
- Picking an interesting and pleasing route for walking or jogging and periodically varying the route
- Alternating "hard" and "easy" days. On some days, exercise may be more intensive than on others. If exercise has been particularly strenuous one day, a less intense exercise session may be planned for the next day
- Preparing for relapses in exercise behavior and developing approaches for dealing with such relapses

Eischens[48] has suggested four approaches for assisting clients to persevere with exercise and conditioning activities. These include intent, regularity, limits capacity, and concentration. The major intent of exercise should be clear to the client, what endurance exercise means personally should be recognized. Is the goal to improve personal health, to reap psychological benefits, to lose weight, or to decrease the risk of coronary disease? Once personal health goals to be attained through physical activity have been identified, setting short-term as well as long-term goals sustains motivation.

Regularity in endurance exercise is also important to optimize positive health effects. As mentioned above, the client may alternate between "hard" and "easy" days. This alternation is considered by some exercise physiologists to lead to more rapid increases in strength than does repetitive strenuous exercise. Options for easy days can be (1) warm-up, stretching, and walking for 20 minutes, or (2) warm-up, stretching, and walk-jog for 15 minutes. For conditioning, 4 days per week are recommended as a minimum.

Clients will discover their physical and psychological limits capacity for endurance exercise; these are subject to change throughout the conditioning

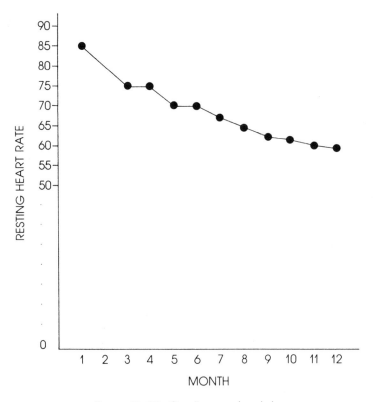

Figure 11–23. Cardiovascular status.

process. Exercise should be a stimulating but manageable challenge for the client; it should not result in excessive stress or discomfort.

Discovering personal capacities through exercise or physical activity is an important expression of the actualizing tendency. Increased awareness of breathing, muscle movement, relationship to terrain, body temperature, and skin sensations through concentration can be an exciting experience for the client. A different part of endurance exercise can be focused on each time. At one time the focus may be on breathing, at another on sensations and positions of legs and feet, still another on skin sensations. Concentration or fully experiencing endurance exercise can provide short-term benefits that are highly reinforcing to the client.

In addition to the above, depicting progress in physical fitness on a graph can provide motivation for continuation of exercise and conditioning activities on the part of the client. Awareness of progress in itself can make exercise rewarding; there may be no need for tangible or social reinforcement. A graph of cardiovascular status in terms of resting heart rate that can be used to chart progress is depicted in Figure 11–23. Other parameters of fitness may also be charted in a personal-growth notebook kept by the client, with assistance from the nurse. Recognizing tangible progress toward desired health goals can support continuation of exercise and physical fitness activities.

EXERCISE FOR SPECIAL GROUPS OF INDIVIDUALS

Diabetics, postcoronary patients, the obese, individuals with chronic illnesses that limit mobility, and older adults need special assistance in structuring exercise programs. While these clients present unique considerations in prescribing an exercise program, few such individuals are restricted from engaging in some form of systematic physical activity. Almost always, they can improve their health by doing so. Close supervision by a physician or nurse is essential for these individuals during the time that an exercise program is being planned, initiated, and stabilized. The program of physical activity must also be reevaluated periodically to ensure that it is within the capabilities of the client.

Diabetics

David Costill, director of the Human Performance Laboratory, Ball State University, has observed that a diabetic who exercises for 30 minutes or more daily may show as much as a 30 to 40 percent decreased need for insulin.[49] Glucose uptake is increased 7 to 20 times during exercise. When exercise stops, blood flow to muscles decreases, but uptake of glucose remains 3 to 4 times that of resting level for an hour.[50] During exercise, insulin levels decrease, while muscle intake of glucose increases. This appears to indicate that during exercise, muscles can take glucose from the blood stream without requiring insulin. This effect is primarily responsible for the reduced insulin requirements and improved glucose tolerance in exercising diabetics. Exercise not only burns calories but lowers blood glucose without insulin. The insulin-dependent diabetic runs a risk of hypoglycemia if he or she does not decrease intake of insulin or increase intake of carbohydrates before strenuous exercise.[51]

Exercise for the diabetic is likely to retard vascular complications and is mandatory for optimum control of the disease. The cardiovascular system of the diabetic can be conditioned to the same extent as that of the nondiabetic. While there are no major limitations on exercise, special precautions that should be kept in mind, including the following:

- Care of feet: good shoes and wrinkle-free socks are a must for the diabetic, to prevent trauma to lower extremities
- Ingestion of a controlled amount of carbohydrates before exercise prevents hypoglycemia
- The physician will most likely have to adjust (decrease) the insulin dosage to accommodate exercise
- Incremental steps in the conditioning program should be more gradual to accommodate any existing cardiovascular impairment
- Becoming overly fatigued should be avoided

Current approaches to the treatment of diabetes recognize the critical role of systematic exercise in therapy, health protection, and health promotion.

Postcoronary Patients

The recovery of many coronary patients has been facilitated through regular systematic exercise. Before beginning an exercise program, the patient should be carefully evaluated by the physician to determine the potential effects of exercise on cardiac status. A step test, bicycle ergometer test, or exercise stress test may be used for this purpose. Through these diagnostic procedures, the physician may be able to detect ischemia not evident during rest (depressed ST segment of EKG), heart rate during activity, and arrhythmias or conduction defects.

Strenuous exercise should be avoided during the first 6 months after myocardial infarction. Under a physician's supervision, walking or bicycling can begin during this time. By the 12th week of walking, the patient may be able to begin a slowly graduated jogging program. Cantu[52] describes postheart attack conditioning programs for individuals under 45 years of age and 45 years of age or older at the time of the attack. The reader is referred to this excellent source for detailed description of such programs. Kuntzleman[53] describes a walking program for cardiacs; this source can provide helpful information for the nurse working with clients following myocardial infarction.

The only contraindications for beginning a postcardiac patient on an exercise regimen are the following:[54]

- Heart muscle damaged to extent of aneurysm or weakness in heart muscle wall
- Acute heart failure
- Myocarditis
- Grossly irregular heartbeats (multifocal ectopic arrhythmias)
- Progressive or sudden onset of severe chest pain with exertion
- Some types of congenital or valvular heart disease
- Recent pulmonary embolism or thrombophlebitis
- Complete heart block

In summary, the importance of systematic exercise to the postcoronary client cannot be overemphasized. The client will reap both physical and psychological benefits that are critical to full recovery. The exercise program for such a client must be carefully monitored by the physician and the nurse and cooperatively planned and modified as needed to meet individual needs.

The Obese

The individual who is markedly overweight presents special needs that must be considered in structuring an exercise program. A stress electrocardiogram or step test is essential before beginning systematic exercise. Increased body weight results in greater stress on the heart, muscles, and joints than in a person of normal weight. Body size may also decrease mobility and flexibility. While description of a complete physical activity program for the obese is beyond the scope of this book, a number of suggestions for modifying exercises for overweight individuals will be provided:

- Correct breathing should be stressed as critical to maximize ventilatory efficiency during exercise
- Warm-up exercises should be selected that can be done in a standing position or in a chair, since obese individuals may have difficulty with floor exercises
- Incremental steps in exercise program should be more gradual than for normal-weight individuals
- Weight loss should be the primary goal of endurance exercise
- Jogging is not recommended for the obese individual
- Swimming is an excellent endurance exercise for the obese person, since water provides buoyancy and weight support

The obese individual can gain major health benefits from a well-planned exercise program. The intent of exercise must be clearly identified by the obese client in order to provide continuing motivation toward physical fitness over an extended period of time. Short-term and long-term goals should be realistic and reinforcement carefully planned to facilitate persistence in exercise and physical activity. The support of a significant other during initiation and stabilization of an exercise program is particularly important to obese individuals, as they are more likely to discontinue exercise than normal-weight people.

The Chronically Ill

Chronically ill clients with limited mobility or decreased tolerance for exercise should be encouraged to develop a physical activity program to meet their special needs. Clients with multiple sclerosis, Parkinson's disease, arthritis, paralysis, and chronic obstructive pulmonary disease all fit into this category. While the pathology may differ, the need for exercise in spite of physical limitations is characteristic of all clients with disabling health problems.

The nurse, in caring for clients with a physical disability, should promote the use of active exercise to the extent possible. Passive range of motion can supplement active exercise as needed. Active exercise of unaffected body parts maintains muscle tone, coordination, and flexibility, while passive range of motion facilitates joint mobility and prevents muscle atrophy. Guidelines for structuring exercise programs for the chronically ill include the following:

- Begin physical activity program gradually, since clients tire easily
- Teach clients relaxation skills to reduce muscle tension or anxiety during exercise
- Avoid excessive force against joint or muscle resistance during exercise
- Provide feedback as needed to facilitate the correct sequence of movements
- Maintain good posture and body alignment during exercise
- Provide positive reinforcement to encourage persistence despite difficulties and slow pace of progress

Maintaining optimum fitness in the chronically ill is an important part of illness prevention and health promotion. While detailed discussion of special exercise techniques is beyond the scope of this book, the reader is referred to additional sources for assistance.[55-59]

Older Adults

The purposes of physical activity for older adults are to enhance the quality of life, aid them in activities of daily living, and assist them in maintaining their independence. Physical activity for the older adult must be geared to the individual's capacity and must contain the necessary components of fitness, exercising all muscles and joints within tolerable limits. Chair exercises, water-supported activities, and fitness nature trails are programs that should be encouraged for older adults, particularly those who have sedentary life styles or those who are over 75 years of age.[60]

Exercise should be an aesthetically pleasing experience for older adults as well as fun, to encourage continuing participation. Low-intensity exercises should be planned initially so clients do not experience excessive fatigue. Walking is a convenient and adaptable form of exercise for older adults. In inclement weather, gyms and shopping malls offer areas for walking that are protected from the elements.

Because of visual changes in older adults, exercise areas should be well

TABLE 11–5. SUMMARY OF SUGGESTED PHYSICAL ACTIVITIES

Warm-Up	Stretching	Endurance	Cool-Down
Walk briskly (1 min)	Back stretch	Walk-jog	Walking and deep breathing
Jog (45 sec)	Leg overs	Jog	Straight arm and leg stretch
Walk briskly (30 sec)	Hamstring stretcher	Walking	
Arm circles	Trunk rotator	Swimming*	Achilles stretcher
Jumping jacks	Cat's arch	Running*	Half knee bend
Lateral bend	Stretching exercises for feet and ankles	Bicycling*	Bent-knee half-curl
Head rotation		Rope skipping*	
Side leg raises			
Single leg raise and knee hug			
Wall push-ups			

*Not discussed in text

lighted. Hearing impairments require that the nurse working with older adults in structured exercise programs look directly at them when giving exercise instructions. The nurse should speak clearly and slowly. Extraneous noises should be minimized to facilitate accurate nurse–client communication. Nonskid surfaces should be provided in exercise areas and locker rooms to prevent slips and falls.

Weakness or stiffness of postural muscles can cause much of the disability observed with aging. Thus, appropriately paced development of systematic exercise programs is critical for the well-being of older adults of all ages.[61]

SUMMARY

The purpose of this chapter has been to provide an overview of the conditioning process for physical fitness. Nurses as key health professionals will need to assume responsibility in many instances for assisting individuals and families in structuring and implementing exercise programs. The skill with which nurses, either singly or in collaboration with exercise physiologists, are able to accomplish this will determine their contribution to clients' optimum health and wellness.

In conclusion, Table 11–5 provides a summary of suggested warm-up, stretching, endurance, and cool-down exercises. This list can be further expanded by the individual nurse to include physical activities described by other authors.

REFERENCES

1. Cantu, R. C. *Toward fitness: Guided exercise for those with health problems.* New York: Human Sciences Press, 1980, p. 12.
2. Fielding, J. E. Successes of prevention. *Milbank Memorial Fund Quarterly/Health and Society.* 1978, *56*, 274–302.
3. Godin, G., & Shephard, R. J. Normative beliefs of school children concerning regular exercise. *Journal of School Health*, December 1984, *54* (11), 443–445.
4. Cantu, op. cit., p. 14.
5. Dishman, R. K., Sallis, J. F., & Orenstein, D. R. The determinants of physical activity and exercise. *Public Health Reports*, March–April 1985, *100* (2), 158–171.
6. Paffenbarger, R. S., Hyde, R. T., Wing, A. L., & Hsieh, C. Physical activity, all-cause mortality, and longevity of college alumni. *New England Journal of Medicine*, 1986, *314*, 605–613.
7. Greist, J. H., Klein, M. H., Eischens, R. R., & Faris, J. W. Running as a treatment for non-psychotic depression. *Behavioral Medicine*, 1978, *6*, 19–24.
8. Greist, J. H., Klein, M. H., Eischens, R. R., et al. Running as a treatment for depression. *Comprehensive Psychiatry*, 1979, *1*, 41–54.
9. Morgan, W. P. Influence of acute physical activity on state anxiety. *NCPEAM Proceedings*, 1973, 113–121.
10. Sidney, K. H., & Shephard, R. J. Attitudes toward health and physical activity in the elderly. Effects of a training program. *Medicine and Science in Sports*, 1976, *8*, 246–252.
11. Blumenthal, J. A., Williams, R. S., Needels, T. L., & Wallace, A. G. Psychological changes accompany aerobic exercise in healthy middle-aged adults. *Psychosomatic Medicine*, December 1982, *44* (6), 529–535.
12. deVries, H. A. Tranquilizer effect of exercise: A critical review. *The Physician and Sports Medicine*, November 1981, *11* (9), 47–55.
13. Haskell, W. L., & Superko, R. Designing an exercise plan for optimal health. *Family and Community Health*, May 1984 (7), 72–88.
14. Haskell, W. M. Overview: Health benefits of exercise. In J. D. Matarazzo, S. M. Weiss, J. A. Herd, et al. (Eds.), *Behavioral health: A handbook of health enhancement and disease prevention.* New York: Wiley, 1984, pp. 409–423.
15. Kirchman, M. M. The preventive role of activity: myth or reality—a review of the literature. *Physical and Occupational Therapy in Geriatrics*, Summer 1983, *2* (4), 39–47.
16. Sime, W. E. Psychological benefits of exercise training in the healthy individual. In J. D. Matarazzo, S. M. Weiss, J. A. Herd, et al. (Eds.), *Behavioral health: A handbook of health enhancement and disease prevention.* New York: Wiley, 1984, pp. 488–508.
17. Getchell, b. *Physical fitness: A way of life* (2nd ed.). New York: Wiley, 1979, pp. 10–13.
18. Ibid., pp. 22–29.
19. Borgman, M. I. Exercise and health maintenance: A teaching program with competence based objectives. *Journal of Nursing Education*, January 1977, *16*, 6–10.

20. Blair, S. N. How to assess exercise habits and physical fitness. In J. D. Matarazzo, S. M. Weiss, J. A. Herd, et al. (Eds.), *Behavioral health: A handbook of health enhancement and disease prevention.* New York: Wiley, 1984, pp. 424–447.
21. Ribisl, P. M. Developing an exercise prescription for health. In J. D. Matarazzo, S. M. Weiss, J. A. Herd, et al. (Eds.), *Behavioral health: A handbook of health enhancement and disease prevention.* New York: Wiley, 1984, pp. 448–466.
22. Cantu, R. C., op. cit., pp. 154–155.
23. Isaacs, B., & Kobler, J. *What it takes to feel good: The Nickolaus technique.* New York: Viking Press, 1978, pp. 47–49.
24. Everly, G. S., Jr., & Girdano, D. A. *The stress mess solution.* Bowie, Md.: Brady, 1980, pp. 121–122.
25. Kirschner, M. J. *Yoga all your life.* New York: Schocken Books, 1977.
26. Cantu, op. cit. p. 29.
27. Cooper, K. H. *The aerobics way.* New York: Evansand, 1977.
28. Getchell, op. cit., p. 121.
29. Bushman, M. *Stretching.* A manual prepared for employees at CF Industries Fitness Center, Long Grove, Ill.
30. Ellfeldt, L., & Lowman, C. L. *Exercises for the mature adult.* Springfield, Ill.: Thomas, 1973.
31. Ibid., p. 108.
32. Simon, R. B. *Relax and stretch.* New York: Walker, 1973, p. 42.
33. Pipes, T. V., & Vodak, P. A. *The Pipes fitness test and prescription.* Los Angeles: Tarcher, 1978.
34. Ibid., p. 85.
35. Kuntzleman, C. T. *The complete book of walking.* New York: Simon & Schuster. 1979, p. 138.
36. Borgman, op. cit., p. 8.
37. Getchell, B., & Cleary, P. The caloric costs of rope skipping and running. *The Physician and Sports Medicine,* February 1980, *8,* 56–60.
38. Glasser, W. *Positive addiction.* New York: Harper & Row, 1976.
39. Geline, R. J. *The practical runner.* New York: Collier Books, 1978.
40. Bridge, R. *The runner's book.* New York: Scribner's, 1978.
41. Sheehan, G. *Dr. George Sheehan's medical advice for runners.* Mountain View, Calif.: World Publications, 1978.
42. Kuntzleman, op. cit., p. 53.
43. DeVries, H. A. Electromyographic comparison of single doses of exercise and meprobamate as to the effects on muscular relaxation. *American Journal of Physical Medicine,* 1972, *51,* 130–141.
44. Fair, J., Rosenaur, J., & Thurston, E. Exercise management. *Nurse Practitioner,* 1979, *4,* 13–18.
45. Kuntzleman, op. cit., p. 161.
46. Anderson, J. L., & Cohen, M. *The West Point fitness and diet book.* New York: Rawson Associates, 1977, p. 171.
47. Ibid., pp. 156, 162.
48. Eischens, R. R. Five easy steps for exercise regimen compliance: A new precise guide to running. *Behavioral Medicine,* June 1979, *2,* 14–17.
49. Getchell, op. cit., p. 263.
50. Cantu, op. cit., p. 78.
51. Ibid., p. 80.
52. Cantu, op. cit., pp. 134–151.

53. Kuntzleman, op. cit., pp. 189–201.
54. Cantu, op. cit., p. 138.
55. Ibid.
56. Nashelsky, G. M. *Redaptor guides for rehabilitation.* Hagerstown, Md.: Harper & Row, 1978.
57. Covalt, N. K. *Bed exercises for convalescent patients.* Springfield, Ill.: Thomas, 1968.
58. Stryker, R. *Rehabilitative aspects of acute and chronic nursing care* (2nd ed.). Philadelphia: Saunders, 1977.
59. Basmajian, J. V. *Therapeutic exercise* (3rd ed.). Baltimore: Williams & Wilkins, 1978.
60. Smith, E. L. Special considerations in developing exercise programs for older adults. In J. D. Matarazzo, S. M. Weiss, J. A. Herd, et al. (Eds.), *Behavioral health: A handbook of health enhancement and disease prevention,* New York: Wiley, 1984, pp. 525–546.
61. Council on Scientific Affairs. Exercise programs for the elderly—Council report. *Journal of the American Medical Association,* July 27, 1984, *252* (4), 544–546.

CHAPTER 12

Nutrition and Weight Control

Adequate nutrition is a critical element in the nurturance of health. Not only is diet believed to play a major role in the prevention of disease, but it also contributes to alertness and energy essential for full and productive living. Unfortunately, dietary inadequacies (malnutrition) in the guise of overnutrition or undernutrition plague 30 to 50 percent of Americans and are found at all socioeconomic levels. Affluent and poor alike often exhibit nutritional habits that are a direct threat to health and well-being.

The complexity of American life complicates the development and maintenance of health-promoting nutritional practices. It has been estimated that 30 percent of meals are eaten outside the home, and convenience foods constitute 60 percent of the American diet. Such foods are frequently high in fat, salt, and refined carbohydrates and low in fiber. By the fifth decade of life, one-third of the men and one-half of the women in the United States are more than 20 percent overweight.[1] This is not surprising, considering that the mean sugar consumption within the population is 125 pounds per person per year and that fats constitute 42 percent of dietary intake. The overconsumption of saturated fats, cholesterol, sugar, and salt has been linked to a number of chronic diseases that are the major causes of death and disability in the United States. Chronic diseases that fall into this category include cardiovascular disorders, hypertension, diabetes mellitus, cancer of the breast, and cancer of the gastrointestinal tract. Links with diet have been suggested for many other health problems.

Undernutrition is also a problem in many segments of the population despite excess caloric consumption among Americans. A dietary survey of low-income rural families in Iowa and North Carolina indicated that calcium intake is often inadequate, followed in frequency by deficiencies in vitamin A, vitamin C (ascorbic acid), and iron.[2] These deficiencies, as well as inadequate nutritional habits that usually accompany them, are the precursors of many health problems in individuals of all ages.

Families often experience limited options in food choices as a result of cost or a confusing array of products for which nutrient content is unclear. The challenge of integrating healthful nutritional practices into individual and family life styles can seem overwhelming.

Since nurses are the health professionals most often in extended contact with clients, they serve as a valuable resource to individuals, families, and communities in providing information and assistance in regard to nutrition and weight control. Dietary counseling should be an integral part of nursing practice in all settings. The professional nurse must be able to deal not only with therapeutic aspects of nutrition but also with nutrition as a critical element in prevention and health promotion. Nutritionists and psychologists are valuable colleagues of the nurse in planning sound nutrition education programs.

THE ROLE OF NUTRITION IN PREVENTION

The role of nutrition in prevention has been most vividly illustrated in relation to cardiovascular disease. The Framingham, Massachusetts, Heart Study, conducted by the National Heart, Lung, and Blood Institute of more than 5000 men and women between 30 and 62 years of age, showed, particularly in males, a substantial increase in the incidence of coronary heart disease with serum cholesterol levels greater than 220 mg. Further studies indicated that 80 percent of heart disease victims were characterized by hyperlipoproteinemia, hypertension, and cigarette smoking.[3]

Hyperlipoproteinemia may be to some extent genetic or secondary to other diseases, such as diabetes, hypothyroidism, nephrosis, and obstructive liver disease, but is more frequently caused by environmental factors over which the individual has control, e.g., factors such as diet, alcohol intake, and sedentary life style.[4] Both cholesterol and triglycerides (serum lipids) have been indicted in the health literature as contributing to the process of atherosclerosis, which leads to cardiovascular disease. Each results in a different type of lipoproteinemia.[5] While the body itself synthesizes cholesterol and triglycerides, dietary fat serves as an exogenous source of both. A 600-mg increase in cholesterol per 3000 calories can account for an 800-mg increase in serum cholesterol. For that reason, a decrease in total fat in the diet, particularly saturated fats and cholesterol, is recommended to prevent cardiovascular deterioration.

Modification of dietary habits recommended to decrease serum lipid levels and the associated threat of cardiovascular disease include the following:[6]

1. Decrease total fat intake to 30 percent of diet
2. Decrease proportion of saturated fats to 10 percent of diet; increase proportion of monounsaturated fats to 10 percent and proportion of polyunsaturated fats to 10 percent of diet. Dietary cholesterol should not exceed 300 mg per day
3. Reduce weight if obese
4. Adjust carbohydrate intake to meet energy needs by increasing complex carbohydrates to 48 percent of diet and decreasing refined and processed sugars to 10 percent of diet
5. Decrease intake of alcohol
6. Maintain but do not exceed adequate protein level at 12 percent of diet

A recent development in understanding the relationship between diet and cardiovascular disease has been the identification of five distinct types of lipoproteins; chylomicrons, very low-density lipoproteins, intermediate-density lipoproteins, low-density lipoproteins, and high-density lipoproteins. It appears that high-density lipoproteins predominate when triglyceride level is normal and actively retard the atherosclerotic process by transporting cholesterol out of tissue to the liver for breakdown. When triglycerides are elevated, low-density lipoproteins predominate, increasing the risk of cardiovascular disease by their transporting of cholesterol to tissues.[7] Total body weight and level of physical activity may also be related to the level of high-density proteins. Combining a diet low in saturated fats with participation in regular exercise appears to be a prudent approach to decreasing both serum cholesterol and triglyceride levels.[8]

While much controversy still surrounds the importance of dietary practices in the prevention of cardiovascular disorders, the preponderance of evidence supports both a direct and indirect relationship between diet and cardiovascular health. The professional nurse exercises good judgment in assisting clients to modify eating behaviors in order to decrease total fat intake, particularly the proportion of unsaturated fats in the diet.

The role, if any, of caffeine, a xanthine drug, in the etiology of cardiovascular disease has not been determined. While caffeine stimulates the sympathetic nervous system, increases cardiac and skeletal muscle contractility, increases excretory functions of the kidneys, increases respiration rate and depth, and stimulates the adrenal glands,[9] a definite link between coffee intake and cardiac disorders has not been identified. Preliminary studies briefly reviewed by Jean Mayer at a conference in Milwaukee on occupational health provide evidence that the combination of frequent smoking and high caffeine intake may synergistically increase the risk of cardiovascular disease.

Still another major chronic health problem in which diet is assumed to play a role is cancer. It has been estimated that diet is related to 35 percent of all cancer deaths, a percent as great as that of smoking. One report estimates that diet is responsible for 30 to 40 percent of cancers in men and 60 percent of cancers in women.[10] Aspects of the diet that are suspect include intake of fats, vitamin deficiencies, surplus or deficiency of trace elements, degree of food processing, methods of food storage, techniques for food preparation, and food additives.[11] There is growing evidence that a high-fat diet contributes to the development of cancer of the colon, rectum, breast, and prostate gland.[12] While the mechanisms for explaining this apparent relationship have not been identified, it is possible that a high level of dietary fat and subsequent serum lipid elevation increases the activity of various carcinogens. It is interesting to note that a correlation of 0.64 between sugar consumption and incidence of breast cancer has been reported.[13] A relationship between a high intake of synthetic sweeteners (saccharin, cyclamate) and bladder cancer has also been reported from laboratory studies. Since many of these results have been obtained from animal studies or epidemiological surveys of specific populations, the extent to which these findings can be generalized to the broader population has not been determined. Other studies have implicated the level of fiber, which is low in the American diet, as a possible precursor or risk factor for cancer of the colon and rectum. Research results on the impact of dietary fiber on health are less definitive than those on dietary fat, but increasing fiber intake by eating fruits, vegetables, and unrefined whole-grain products is recommended.

The protective or preventive effects of vitamins and minerals have been addressed in cancer studies on animals. Some evidence exists that selenium (an antioxidant found in brewer's yeast, garlic, and liver), vitamin C, and vitamin E may provide protection against breast cancer. At present, these results are equivocal, with much debate surrounding their validity.[14]

In light of current evidence on the link between diet and cancer, it appears that the prudent individual ought to decrease the amount of fat in the diet to 30 percent. That is the recommendation of the Senate Select Committee on Nutrition and Human Needs in the Dietary Goals for the United States. In addition, the intake of refined and processed sugars should be decreased, and the intake of complex carbohydrates and fiber increased.

At this point, the threat to health posed by chronic obesity will be mentioned; the subject will be discussed more fully under the section of this chapter on Weight Control. Studies have shown that the death rate among obese adults is 50 percent greater than that of normal-weight adults. Middle-aged males who are 30 percent overweight have four times as many myocardial infarctions as men of normal weight, and are seven times more likely to suffer a cerebrovascular accident.[15] Obesity is a health problem of epidemic proportions that the professional nurse will repeatedly encounter as she provides illness–prevention and health-promotion services to clients. Permanent modification of dietary behaviors and increased physical activity must be the long-term goals for overweight clients if excess weight is to be lost and the risk of obesity to health reduced.

The role of diet in prevention is well recognized in *Objectives for the Nation*. Seventeen nutrition-related goals are identified for accomplishment by 1990. The goals are organized into the following categories: improved health status, reduced risk factors, increased public–professional awareness, improved services-protection, and improved surveillance–evaluation system. While a complete discussion of national nutrition goals and related federal initiatives is beyond the scope of this chapter, the reader is referred to *Public Health Reports Supplement*, September–October 1983, for a comprehensive overview of nutrition goals and related government programs.[16]

FACTORS INFLUENCING EATING BEHAVIOR

A wide variety of factors influence overt eating behavior. These factors can be classified as biological, psychological, sociocultural, and environmental. The multicausal nature of eating behavior makes it highly complex and resistant to change. Eating behaviors are an integral part of individual and family life style. Effective modification requires consideration of the factors that determine eating behavior and the use of appropriate change techniques. In order to select effective intervention strategies, the nurse must understand the determinants of eating behavior and their impact on nutritional status.

Biological Factors

Eating behaviors are determined biologically by nutrient requirements. Nutrients are the chemicals that are essential for proper body functioning. To date, approximately 50 macronutrients (e.g., fats, carbohydrates, and proteins) and micronutrients (e.g., vitamins and minerals) have been identified as essential for human growth and maintenance.[17] Nutrients have one or more of the following functions: (1) providing energy necessary for metabolic processes and movement, (2) providing structural components for bones and tissues, and (3) catalizing or regulating physiological processes. Nutrient needs of individuals vary according to metabolic rate, stage of growth, age, level of physical activity, excretory functions (menstruation, heavy perspiration), and reproductive functions (in women, i.e., pregnancy and lactation).

Metabolic rate is expressed as basal metabolism, that is, the number of kilocalories needed to maintain the body at rest. Basal metabolism rate declines sharply between 5 and 25 years of age and gradually thereafter. A rough guide for determining daily basal energy requirements for adults is to multiply ideal body weight by 10. For example, a woman weighing 120 pounds (recommended weight) would require 1200 calories to maintain body functions at complete rest. Obviously, activity increases the need for calories. Depending on the level of activity, caloric intake should be appropriately modified to maintain current weight or achieve desired weight.

During periods of rapid growth in childhood and adolescence, caloric and nutrient needs are increased. Throughout adulthood, nutrient needs re-

TABLE 12–1. AVERAGE RECOMMENDED CALORIC INTAKE FOR MEN AND WOMEN OF DIFFERENT AGES: MODERATE ACTIVITY (in kilocalories)

Age	Men		Women	
	MEAN	RANGE	MEAN	RANGE
19–22	2900	2500–3000	2100	1700–2500
23–50	2700	2300–3100	2000	1600–2400
51–75	2400	2000–2800	1800	1400–2200
over 75	2050	1650–2450	1600	1200–2000

main relatively stable, but caloric needs gradually decline. The decrease in caloric needs generally reflects the lower basal metabolic rates of the elderly and decreases in activity because of physical limitations. Decreased energy requirements with aging may also reflect an increase in fat and a decrease in lean-tissue mass. Recommended caloric levels for individuals of different ages with moderate physical activity are presented in Table 12–1.

Energy requirements rather than nutrient needs appear to be the most salient biological determinants of eating behavior. In general, individuals exhibit awareness and sensitivity to low energy levels. Fatigue, listlessness, and apathy can indicate a caloric intake that is inadequate to meet energy needs.

While overall nutrient requirements remain relatively stable throughout adulthood, selected nutrients may have to be increased because of physiological changes, e.g., diminished gastric secretions and decreased gastric motility that occur with aging. For example, decreased gastric secretions can result in limited absorption of iron, calcium, and vitamin B_{12}. Decreased gastric motility augments the need for foods high in fiber (fresh fruits, raw vegetables, whole-grain breads, and cereals) and increases the importance of water consumption to promote regularity in bowel evacuation.

It should be noted that the hypothalamus is an important biological determinant of eating behavior. The lateral nucleus of the hypothalamus is stimulated by hunger, initiating food-seeking behavior, while the ventromedial hypothalamus signals satiety and results in the urge to cease food consumption.[18] One theory of obesity is based on the malfunctioning of the hypothalamus in the biological regulation of food intake.

Psychological Factors

Major psychological factors that affect eating behavior include emotions, habits, self-esteem, perceptions of control, and perceived benefits of good dietary practices. People frequently engage in eating behavior because of the emotions of enjoyment, peace, and tranquility aroused. On the other hand, negative emotions, such as anger, frustration, and insecurity, can lead to disturbances in eating behavior (overeating or anorexia nervosa) that are indicative of a personal search for comfort, security, and nurturance through food intake.

Habits constitute another important determinant of eating behavior. A habit can be defined as a behavior that occurs often and is performed automatically or with little conscious awareness.[19] Habits are performed so frequently that many cues within the environment serve as signals for the behavior. They often result in a psychological addiction to certain behaviors because they become a pervasive part of life style. Such behaviors are known as consummatory because the response itself (eating) provides the reinforcement. People can also become psychologically addicted to the consequences of habitual behaviors such as the "energy spurt" experienced after the ingestion of highly refined sugars at midmorning (doughnuts or sweet rolls), late afternoon, or evening (snack foods). Habits can result in poor dietary practices because little or no conscious thought is given to eating behavior. Habits also depend on the availability of foodstuffs that can be readily consumed without preparation. Fast foods that are high in fats and refined carbohydrates and low in protein, minerals, and vitamins often meet this requirement.

Level of self-esteem and nutrition knowledge have also been shown to be significantly correlated with eating behavior. Schafer[20] selected 116 married women under 36 years of age to test in relation to self-concept and diet quality. Self-concept was measured by 10 adjective pairs selected from Gough and Heilbrim's adjective checklist, while diet quality was determined by the frequency of consumption and serving sizes for 67 different food items. Food items were converted to percentage of recommended daily allowances for six nutrients: protein, calcium, iron, vitamin A, thiamin, and ascorbic acid. Self-concept correlated 0.20 ($p < 0.01$) with diet quality, which is a low correlation but a statistically significant one. Consumption of "junk food" or empty calories was negatively correlated with self-concept (-0.16, $p < 0.05$). Previous involvement in nutritional courses correlated at 0.41 with self-concept.

Perceived control of nutritional status and belief in the benefits of good nutrition have also been shown to increase the quality of dietary behavior. In the Stanford three community study,[21] a mass-media campaign informed citizens of two communities about the impact of a diet low in cholesterol and saturated fats on risk for cardiovascular disease. Results revealed that awareness of actions to be taken and the benefits of a low-fat diet within the target communities decreased the cholesterol and fat consumption among both men and women 20 to 40 percent.

Sociocultural Factors

Ethnic and cultural backgrounds serve as important influences on eating behavior. Ethnic foods are a source of pride and identity for many groups. Ethnic foods often have deep emotional meanings for individuals because of their association with the "mother country" or because of fond childhood memories of holidays or special occasions on which particular foods were served. Recognition of and respect for individual food preferences is important for professional nurses in dealing with adults from a wide variety of cultural backgrounds. The nurse should become acquainted with food behaviors of different sociocultural groups in order to evaluate their beneficial, neutral, or harmful effects on health.[22]

Boykin[23] has made a number of helpful suggestions in dealing constructively with the food preferences of various ethnic and cultural groups:

- Food habits and preferences should be recognized
- Consumption frequency for various ethnic foods should be ascertained
- Positive attributes of ethnic foods should be recognized and reinforced
- Nutrition information relevant to ethnic–cultural foods should be provided to clients
- The client should be an active member of the dietary-planning team
- Changes recommended in food preparation and consumption should be tailored as much as possible to ethnic–cultural patterns. Ethnic foods can serve as important sources of nutrients and as the basis for a well-balanced and nutritious diet. Every effort should be made by the nurse to incorporate ethnic–cultural food preferences in diet planning. Only when foods are clearly hazardous to health should clients be encouraged to make major changes in ethnic dietary habits.

Environmental Factors

The major environmental factors influencing eating patterns appear to be accessibility, convenience, and cost. These factors can present barriers to positive nutritional practices during the action phase of health behavior. Seasonal variation in availability of foods such as raw vegetables and fresh fruits determines both accessibility and costs. The types of fruits and vegetables used by clients need to follow seasonal patterns in order to maximize nutrient quality and minimize cost. Use of frozen fruits and vegetables rather than canned during off-season is recommended to decrease the intake of sugar and salt. Home-frozen products can also be an important source of nutrients at reasonable cost.

Convenience foods constitute a significant portion of dietary intake in the American population. Unfortunately, the nutrient quality of many fast foods is questionable. Vending machines often have only foods high in fats and starch. If access to more nutritious foods is inconvenient, individuals often select the easiest option. Ease of preparation plays an important role in food selection. Quick and effortless preparation techniques appeal to many families because of busy work schedules. In addition, attractiveness of prepared foods is an important consideration. Assisting the client in selecting nutritious foods that are quickly prepared and esthetically appealing increases the likelihood of sustained changes in eating behavior.

With inflationary trends in the economy, cost of food is an important consideration for the majority of families. Sources of complex carbohydrates (fruits, vegetables, and grains) may exceed the cost of highly refined sugar products. Proteins also vary greatly in per-unit cost. An important approach to optimizing nutritional quality of the diet at minimum cost is to calculate the per-unit cost of given nutrients in food products. An example of a method for such calculations that is relatively easy for the client to use is presented in the next section of this chapter.

HEALTH PROMOTION THROUGH POSITIVE NUTRITION PRACTICES

Many individuals engage in eating because of the pleasurable sensations experienced and the esthetic enjoyment of well-prepared and attractive foods. Interest in foods rather than concern about nutrients and health may largely determine patterns of food consumption. Visual appearance of foods as well as internal sensations of hunger provide powerful cues that initiate eating behavior. The mass media influence the types and variety of foods consumed through the presentation of information on various food products. Within recent years, changes have occurred in the eating habits of Americans. Favorable changes include increased use of fish, poultry, and frozen vegetables, and decreased use of butter. Unfavorable changes include decreased use of fresh fruits and increased use of synthetic sweeteners.[24]

Meal planning is an important activity that facilitates preparation of well-balanced meals. In assisting clients with planning, the nurse must take into consideration food preferences, preparation time, purchasing practices, cost, and daily meal patterns (three or more meals per day). Variation in color, texture, and temperature are also important considerations to make meals attractive and appealing. Since meal planning and food preparation take place in the home, this provides an excellent environment for nutrition education. The nurse in using the home as a learning center capitalizes on environmental cues relevant to positive nutritional practices.[25]

Guide to Good Eating

A simple guide to healthful eating for children, teenagers, and adults has been provided in Table 12-2. The milk group is a rich source of calcium, phosphorus, protein, riboflavin, vitamin A, vitamin B_{12}, and vitamin D (if fortified). The meat group provides protein, B-complex vitamins, and minerals. Vegetable equivalents for meat, such as beans, dried peas, lentils, and nuts, do not contain significant amounts of vitamin B_{12}. The fruit and vegetable group provides vitamins A, C, E, K, and B-complex (except B_{12}), as well as minerals and fiber. Grains contain protein, B-complex vitamins, minerals, and fiber.[26] Appendix A, developed from a variety of information sources, presents an overview of the biological importance, sources, deficiency symp-

TABLE 12–2. GUIDE TO GOOD EATING: A RECOMMENDED DAILY PATTERN*

Food Group	Recommended Number of Servings†				
	CHILD	TEENAGER	ADULT	PREGNANT WOMAN	LACTATING WOMAN
Milk	3	4	2	4	4

1 cup milk or yogurt OR calcium equivalent:

   $1\frac{1}{2}$ slices ($1\frac{1}{2}$ oz) cheddar cheese‡
   1 cup pudding
   $1\frac{3}{4}$ cups ice cream
   2 cups cottage cheese‡

Meat	2	2	2	3	2

2 oz cooked, lean meat, fish, or poultry OR protein equivalent:

   2 eggs
   2 slices (2 oz) cheddar cheese‡
   1 cup dried beans, peas
   4 tbs peanut butter

Fruit–Vegetable	4	4	4	4	4

   $\frac{1}{2}$ cup cooked or juice
   1 cup raw
Portion commonly served, such as a medium-size apple or banana

Grain	4	4	4	4	4

Whole grain, fortified, enriched:

   1 slice bread
   1 cup ready-to-eat cereal
   $\frac{1}{2}$ cup cooked cereal, pasta, or grits

*The recommended daily pattern provides the foundation for a nutritious, healthful diet. Amounts should be further modified by individual caloric needs.
†The recommended servings from the four food groups for adults supply about 1200 calories. The chart gives recommendations for the number and size of servings for several categories of people.
‡Count cheese as serving of milk or meat, not as belonging to both simultaneously.
Courtesy of National Dairy Council, Rosemont, Illinois. Copyright © 1977. All rights reserved.

toms, and toxicity levels of a wide variety of nutrients. Table 12–3 presents the National Research Council Recommended Daily Dietary Allowances as revised in 1979 for selected nutrients. The use of a variety of foods from each group and an adequate intake of water (the most basic human nutrient) assist in maintaining a desired level of nutrient quality within the diet.[27]

Nutrient and Caloric Density. Important considerations in food selection are nutrient density and caloric density. Nutrient density refers to the content of specific nutrients in given amounts of food in relation to the kilocalories provided by that same amount.

$$\text{Nutrient density} = \frac{\text{Percent of RDA of nutrient provided by food}}{\text{Percent of mean energy requirements provided by food}}$$

Caloric density can be defined as the number of kilocalories provided per unit of food.[28] Fats, oils, and alcohol have the highest caloric density of all food substances, yet they are low in essential nutrients. The caloric density of fats is 9 kcal per gram and of alcohol 7 kcal per gram. The caloric density of protein is 4 kcal per gram. Vegetables, fruits, milk products, and meat vary greatly in caloric density, while grain products are relatively similar for equivalent weights. Nutritive sweeteners, such as sugar, honey, corn syrup, fructose, and sorbitol, have comparable but high caloric densities, approximately 20 kcal per teaspoon. For this reason, fruit as a natural sweetener should be used as frequently as possible to decrease caloric intake and intake of highly refined sugar.

The nutrient and caloric densities of foods can be calculated from food-value tables, but the bioavailability of nutrients depends on the metabolic characteristics of the client, existing illnesses that may affect metabolic processes, the form of the nutrient present in food, and the presence or absence of other interacting nutrients. For example, "heme" iron available in meats is more bioavailable than is iron from vegetables. As another example, the presence of vitamin C increases the absorption of iron and the presence of vitamin D increases the absorption of calcium. The concept of bioavailability may be difficult for the client to grasp, but the nurse should be aware of these parameters in order to teach effective meal planning.

The seven nutrients, often referred to as index nutrients, that serve as the best overall indicators of diet and nutrient adequacy are calcium, iron, magnesium, vitamin A, vitamin B_6, pantothenic acid, and folacin. A rough estimate of the extent to which these nutrients are included in the diet can be obtained for any individual by nutritional analysis using manual or computerized tables of food composition.

Loss of Nutrients in Food Preparation. Nutrients available to the client in foodstuffs can be lost through inadequate methods of preparation. Nutrients may be lost in the following ways:[29]

- Trimming (e.g., peeling potatoes, fruits, and vegetables)
- Solution loss (e.g., particularly water-soluble vitamin C, B complex, and minerals by cooking foods in water)
- Heat and exposure to air (e.g., in the case of carotene, vitamin C, thiamin, and folacin)

Loss of nutrients can be avoided by decreasing the amount of water in

TABLE 12–3. RECOMMENDED DAILY DIETARY ALLOWANCES,* DESIGNED FOR THE MAINTENANCE OF GOOD NUTRITION OF PRACTICALLY ALL HEALTHY PEOPLE IN THE UNITED STATES, REVISED 1979

	Age (years)	Weight (kg)	Weight (lb)	Height (cm)	Height (in.)	Protein (gm)	Vitamin C (mg)	Thiamin (mg)	Riboflavin (mg)	Niacin (mg N.E.)†	Vitamin B_6 (mg)	Folacin‡ (µg)	Vitamin B_{12} (µg)
Infants	0.0–0.5	6	13	60	24	kg × 2.2	35	0.3	0.4	6	0.3	30	0.5§
	0.5–1.0	9	20	71	28	kg × 2.0	35	0.5	0.6	8	0.6	45	1.5
Children	1–3	13	29	90	35	23	45	0.7	0.8	9	0.9	100	2.0
	4–6	20	44	112	44	30	45	0.9	1.0	11	1.3	200	2.5
	7–10	28	62	132	52	34	45	1.2	1.4	16	1.6	300	3.0
Males	11–14	45	99	157	62	45	50	1.4	1.6	18	1.8	400	3.0
	15–18	66	145	176	69	56	60	1.4	1.7	18	2.0	400	3.0
	19–22	70	154	177	70	56	60	1.5	1.7	19	2.2	400	3.0
	23–50	70	154	178	70	56	60	1.4	1.6	18	2.2	400	3.0
	51+	70	154	178	70	56	60	1.2	1.4	16	2.2	400	3.0
Females	11–14	46	101	157	62	46	50	1.1	1.3	15	1.8	400	3.0
	15–18	55	120	163	64	46	60	1.1	1.3	14	2.0	400	3.0
	19–22	55	120	163	64	44	60	1.1	1.3	14	2.0	400	3.0
	23–50	55	120	163	64	44	60	1.0	1.2	13	2.0	400	3.0
	51+	55	120	163	64	44	60	1.0	1.2	13	2.0	400	3.0
Pregnant						+30	+20	+0.4	+0.3	+2	+0.6	+400	+1.0
Lactating						+20	+40	+0.5	+0.5	+5	+0.5	+100	+1.0

	Age (years)	Weight (kg)	Weight (lb)	Height (cm)	Height (in.)	Protein (gm)	Fat-Soluble Vitamins			Minerals					
							Vitamin A (µg R.E.)‖	Vitamin D (µg)#	Vitamin E (mgα T.E.)**	Calcium (mg)	Phosphorus (mg)	Magnesium (mg)	Iron (mg)	Zinc (mg)	Iodine (µg)
Infants	0.0–0.5	6	13	60	24	kg × 2.2	420	10	3	360	240	50	10	3	40
	0.5–1.0	9	20	71	28	kg × 2.0	400	10	4	540	360	70	15	5	50
Children	1–3	13	29	90	35	23	400	10	5	800	800	150	15	10	70
	4–6	20	44	112	44	30	500	10	6	800	800	200	10	10	90
	7–10	28	62	132	52	34	700	10	7	800	800	250	10	10	120
Males	11–14	45	99	157	62	45	1000	10	8	1200	1200	350	18	15	150
	15–18	66	145	176	69	56	1000	10	10	1200	1200	400	18	15	150
	19–22	70	154	177	70	56	1000	7.5	10	800	800	350	10	15	150
	23–50	70	154	178	70	56	1000	5	10	800	800	350	10	15	150
	51+	70	154	178	70	56	1000	5	10	800	800	350	10	15	150
Females	11–14	46	101	157	62	46	800	10	8	1200	1200	300	18	15	150
	15–18	55	120	163	64	46	800	10	8	1200	1200	300	18	15	150
	19–22	55	120	163	64	44	800	7.5	8	800	800	300	18	15	150
	23–50	55	120	163	64	44	800	5	8	800	800	300	18	15	150
	51+	55	120	163	64	44	800	5	8	800	800	300	10	15	150
Pregnant						+30	+200	+5	+2	+400	+400	+150	††	+5	+25
Lactating						+20	+400	+5	+3	+400	+400	+150	††	+10	+50

*The allowances are intended to provide for individual variations among most normal persons as they live in the United States under usual environmental stresses. Diets should be based on a variety of common foods in order to provide other nutrients for which human requirements have been less well defined.

†1 NE (niacin equivalent) is equal to 1 mg of niacin or 60 mg of dietary tryptophan.

‡The folacin allowances refer to dietary sources as determined by *Lactobacillus casei* assay after treatment with enzymes ("conjugases") to take polyglutamyl forms of the vitamin available to the test organism.

§The RDA for vitamin B₁₂ in infants is based on average concentration of the vitamin in human milk. The allowances after weaning are based on energy intake (as recommended by the American Academy of Pediatrics) and consideration of other factors, such as intestinal absorption.

‖Retinol equivalents. 1 retinol equivalent = 1 µg retinol or 6 µgβ carotene.

#As cholecalciferol. 10 µg cholecalciferol = 400 I.U. vitamin D.

**α tocopherol equivalents. 1 mg d α – tocopherol = 1 α T.E.

††The increased requirement during pregnancy cannot be met by the iron content of habitual American diets nor by the existing iron stores of many women; therefore the use of 30 to 60 mg of supplemental iron is recommended. Iron needs during lactation are not substantially different from those of nonpregnant women, but continued supplementation of the mother for 2 to 3 months after parturition is advisable in order to replenish stores depleted by pregnancy.

From Food and Nutrition Board, National Academy of Sciences, National Research Council. *Recommended dietary allowances, revised 1979.* Washington, D.C.: Government Printing Office.

which foods are cooked, decreasing the length of time foods are in water (i.e., by using a pressure cooker), avoiding the peeling or soaking of foods before cooking, refraining from adding salt to cooking water (draws out water-soluble nutrients), and decreasing food-cooking surface exposed to water by cutting food into large pieces.

Maintaining Optimum Energy Balance. For every 3500 excess kilocalories consumed that are not utilized for energy, 1 pound of fat is formed. This means that 100 unburned calories each day for 35 days will result in 1 pound of fat and in a 10-pound weight gain per year (350 days).[30] The same level of deficit in calories (100 per day for 35 days) can result in a 1-pound loss that, if continued over a year, would result in the loss of 10 pounds. The factors that determine energy balance include basal metabolism, level of physical activity, and food intake. Energy balance is maintained by burning all calories ingested. If excess calories are being consumed and undesirable weight gain is occurring, this can only be remedied by decreasing food intake or increasing exercise.

Some individuals express concern that if they exercise more, their appetite will increase. This has been found not to be true. Appetite is actually decreased following exercise because of lowered blood supply to the gastrointestinal tract. Few avid physical fitness enthusiasts wish to eat before exercising, since this makes physical activity more difficult and less comfortable. In addition, exercise may decrease stress and tension; as a result, there will be less frequent eating for nonnutritive purposes.[31]

IMPORTANT NUTRIENTS

Protein

The body's requirement for protein can be easily met if foods are properly combined to provide usable protein. Some foods, such as milk, milk products, eggs, and meat of all types, contain protein of high biological value. Such proteins, sometimes called *complete proteins*, support growth. Other proteins, if used as the sole source of protein, can support life but not growth. They are referred to as *partially complete* or *incomplete* proteins.

Proteins are composed of amino acids. There are 22 amino acids, 8 to 9 of which are essential; that is, they must be ingested since they cannot be biologically synthesized. The essential amino acids are tryptophan, leucine, lycine, methionine, phenylalanine, isoleucine, valine, theonine, and histidine (for children). The bioavailability of protein depends on proper balance of essential amino acids. Amino acids can only be properly used when all of them are available at the same time.[32]

Meat, fish, poultry, and dairy products (complete proteins) contain good proportions of all essential amino acids, while vegetables and fruits (incomplete proteins) may be low or missing some amino acids, thus limiting protein use. The amino acid present in the smallest amount (LAA) limits the bio-availability of others. For example, if a food contains 100 percent of the daily lycine requirement but only 20 percent of the methionine requirement, only 20 percent of the protein in that food is used as protein; the rest is used for fuel rather than for replenishing or building tissues. The following illustration of bioavailability vividly illustrates this point:[33]

	Percent of Daily Protein Requirement (160-lb man)
2 poached eggs	54% LAA
2 pieces dry whole wheat toast	10% LAA
Orange juice	0% LAA
Total % of daily requirement	64%

Following the breakfast described, only 36 percent of the daily requirement of protein remains to be ingested. Thus, protein needs are easily met when incomplete proteins (whole-grain breads) are complemented by complete proteins (eggs) in the diet.

If incomplete proteins are the primary source of amino acids, as in a vegetarian diet, complementarity of proteins is particularly important. *Complementing proteins* is the term used for combining incomplete proteins with opposite amino acid strengths and weaknesses. For example, peanut butter or chili beans (high in lysine but low in methionine) can be served with whole wheat bread or corn bread (low in lysine but high in methionine). Balancing the amino acid strengths and weaknesses of foods can result in good biological availability of proteins.

The cost of protein foods can also pose a problem for clients. The cost of adequate nutrition can be decreased by serving small portions of fish, poultry, or lower-grade, less tender cuts of meat that are cooked slowly to tenderize and enhance flavor. Milk, eggs, and vegetable sources of protein may be used as substitutes for meat products, but consumption of some red meat is desirable to obtain vitamin B_{12}.

As a cost-comparison example, 4 ounces of lean ground beef supplies approximately 20 grams of protein, while 3.5 hot dogs must be eaten for the same amount of protein. Williams and Justice[34] have developed a guide for calculating protein costs (Figure 12–1). Foods that are good sources of protein are listed along with the amount that contains 14 grams, or one-fourth to one-third of RDA. The number of grams of protein in a 1-pound edible portion of food has been taken from tables of food composition and divided by 14, giving a factor that, when multiplied by price per pound of the target food, gives the cost of 14 grams of protein. Remember that 14 grams constitute approximately 17 to 25 percent of the RDA for children between 1 and 10 years of age; 32 percent of the RDA for women; and 25 percent of the RDA for men. By use of the multiplication factors with current retail price of foods, protein costs can be calculated.

346

Item	Serving Size to Provide 14 gm Protein	Multiplication Factor	Current Retail Price per Pound	Cost of 14/gm Protein
Dry beans	1 cup cooked	0.128	× _____	= _____
Peanut butter	3½ tbs	0.123	× _____	= _____
Eggs	2 eggs	0.269	× _____	= _____
Bologna	4–5 slices (if 18 slices/lb)	0.255	× _____	= _____
Beef liver	(6–7 servings/lb)	0.155	× _____	= _____
Milk	1¾ cup	0.881	× _____	= _____
Dry milk	9 tbs dry	0.086	× _____	= _____
Cottage cheese	(4–5 servings/lb)	0.227	× _____	= _____
Hamburger	(5–6 servings/lb)	0.172	× _____	= _____
Ocean perch, fillet, frozen	(6 servings/lb)	0.160	× _____	= _____
Tuna fish	(3 servings to a 6-oz can)	0.128	× _____	= _____
American processed cheese	2½ slices (if 16–18 slices/lb)	0.133	× _____	= _____
Chicken, whole	(4 servings/lb)	0.244	× _____	= _____
Ham, whole	(4–5 servings/lb)	0.228	× _____	= _____
Pork sausage links	6 links (if 16 links/lb)	0.329	× _____	= _____
Frankfurters	About 2½ (if 10/lb)	0.247	× _____	= _____

Figure 12–1. Guide for calculating protein costs. To figure the cost per pound for large eggs, multiply ⅔ times the price per dozen; for milk, divide the cost per gallon by 8.6; for dry milk, calculate the cost of 5 quarts of reconstituted milk; and for tuna, multiply 2⅔ times the cost of a 6-ounce can (continued on next page). *(Reprinted with permission from Williams, F. L., & Justice, C. L., A ready reckoner of protein costs.* Journal of Home Economics, *1975, 67, pp. 20–21. With permission.)*

Item	Serving Size to Provide 14 gm Protein	Multiplication Factor	Current Retail Price per Pound	Cost of 14/gm Protein
Pork chops, with bone	(4 servings/lb)	0.239	× _____	= _____
Bacon, sliced	5½ slices (if 20 slices/lb)	0.403	× _____	= _____
Sirloin steak, choice grade	(4⅓ servings/lb)	0.229	× _____	= _____
Rib roast of beef	(4–5 servings/lb)	0.227	× _____	= _____
Round pot roast	(6–7 servings/lb)	0.158	× _____	= _____

Figure 12–1. (continued)

Fats

Fats are essential for the absorption of fat-soluble vitamins and serve as an energy source. In the average American diet, fats compose roughly 42 percent of total caloric intake. Fats are needed in limited amounts; a total of 30 percent fat in the diet is recommended, with 10 percent being saturated fats and 20 percent unsaturated fats. Intake of meats high in saturated fats, such as beef and pork, can be avoided if fish, poultry, or veal are used frequently. In addition, low-fat or skim milk and low-fat dairy products can be substituted for those higher in fat content. Consumption of butter, eggs, shellfish, non-dairy creamers, and other high-cholesterol sources should be limited. Animal fats are generally saturated, while vegetable sources of fat are unsaturated. Cholesterol consumption should not exceed 300 mg per day.

Abraham et al.[35] have shown that changes occur in total serum cholesterol from youth to old age. Median level of 18- to 24-year old males and females is approximately 180 to 190 mg per 100 ml. In men, levels rise sharply from 25 to 44 years of age and stabilize at 230 to 235 mg per 100 ml from 45 to 74 years. In women, the rise is steepest after 45 years of age, reaching a median of approximately 250 mg per 100 ml by 65 to 75 years of age. Upon autopsy following accidental death, studies have shown that in individuals with a cholesterol level of 180 mg per 100 ml or below, little atherosclerosis is present, while in individuals with a serum cholesterol above 220 mg per 100 ml, definite atherosclerotic changes have occurred.

The American Heart Association has made the following suggestions for controlling cholesterol and total fat intake:[36]

To control your intake of cholesterol-rich foods:
- Eat no more than three egg yolks a week, including eggs used in cooking. Commercial egg substitutes or egg whites may also be used
- Limit your use of shellfish and organ meats

To control the amount and type of fat you eat:
- Eat 6 to 8 ounces of lean meat, fish, or poultry daily. (Fish, poultry, and veal are low in saturated fat, so should be eaten more frequently than beef, lamb, or pork.)
- Choose lean cuts of meat, trim visible fat, and discard the fat that cooks out of the meat
- Avoid deep fat frying; use cooking methods that help to remove fat—baking, boiling, broiling, roasting, stewing
- Restrict your use of "luncheon" and "variety" meats like sausages and salami
- Instead of butter and other cooking fats that are solid or completely hydrogenated, use liquid vegetable oils and margarines that are rich in polyunsaturated fats
- Instead of whole milk and cheeses made from whole milk and cream, use skimmed or low fat milk and cheeses

Carbohydrates

The main function of carbohydrates is as an energy source for metabolic processes and activity. While 46 percent of the current American diet consists of carbohydrates, the Dietary Goals of the United States recommend an increase to 58 percent, with changes made in the types of carbohydrates consumed. In the average American diet, 18 percent of the carbohydrate intake consists of refined and processed sugars having high caloric density but low nutritional value. The Senate Select Subcommittee on Nutrition and Human Needs has suggested that this be reduced to 10 percent and that complex carbohydrates and naturally occurring sugars be increased to 48 percent of caloric intake. Fruits, vegetables, and whole-grain cereals and breads are sources of complex carbohydrates that are much richer in vitamins and minerals than are foods containing highly processed sugars. Suggestions for changing the nature of carbohydrate intake include the following:

- Carbonated beverages should be replaced with fruit juices or ice water
- Fruit should be substituted for high-caloric desserts
- Dried and fresh fruits should be used as natural sweeteners
- Snacks should consist of fruit, raw vegetables, whole-grain breads or cereals, cheese (low-fat skim), milk (low-fat or skim), fruit juices, or nuts (unsalted)

Vitamins

Vitamins and minerals serve many functions within the human body, as is indicated in Appendix A. Since vitamin A is stored in the liver, a good source of this vitamin each day or every other day is sufficient. Vitamin D, like vitamin A, is stored in the body, so large supplemental doses should be avoided. Vitamin C and the B-complex vitamins are not stored; therefore, several sources of these important vitamins should be consumed daily. Insofar as bioavailability is concerned, there is no apparent difference between natural and synthetic vitamins. However, if an adequate diet is maintained, the need for supplementation is minimized.

Sodium

Numerous minerals are critical to proper functioning of the body; information on many of them will be summarized in Appendix A. Sodium is the only mineral discussed in this chapter in more detail. The level of sodium intake has been related to systolic and diastolic blood pressures, even though the cause of hypertension is unknown. Therefore, in a prudent diet, even in the absence of hypertension, moderate salt restriction is recommended. Guidelines for restricting salt include:

- Do not add salt to foods at the table
- Use herbs, spices, and lemon in place of salt or monosodium glutamate
- Do not use baking soda as an antacid
- Use fresh or frozen vegetables as opposed to canned vegetables, which may be high in salt
- Avoid foods prepared in brine, such as ham, bacon, pickles, corned beef, and sauerkraut
- Restrict use of carbonated low-calorie beverages which contain sodium saccharin
- Do not add salt during cooking
- Avoid snack foods with visible salt, such as pretzels, potato chips, and cheese curls

Salt substitutes can be used to enhance the flavor of food if, after allowing a period of adjustment to low-sodium foods, the client finds such foods unpalatable.

Fiber

Fiber is not a nutrient but plays an important role in the diet. Fiber is important to the efficient functioning of the gastrointestinal tract. A high-fiber diet has been suggested by some studies as being important in the prevention of colon and rectal cancer because it facilitates the movement of waste products out of the body before toxic products have a chance to accumulate. The difference in fiber between whole grains and processed grains can be seen in Figure 12–2. When grain is refined, little more than the endosperm is left. This refined product is primarily starch and protein and lacks many of the vitamins and minerals found in whole grains. Both because of their fiber and nutrient content, whole grains are an important part of a nutritious diet.

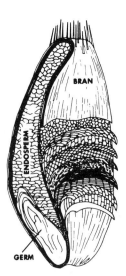

Whole grain. May be eaten as is (e.g., brown rice) or may be flaked into whole-grain cereal (e.g., oatmeal) or ground into whole-grain cereal or flour.

Endosperm. (refined white grains contain little else.) Mainly starch and protein.

Germ. High in vitamin E, many B vitamins, minerals, and protein; a source of polyunsaturated fat.

Bran. High in fiber, many B vitamins, and minerals.

Figure 12–2. Nutrient content of whole and refined grains. *(Reprinted with permission from Suitor, C. W., & Hunter, M. F., Nutrition: Principles and application in health promotion. Philadelphia: Lippincott, 1980, p. 15. With permission.)*

FOOD ADDITIVES

In modern society, food additives are necessary to retard spoilage and prevent deterioration of quality. However, additives are also used for other purposes, such as to improve nutritional value, to enhance consumer acceptability, and to facilitate preparation. Currently, food processors can add more than 10,000 chemicals to food products. Types of additives include preservatives, acids, alkalies, buffers, neutralizers, moisture-content controls, coloring agents, flavorings, physiological–activity controls, bleaching and maturing agents and bread improvers, processing aids, and nutrition supplements.[37]

By law, labels of many products must list the manufacturer, packer, and distributor, and the amount of each ingredient, and they must present the ingredients in order according to predominance; U.S. RDA (recommended daily allowance) may also be listed. However, for more than 300 standard foods (products made according to standard recipes issued by the federal government), including ice cream, catsup, and mayonnaise, no ingredients need be listed. Even when ingredients are listed, information on the products is often insufficient in and of itself to guide knowledgeable food selection.

Not only are potentially carcinogenic additives used in preparation of foods, e.g., nitrosamines in bacon and saccharin in low-calorie carbonated beverages, but unintentional food additives such as pesticides and other agricultural chemicals may appear in foods. A great deal of research must be done on the safety of large numbers of food additives. While studies are under way, the synergistic, cumulative, and long-term effects of many additives will only be determined after years of use and exposure within human populations.

FOOD–DRUG INTERACTIONS

A word needs to be said about the interaction of foods and drugs. Foods and drugs can interact, increasing the absorption of some foods and drugs and decreasing the absorption of others. The rate of absorption or the total level of absorption of drugs or nutrients may be affected. For example, crackers, dates, jelly, and other carbohydrates may slow down the rate of absorption of analgesics such as Tylenol and limit their effectiveness in reducing pain. Milk, eggs, cereals, and dairy products can inhibit the absorption of iron. Antibiotics such as tetracycline are less readily absorbed when milk, dairy products, or iron supplements are taken. Prune juice, bran cereal, and high-fiber foods can increase intestinal emptying time to the point where drugs such as digoxin cannot be adequately absorbed.[38]

Some medications increase the need for nutrients. Interesting findings have resulted from intensive studies of women on oral contraceptive medications. It appears that such medications lower levels of folacin, vitamin B_6, pyridoxine, riboflavin, and ascorbic acid in women; there is a need for further exploration of this and other food–drug interactions.

WEIGHT CONTROL

It has been estimated that two out of every five Americans in the United States are 20 percent or more overweight.[39] At least 60 to 70 million individuals weigh more than they should for optimum health. In terms of prevention of disease and maintenance of health, maintaining recommended weight appears to have a powerful impact. Men 45 to 55 years of age appear to increase mortality rate by 1 percent for each pound that they are overweight.[40] The incidence of cardiovascular disease, hypertension, diabetes mellitus, and cancer, major causes of disability and death, is higher among the obese.

Obesity is generally defined as being 20 percent or more overweight by standard height and weight tables. While a large amount of muscle mass in individuals can make these tables inaccurate, they represent the most accessible and convenient way of determining obesity. Since obesity almost always results in excessive amounts of nonessential subcutaneous fat, measurement of skinfold thicknesses has also been used as a convenient and nonintrusive measure of obesity.[41] Both of these approaches to assessment have been discussed in Chapter 6 on Health Assessment.

While the physical basis for obesity is relatively simple and straightforward, that is, the ingestion of more calories than needed for energy expenditure, the actual causes of obesity are complex. Proposed causes of obesity include:

1. Heredity
2. Cognitive factors (e.g., unrealistic personal standards and expectations)
3. Affective factors (e.g., emotional problems such as anxiety, boredom, and feelings of powerlessness)
4. Interpersonal factors (e.g., family problems, difficulties with fellow workers or colleagues)
5. Sociocultural factors (food selection, food preparation, and food consumption practices)
6. Environmental factors (e.g., salient cues for eating behavior and level of environmental sensitivity)

At this point, results of numerous studies suggest that it is more important to deal with personal, social, and environmental influences, rather than biochemical causes of obesity. Research has yielded little definitive information on biochemical etiology except in relation to a limited number of metabolic disorders.

Types of obesity have been classified to facilitate description of the problem and application of appropriate treatment strategies. Specific types include juvenile or adolescent-onset obesity (chronic obesity), adult-onset obesity (acute or chronic), reactive obesity (acute, sudden weight gain), and obesity secondary to a metabolic disorder.[42] Prevention is always the approach of choice, since treatment of obesity after it develops has met with limited success. Juvenile-onset obesity appears to be the type most resistant to treatment.

The primary goal of interventions for obesity is the permanent alteration of eating patterns and physical activity rather than weight loss only. In counseling clients, the term *dieting* should be avoided since it has a negative connotation. Actually, adopting more healthful eating behaviors is directed toward increasing rather than decreasing the pleasures derived from eating. New awareness of taste, texture, and form of foods allows the individual to participate to the fullest in the eating experience, totally involving gustatory, visual, olfactory, and tactile senses. Eating that promotes optimum health can be fulfilling, self-actualizing, and totally enjoyable.

Positive Effects of Maintaining Recommended Weight
The individual who maintains desired weight has taken a major step in decreasing risk for many chronic health problems. The Framingham study sponsored by the National Heart, Lung, and Blood Institute found that a 15-percent loss in weight among males corresponded to a 10-percent drop in systolic blood pressure and a slightly lower percentage drop in diastolic blood pressure.[43] Many hypertensive individuals become normotensive through weight loss. Not only does weight loss decrease the risk of chronic disease,

it has been shown to increase self-esteem, perceptions of control, and feelings of social desirability and acceptance. Individuals of normal weight are more active than their obese counterparts, and this further promotes health and decreases risk for health problems.

Maintaining weight has also been shown to result in a more consistent level of serum cholesterol. Frequent fluctuations in weight may be detrimental to health, since serum cholesterol is elevated during weight loss. Frequent elevations predispose individuals to more rapid progress of atherosclerosis. Adipocytes are the fat cells within the body that increase in lipid content with weight gain. In the obese, the size of fat cells can increase from 50 to 100 percent. Weight reduction is achieved though decrease in size of cells. As increased by-products of fat metabolism enter systemic circulation, precautions must be taken to prevent their deposit in the lining of vessels and their detrimental effects to internal organs such as liver and kidneys. Stability of weight can prevent many of these potential hazards.

Points To Consider Before Initiating a Weight-Reduction Program

The individual who desires to lose more than 20 pounds should have a medical history, physical examination, blood lipid and glucose analysis, and electrocardiogram before beginning a weight-loss program. Also, careful assessment of current dietary habits is essential in order to develop an individualized, effective program.

Other points to consider include the following:

- Are there weight-reduction measures that offer the individual a good chance of success?
- Is the person well adjusted to his or her weight or strongly motivated to change?
- Are there health conditions that make weight reduction a high priority?
- If change is desired, are expectations realistic?
- Will weight loss and weight maintenance be compatible with continuance of valued social relationships?
- Does the person have a support system within or outside of the family to facilitate weight loss?
- Does the person have a history of repeated failure in either achieving or maintaining weight loss?

These considerations are important in estimating the client's chances for success in weight loss. Studies have shown that individuals who derive the greatest benefits from a weight reduction program exhibit adult-onset rather than adolescent-onset obesity, report few previous attempts to achieve weight loss, cite numerous reasons for wanting to lose weight, are more adept at self-reinforcement, and have a social support system readily available.[44] The extent to which these conditions exist for any given client should be evaluated carefully by the nurse to estimate potential for successful weight loss.

General Guidelines for Healthy Weight Loss

It is critical that health be maintained during periods of weight loss. Inappropriate approaches to changing eating patterns can threaten nutritional, psychological, and physical health status. The following guidelines should be followed:[45]

- Diet should be deficient in calories only, not in nutrients
- Diet should be realistic
- Foods should be used in the diet rather than vitamins, weight-loss pills, or prepared liquids
- The diet should supply all vitamins and minerals needed for proper body functioning
- Adequate fiber should be ingested for proper functioning of the GI tract
- Enough fat should be ingested to supply the essential fatty acid, linoleic acid
- Food servings should be small
- A wide variety of high-nutrient foods should be included
- Regular meals should be eaten and snacks avoided

TABLE 12–4. SAMPLE OF A ONE-DAY MENU: NUTRITIOUS WEIGHT-LOSS PLAN, PROVIDING 1200 CALORIES

Breakfast
    1 serving fruit high in vitamin C
    1 serving enriched or whole-grain cereal
    1 serving whole wheat bread
    1 teaspoon liquid corn oil margarine
    $\frac{1}{2}$ cup skim milk

Lunch
    2 slices whole wheat bread or 1 cup cooked enriched pasta
    1 teaspoon liquid corn oil margarine
    1 slice cheese
    1 serving vegetable or salad
    1 serving fruit
    $\frac{1}{2}$ cup skim milk

Dinner
    Meat, fish, or poultry, $3\frac{1}{2}$ oz
    Half a freshly cooked potato
    1 serving vegetable high in vitamin A
    1 serving other vegetable or salad
    1 teaspoon liquid corn oil margarine or salad dressing
    1 serving fruit

Reprinted from McGill, M., & Pye, O. *The no-nonsense guide to food and nutrition.* New York: Butterick, 1978, p. 215. With permission.

- A gradual decline in weight of no more than 2 to 3 pounds per week is desirable and more likely to be permanent than is rapid weight loss
- Taking personal control is important; eating habits can be changed
- Eating nutritious and attractive low-calorie foods should be made a way of life

A sample of a good, nutritious weight-loss plan is provided in Table 12–4. Caloric and nutrient intake should be modified according to current age, weight, sex, and health status of the client. The sample daily weight-loss plan provides 1200 calories, maintenance calories for a person weighing 120 lbs. The reader is referred to other excellent texts on nutrition for further specific information.[46–48]

Behavioral Approaches to Changing Eating Behavior

The presentation of a comprehensive overview of behavioral strategies for the promotion of weight loss is beyond the scope of this chapter. Many appropriate approaches for behavior change have already been discussed in Chapter 10. An attempt will be made here to summarize the behavioral approaches to weight loss that have been reported in professional literature. All behavioral approaches focus on either the antecedents of eating, eating behavior itself, or the consequences of eating behavior as the points for professional intervention or self-control by the client.[49] Meaningful application of strategies to change eating behaviors requires consideration of the client's personality, life style, and environment if chances for success are to be optimized. Long-term and short-term goals should be carefully selected to provide a framework for behavior change that is realistic yet structured.

Nutrition education is an integral part of all behavioral approaches to weight control. Clients must have information to use in understanding and structuring dietary practices and in assessing the potential effects of behavior change. They must also develop awareness of the adverse effects of quick weight loss and fad diets. Educational activities may be designed for individuals or groups. Families should be the target for nutrition education efforts since family eating patterns play a pivotal role in both the creation and control of obesity among children and adults.[50]

The following four behavioral approaches to weight control have been used with clients and are reported in the literature to be effective for short-term weight loss:

1. Self-monitoring
2. Operant conditioning
   - Aversive conditioning and punishment
   - Self-reinforcement
   - Reinforcement by therapist
   - Reinforcement by significant others
   - Contingency contracting
   - Coverant conditioning

3. Stimulus control
   • Cue reduction
   • Cue expansion
4. Exercise

With the many approaches available for intervention, the nurse and client should select the approach or combination of approaches that best fits each individual's needs.

Self-Monitoring. Most obese people are not aware of why they overeat, how much they eat, or how frequently they eat. Awareness can be increased by use of food diaries and frequency graphs of eating behavior. Through self-monitoring, the client may become more aware of internal cues that initiate eating behavior as well as cues that indicate satiety. Bellack[51] compared the effects of two different types of self-monitoring on weight loss. One group used premonitoring (recording food intake before consumption) while a second experimental group used postmonitoring (recording food after consumption). The premonitoring group was superior to both the postmonitoring group and the control group in the weight loss.

It is possible that premonitoring makes eating less of an automatic behavior. Food intake is more carefully considered and planned. Gaining conscious awareness of eating behavior so that actions are more deliberate and under personal control can facilitate weight loss. However, few studies have shown major changes in weight with monitoring alone. It appears that this approach must be combined with others if it is to be effective. It is also possible that the studies that have shown little effect from monitoring have used postmonitoring rather than premonitoring, thus decreasing the possible effectiveness of monitoring activities.

Operant Conditioning. Positive reinforcement of desirable eating behaviors has been used successfully in a variety of studies. One thing that appears to be clear is that aversive conditioning through use of negative reinforcement or punishment is much less effective than conditioning of eating behaviors through positive reward or reinforcement. Mahoney, Moura, and Wade[52] had subjects either reward themselves for weight loss or fine themselves for weight gain from money that they had deposited to be used in that way. Individuals who rewarded themselves for weight loss rather than fined themselves for failure to lose weight were more successful.

In a subsequent study, Mahoney[53] compared a self-monitoring treatment with self-reward for weight loss. He also compared self-reward for weight loss with self-reward for positive changes in eating behavior. Self-reward was more effective than self-monitoring (premonitoring) and self-reward for changes in eating behavior was more effective than self-reward for weight loss in terms of pounds. This indicates the importance of proper selection of the target behavior to maximize the effects of positive reinforcement techniques.

Bellack[54] demonstrated the superiority of self-reinforcement to self-monitoring in promoting weight loss. Self-reinforcement has a number of advantages over reinforcement by the nurse or significant others. Reinforcement can be immediately contingent on appropriate eating behavior since the source of action and reward are the same. In addition, self-reward gives individuals a means of controlling their own behavior, thus supporting independence, autonomy, improved self-concept, and perceptions of control.

Saccone and Israel[55] studied seven treatment groups, each with different target behaviors to be reinforced (eating behavior versus weight loss) and differing sources of reinforcement (experimenter versus significant other). They found that the greatest weight loss occurred in the group reinforced by a significant other for positive changes in eating behavior. Family members or significant others are likely to be aware of effective sources of reward and environmental contingencies of reinforcement because of intimate contact with the client. Involvement of family members in applying reinforcement contingencies for behavioral change provides a continuing support system for the client.

In operant conditioning, rewarding new behaviors that are incompatible with health-damaging behaviors (in this case unhealthy eating patterns) assists in extinguishing undesirable behaviors. New behaviors to be learned as substitutes for health-damaging behaviors should be activities that the client enjoys performing and that are readily accessible to the client. For instance, the desire to eat a midday snack could signal the client to call a friend for a telephone visit, go bike riding, or go for a walk. If feelings of frustration provoke eating behavior, learning to relax through imagery, deep breathing, or use of systematic relaxation can be helpful as a replacement behavior for eating. In addition, the client learns to cope more effectively with stressful situations so that there is less need to eat as a coping strategy.

Shaping is an important concept in the application of positive reinforcement to change eating behavior. In shaping, progressive approximations of the desired behavior are rewarded. Initial reinforcements may be given for skipping one between-meal snack or even for cutting down on the amount eaten for a snack or for improving the quality of the snack selected (e.g., for choosing fruit or raw vegetables). Gradually, the client can move toward omitting between-meal snacks entirely.

Contingency contracting has been discussed in detail in Chapter 10. Its application to changing eating behavior has met with considerable success. Contracting makes explicit the parameters of behavior to be engaged in and the conditions or rewards that are to be expected upon fulfillment of the contract. While the promise of tangible reinforcement for changing eating behaviors is undoubtedly of considerable importance, the commitment to behavior change made by the client in contingency contracting also seems to be an important factor in accomplishing desired behaviors.

Lambert and Schwab[56] conducted an intensive nutrition campaign in two communities during a 1-week period. Three weeks later a group of people in one community were asked to sign a pledge card to change a particular eating behavior of their choice. That is, they were asked to make a commitment to behavior change relevant to personal nutrition and diet. Of those who made a pledge to change, 67 percent had fulfilled their commitment 90 to 100 percent of the time after 1 week. Of the sample, 51 percent made a commitment to change an old behavior, while 46 percent made a commitment to adopt a new eating habit. After 1 week, a higher percentage of those who made a commitment to adopt a new behavior were more persistent (69 percent) than of those who made a commitment to change or discontinue an old behavior (52 percent). After 3 months, 59 percent of the individuals who signed a pledge were fulfilling that pledge over more than 50 percent of the time. In the control community exposed to the intensive information program on nutrition but not asked to pledge, only 10 percent had actually changed a nutritional habit for the better. It appears that personal commitment plays a major role in persistence of dietary changes.

Conditioning covert behavior has been espoused as a logical approach to changing overt eating behavior since covert operants (coverants) precede actual operant behavior. For instance, the thought "I should eat an apple instead of a cookie" should be reinforced, since it is a thought that serves as a precursor or intervening variable for desired dietary behavior. By increasing the frequency of such positive thoughts though reinforcement, negative coverants such as "That sundae looks so creamy and delicious" may be decreased in frequency. Reinforcement for coverants can be tangible objects, experiences, praise by others, or self-praise. Since coverants are private events, self-reinforcement is usually more effective than is reinforcement by others to whom coverants have to be reported. Coverant conditioning represents a special instance of operant conditioning. From the research conducted thus far, it appears that covert control of eating behavior can be combined with other strategies and may then act in a synergistic manner to facilitate effective weight loss.

Stimulus Control. Stimulus control consists of modifying the environment to decrease cues for eating behavior and increase cues for positive or neutral behaviors that are incompatible with eating. Schachter[57] proposed the "external cue hypothesis," which states that the obese individual is more under the control of external cues for eating behavior than under internal cues. That is, eating behavior may be controlled by the frequency and availability of food rather than by hunger and satiation. McReynolds et al.[58] found that when two groups were compared, one receiving self-control instruction and the other receiving information about stimulus control, both groups exhibited comparable weight losses at the end of treatment. However, on both 3- and 6-month follow-up, the stimulus-control group was superior to the self-control group. These findings provide support for the importance of changing external as well as internal cues to facilitate change in eating behaviors.

Cues that trigger eating can be reduced. This is referred to as *stimulus reduction.* For instance, the client may reinforce eating only when it occurs in the dining room, i.e., in no other location within the house. This means that snacks cannot be eaten while the client is watching television in the family room, nor can food be consumed while the client is sitting in the kitchen making out a grocery list. By cue reduction or stimulus narrowing for eating behavior, food consumption comes under the control of a restricted number of stimuli that can be controlled and manipulated. Clients can also learn to respond to external food cues with behaviors that are positive but do not involve eating. Reading the paper, sewing, or knitting in environmental situations where food was usually eaten occupy the client with meaningful activity while preventing ingestion of food.

Exercise. Physical activity is also a behavioral intervention that promotes expenditure of energy and can facilitate weight loss. Most obese individuals are less active than their normal-weight counterparts. Exercise is not only useful in burning excess calories; studies have suggested that it also prevents the loss of protein from muscle and minerals from bone that frequently occur when attempts at weight loss are accompanied by inactivity. Exercise in combination with restricted calories also assists in reducing undesirable lipoprotein lipids, increasing work capacity, lowering resting heart rate, and decreasing blood pressure. These positive changes cannot be attained through restricting calories only.[59] Exercise is increasingly recommended in weight reduction programs, for reasons other than increased energy expenditure and improved physical fitness. Increased physical activity generally decreases appetite, increases basal metabolism rate for at least 4 hours after exercise (offsetting reduced metabolic rate that accompanies calorie restriction), and positively affects mood and self-esteem, which may improve long-term compliance with newly acquired eating behaviors. Both programmed activity (bicycling, working out, running) and routine activity (stair climbing, walking, and moving objects) should be significantly increased as a complement to healthy nutritional practices.[60] The reader is referred to Chapter 11 for exercises appropriate for clients who are overweight.

Combining Behavior Approaches to Weight Control

Exercise is often used in combination with other behavioral interventions. Dahlkoetter et al.[61] compared the relative effectiveness of exercise versus eating habit change and both in combination on weight loss. Forty-four subjects were assigned to four groups: exercise, eating habit change, combination, or the control group. Each group met for eight 1-hour sessions. Results indicated significant improvements for all groups on body weight. The combined group of exercise and eating habit change showed the most progress in weight and body circumference measures. At the 8-week follow-up, only the combination group continued to lose weight. These results suggest the desirability of combining exercise and eating habit change in dealing with obesity.

Kelly[62] demonstrated the effectiveness of combining approaches to weight control in working with 53 male officers from the Boston Police Department. The officers participated in a 12-week program during which they did the following:

- Kept record of weight change (monitoring)
- Attended lectures on nutrients, stress, heart disease, food, energy, and respiratory disease (education)
- Engaged in light to moderate physical activity (exercise)
- Completed homework that included behavior modification assignments given at the end of each lecture (reinforcement contingencies)

Immediately following completion of the program, the 53 officers had a mean weight loss of 7.5 kg. One year later, when 26 of the officers responded to a follow-up questionnaire, mean weight loss maintained was 11.4 kg. At completion of the initial program, the mean weight loss for these 26 individuals had been 10.9 kg. Thirteen had lost a mean of 4.4 kg on their own; one maintained weight loss; 12 had a mean weight gain of 3.5 kg. None of the officers had returned to his original weight.

In contrast, some studies have failed to support the superiority of combined approaches over single interventions. Abrahms and Allen,[63] in comparing the effectiveness of stimulus control, financial payoffs, and group pressure in weight reduction, found that stimulus control and monetary reward (contingency contracting) from the therapist were no more effective in achieving weight loss than was stimulus control alone.

Heckerman and Prochaska[64] reported a study of 43 young adults who were randomly assigned to one of four groups for behavioral modification of eating behaviors: standard self-control, self-control plus external control via contingency contracting, self-control plus additional internal control, or the no-treatment control group. The standard self-control program consisted of presenting nutritional information and behavioral principles, including self-monitoring, stimulus control, self-reinforcement, and social reinforcement. The self-control plus external reinforcement group received the standard self-control program with an external reinforcement system by way of a contingency contract. The self-control plus more internal control group received the standard package and additional attempts to increase personal control of eating behavior. All experimental groups differed from the no-treatment control group, but there were no significant differences among the experimental groups.

Failure to find differences among the groups in the studies described, may have been the result of a lack of match between the locus of control of the subjects and type of weight-loss program. Wallston et al.[65] found that externally oriented individuals were more satisfied with a group weight-reduction program where external sanctions and control were used, while internally oriented individuals preferred an individualized program in which they could set their own goals.

Findings as to the differential effects of single versus combined behavioral approaches are equivocal at this point in time. Further research is needed to clarify the usefulness of single and combined interventions in assisting individuals with differing characteristics to change eating behaviors.

Barriers to Changing Eating Behaviors

Obstacles or difficulties that may be anticipated during the action phase in changing eating behaviors include the following:

- Reaching a plateau
- Perception and balance problems with relatively rapid weight loss
- Premature cessation of newly acquired behaviors because of compliments on progress or negative reactions and ridicule of others
- Temptation to reward weight loss with food treats
- Failure to enlist the assistance of family or significant others in weight-loss program
- Lack of "booster sessions" with health professional during stabilization phase for newly acquired eating behaviors (first 6 months to 1 year)
- Heterosexual anxiety aroused by weight reduction and fear or apprehension concerning increased attractiveness to opposite sex
- Interpersonal difficulties with significant others because of physical changes and accompanying psychological adjustments

If at all possible, the client should be alerted to these possible difficulties and preventive measures instituted to avert problems. Professional support of the client by the nurse and suggestions for constructively dealing with barriers when they arise will facilitate the client's efforts to eliminate or minimize obstacles that block attainment of desired nutritional goals.

Maintaining Weight Loss

An important consideration in evaluating the effectiveness of any behavior change program directed at weight loss is the maintenance of weight or continued loss after cessation of the initial program. Hall[66] found that subjects participating in an organized weight-loss program had regained all treatment losses 2 years after cessation of the program. Harris and Bruner[67] report that their experimental and control subjects did not differ in weight loss after a period of 10 months. Beneke et al.[68] report more encouraging results, their subjects gaining a mean of 5.9 pounds after cessation of the behavioral treatment program but maintaining 66 percent of the treatment loss. Stunkard[69] estimated that 80 percent of obese individuals drop out of weight loss programs within the first 3 months and no more than 50 percent adhere to newly acquired eating behaviors to maintain weight loss. This presents a major dilemma for health care professionals providing care to overweight clients and for the clients themselves. Not only are wide fluctuations in weight detrimental to health, but they are psychologically demoralizing. Feelings of hopelessness can result from unsuccessful attempts at weight reduction or from regaining weight that previously had been lost. Assisting clients to develop relapse prevention strategies appears to be one of the more promising approaches to helping them maintain positive eating behaviors.[70]

SUMMARY

An attempt has been made to present an overview of salient principles, concerns, and issues related to effective nutritional care. Since obesity is a health problem of epidemic proportions within the American population, special attention has been given to this difficulty. The reader is encouraged to consult the many references listed at the end of this chapter in order to acquire more information about nutritional care of clients. Promoting good nutrition is a critical concern in illness prevention and health promotion and an important dimension of competent self-care.

REFERENCES

1. Cantu, R. C. *Toward fitness: Guided exercises for those with health problems.* New York: Human Science Press, 1980, p. 60.
2. Inano, M., & Pringle, D. J. Dietary survey of low-income rural families in Iowa and North Carolina. 2. Family distribution of dietary adequacy. Journal of the American Dietetic Association, 1975, *66*, 361–365.
3. Corey, J. E. Dietary factors in atherosclerosis: Prevention should begin early. *Journal of School Health*, November 1974, *44*, 511–513.
4. Suitor, C. W., & Crowley, M. F. *Nutrition: Principles and application in health promotion* (2nd ed.). Philadelphia: Lippincott, 1984, pp. 503–504.
5. DHEW, NIH, National Heart, Lung and Blood Institute. *The dietary management of hyperlipoproteinemia.* DHEW Publ. No. (NIH) 76-110. Bethesda, MD : Government Printing Office, 1976.
6. U.S. Senate Select Committee on Nutrition and Human Needs. *Dietary Goals for the United States.* Washington, D.C.: Government Printing Office, 1977.
7. Suitor & Crowley, op. cit., p. 502.
8. Cantu, op. cit., p. 42.
9. Van Handel, P. J., & Essig, D. *Caffeine.* (Unpublished manuscript.) Muncie, Ind.: Human Performance Laboratory, 1980.
10. Newell, G. R. The provocative role of diet in carcinogenesis. *Consultant*, January 1984, 116–125.
11. Scarpa, I. S., & Kiefer, H. S. (Eds.), *Sourcebook on food and nutrition* (1st ed.). Chicago: Marquis Academic Media, 1978, p. 23.
12. Ibid.
13. Fredericks, C. *Winning the fight against breast cancer: The nutritional approach.* New York: Grosset and Dunlap, 1977.
14. Ibid., p. 59.
15. Cantu, op. cit., p. 61.
16. Improved nutrition. *Public Health Reports Supplement*, September–October 1983, 132–154.

17. Beal, V. A. *Nutrition in the life span.* New York: Wiley, 1980, p. 58.
18. Suitor & Crowley, op cit., p. 83.
19. Martin, R. A., & Poland, E. Y. *Learning to change: A self-management approach to adjustment.* New York: McGraw-Hill, 1980, p. 56.
20. Schafer, R. B. The self-concept as a factor in diet selection and quality. *Journal of Nutritional Education,* 1979, *11,* 37–39.
21. Stein, M. P., Farquhar, J. W., Maccoby, N., & Russell, S. H. Results of a two year health education campaign on dietary behavior: The Stanford three community study. *Circulation,* November 1976, *54,* 826–832.
22. Suitor & Crowley, op. cit., p. 96.
23. Boykin, L. S. Soul foods for some older Americans. *Journal of the American Geriatric Society,* 1975, *23,* 380–382.
24. Hataway, H., Raines, J. L., & Weinsier, R. L. Nutrition: Its ever increasing role. *Family and Community Health,* 1984, 7, 22–35.
25. Kolasa, K., Wenger, A., Paolucci, B., & Bobbit, N. Home based learning implications for nutrition educators. *Journal of Nutrition Education,* 1979, *11,* 19–21.
26. Suitor & Crowley, op. cit., pp. 13–18.
27. Nutrition Search, Inc. *Nutrition almanac* (rev. ed.). New York: McGraw-Hill, 1973.
28. Suitor & Crowley, op. cit., p. 85.
29. Ibid., pp. 123–124.
30. Kuntzlemann, C. T. *The complete book of walking.* New York: Simon and Schuster, 1979, p. 53.
31. Suitor & Crowley, op. cit., p. 88.
32. Ibid., p. 38.
33. *Nutrition almanac,* op. cit., pp. 9–10.
34. Williams, F. L., & Justice, C. L. A ready reckoner of protein costs. *Journal of Home Economics,* 1975, *67,* 20–21.
35. Abraham, S., Johnson, C. L., & Carroll, M. D. Total serum cholesterol levels of adults 18 to 74 years, U.S. 1971–1974. DHEW Publ. No. (PHS) 78-1652. Washington, D.C.: Government Printing Office, 1978.
36. American Heart Association. *Eat well but eat wisely.* New York: The Association, 1973.
37. Winter, R. *A consumer's dictionary of food additives.* New York: Crown, 1978.
38. Wakefern Food Corporation. *Food-drug interactions: Can what you eat affect your medication?* Elizabeth, N.J.: The Corporation, 1978.
39. Kelly, K. L. Evaluation of a group nutrition education approach to effective internal control. *American Journal of Public Health,* August 1979, *69,* 813–816.
40. Abramson, E. E. *Behavioral approaches to weight control.* New York: Springer, 1977.
41. Gain, S. M., & Clark, D. C. Trends in fatness and the origins of obesity. *Pediatrics,* 1976, *57,* 443–456.
42. Suitor & Crowley, op. cit., p. 466.
43. Cantu, op. cit., p. 62.
44. Abramson, op. cit., p. 40.
45. McGill, M., & Pye, O. *The no-nonsense guide to food and nutrition.* New York: Butterick, 1978.
46. Suitor & Crowley, op. cit.
47. Beal, op. cit.
48. *Sourcebook on food and nutrition,* op. cit.
49. Stunkard, A. J. Adherence to medical treatment: Overview and lessons from behavioral weight control. *Journal of Psychosomatic Research,* 1981, *25* (3), 187–197.

50. Frankle, R. T. Obesity a family matter: Creating new behavior. *Journal of the American Dietetic Association,* May 1985, *85* (5), 597–602.
51. Bellack, A. S. A comparison of self-reinforcement and self-monitoring in a weight reduction program. *Behavior Therapy,* 1976, 7, 68–75.
52. Mahoney, M. J., Moura, N. G. M., & Wade, T. C. Relative efficacy of self-reward, self-punishment, self-monitoring techniques for weight loss. *Journal of Consulting Clinical Psychology,* 1973, *40,* 40–47.
53. Mahoney, M. J. Self-reward and self-monitoring techniques for weight control. *Behavior Therapy,* 1974, *5,* 48–57.
54. Bellack, op. cit.
55. Saccone, A. J., & Israel, A. C. Effects of experimenter versus significant other-controlled reinforcement and choice of target behavior on weight loss. *Behavior Therapy,* 1978, *9,* 271–278.
56. Lambert, V. E., & Schwab, L. O. Can we change our food habits? *Journal of Home Economics,* 1975, *67,* 33–34.
57. Schachter, S. Some extraordinary facts about obese humans and rats. *American Psychologist,* 1971, *26,* 129–144.
58. McReynolds, W. T., Lutz, R. N., Paulsen, B. K., & Kohrs, M. B. Weight loss resulting from two behavior modification procedures with nutritionists as therapists. *Behavior Therapy,* 1976, 7, 283–291.
59. Heath, G. W., & Broadhurst, C. B. Effects of exercise training and dietary behavior modification on weight reduction and lipoprotein lipids in female hospital employees. *Heath Values: Achieving High Level Wellness,* November–December 1984, *8,* (6), 3–9.
60. Hataway, Raines, & Weinsier, op. cit., p. 26.
61. Dahlkoetter, J., Callahan, E. J., & Linton, J. Obesity and the unbalanced energy equation: Exercise versus eating habit change. *Journal of Counseling and Clinical Psychology,* 1979, *47,* 898–905.
62. Kelly, op. cit.
63. Abrahms, J. L., & Allen, G. J. Comparative effectiveness of situational programming, financial payoffs and group pressure in weight reduction. *Behavior Therapy,* 1974, *5,* 391–400.
64. Heckerman, C. L., & Prochaska, J. O. Development and evaluation of weight reduction procedures in a health maintenance organization. In Stuart, R. B. (Ed.), *Behavioral self-management: Strategies, techniques and outcomes.* New York: Brunner/Mazel, 1977, pp. 215–229.
65. Wallston, B. S., Wallston, K. A., Kaplan, G. D., & Maides, S. A. Development and validation of the health locus of control (HLC) scale. *Journal of Consulting Clinical Psychology,* 1976, *44,* 580–585.
66. Hall, S. M., Behavior treatment of obesity: A two-year follow-up. *Behavior Research and Therapy,* 1973, *11,* 647–648.
67. Harris, M. B., & Bruner, C. G. A comparison of a self-control and a contract procedure for weight control. *Behavior Research and Therapy,* 1971, 9, 347–354.
68. Beneke, W. M., Paulsen, B., McReynolds, W. T., Lutz, R. N., & Kohrs, M. B. Long-term results of two behavior modification weight loss programs using nutritionists as therapists. *Behavior Therapy,* 1978, *9,* 501–507.
69. Stunkard, op. cit., p. 187.
70. Wilson, G. T. Weight control treatments. In J. D. Matarazzo, S. M. Weiss, J. A. Herd, et al. (Eds.), *Behavioral health: A handbook of health enhancement and disease prevention.* New York: Wiley, 1984, pp. 657–670.

CHAPTER 13

Stress Management

Stress is inevitable in modern society where technological, social, political, environmental, and cultural change occur at an ever-increasing rate. Thousands of articles and books have been written on the subject of stress, yet the complexity of the concept continues to baffle the best scientific minds. Selye, a pioneer in stress research, has defined stress as "the nonspecific response of the body to any demand made on it."[1] The body's response to stress involves the nervous, endocrine, and immunological systems, which in turn affect all organ systems. Stress is an all-too-common human experience that over time can produce health-damaging effects. It is estimated that production loss from stress-induced physical illnesses is $60 billion annually and from stress-induced mental dysfunction, $17 billion per annum.[2]

In nursing literature, stress produced by the experiences of illness and hospitalization has been the most frequent focus of investigation. Less attention has been given to the mechanisms by which reactions to life events and everyday hassles affect neurohormonal functions, often resulting in recurrent and prolonged stress. While the nurse in the hospital setting may actively manage sources of biological and environmental stress for patients who are acutely ill, in the community, the major responsibility for preventing the deleterious effects of stress rests with individuals and families. Consequently, nurses need to assist clients in assessing stress levels and adequacy of coping strategies. In addition, nurses can help clients develop competence in using various approaches for the management of stress.

As an example of what nurses can do in this area, the author of this book

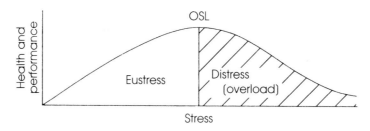

Figure 13–1. Optimum stress level (OSL) and effects of overload on health and performance. (*From Hans Selye.*)

provides training in progressive relaxation and biofeedback to clients with hypertension as part of a comprehensive hypertension control program within the community. Clients contract individually with the author for the 16-week program. Details of the author's stress management practice will be provided in a later section of this chapter. Another nurse actively involved in providing stress management to clients and investigating its effects is Helen Kogan of Seattle, Washington. Through use of biofeedback and other techniques, she and her staff assist clients in learning how to prevent the psychophysiological effects of stress that are detrimental to health.

As a context for the discussion of stress management, two conceptualizations of stress will be presented. In addition, what is currently known about the mechanisms that mediate stress will be summarized briefly.

Selye breaks the stress response down into eustress and distress. Eustress is an agreeable and healthy experience in which, as stress increases, health and performance also increase. Distress is a disagreeable and pathogenic state in which, as stress increases, health and performance decrease.[3] Stress overload is considered by Selye to be the cause of distress. The relationship between eustress and distress is pictured in Figure 13–1. According to Selye, the optimal stress level for any individual is the point on the stress continuum where performance and health are maximized. He proposes that eustress and distress are not qualitatively different; they are only quantitatively different.

Internal and external manifestations of stress are referred to by Selye as the General Adaptation Syndrome (GAS) or the "fight-or-flight" response.

TABLE 13–1. FIGHT-OR-FLIGHT RESPONSE

Dilatation of pupils	Increased muscle tension
Increased respiratory rate	Increased gastric motility
Increased heart rate	Release of adrenalin
Peripheral vasoconstriction	Increased blood glucose level
Increased perspiration	Raising of body hair
Increased blood pressure	Cold and clammy hands

Specific physiological or behavioral changes that occur are presented in Table 13–1. In modern society, the "fight-or-flight" response serves few useful functions since distress seldom results from direct physical threat. The major sources of distress experienced by individuals today originate in interpersonal relationships (communication) and performance demands (action). Since communication and action represent two basic human processes, the potential for stress is always present.

Recent studies of stress appear to support the premise that undesirable life events correlate more highly with subsequent illness than desirable life changes.[4,5,6] Zautra and Sandler[7] have proposed that psychological distress and psychological growth are two separate processes. The Psychological Distress Model is presented in Figure 13–2A and the Psychological Growth Model in Figure 13–2B. While the two models share common structural features, they differ markedly in terms of underlying motivational mechanisms. Zautra and Sandler reject the notion proposed by Selye that distress and growth differ only in the quantity of stress experienced. They propose qualitative differences in the two processes. Underlying the Psychological Distress Model is the basic need to reduce and cope with harmful or otherwise threatening events that arise from person–environment transactions. Defense is the primary orientation. These encounters create personal discomfort or uneasiness. When the pressure is off and stress is decreased, the person no longer has to maintain a defensive posture. The orientation toward events underlying the Psychological Growth Model is very different. This orientation is a need for competency and personal growth. Increased mastery of self and the environment is a positive process that results in greater individuation and self-reliance.

The view of the author of this book agrees with Zautra and Sandler rather than Selye. States of negative tension (distress) are viewed as qualitatively different from states of positive tension (challenge). The former activates the stabilizing tendency; the latter, the actualizing tendency. Within this chapter, the term *stress* denotes states of negative tension or distress. Acquiring the skills needed to prevent stressful situations or to deal constructively with them when they arise, thus minimizing their harmful effects, is critical for individuals and families if they are to maximize their health potential.

MEDIATION OF STRESS

In order to assist clients in managing stress, the health professional should understand the neuroendocrine pathways currently believed to mediate stress. Neuroendocrine pathways believed to be responsible for the stress response are presented in Figure 13–3. The early work of Papez[8] and McLean[9] indicated that emotional states or responses are correlated with electrophysiological activity in the limbic system of the brain. This activity is then transmitted to the sympathetic network of the autonomic nervous system, the hypothalamus, the pituitary gland, the adrenal cortex, and the adrenal medulla, re-

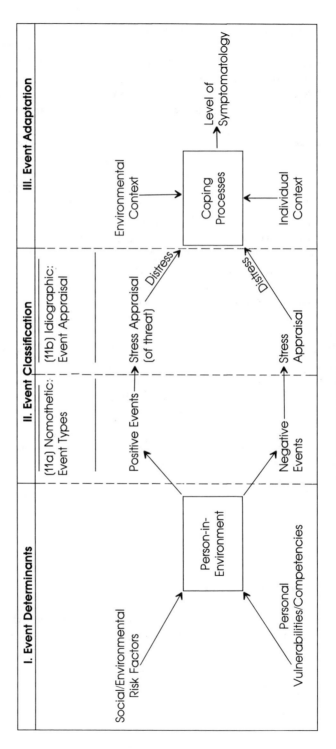

A. PSYCHOLOGICAL DISTRESS MODEL

| I. Event Determinants | II. Event Classification | III. Event Adaptation |

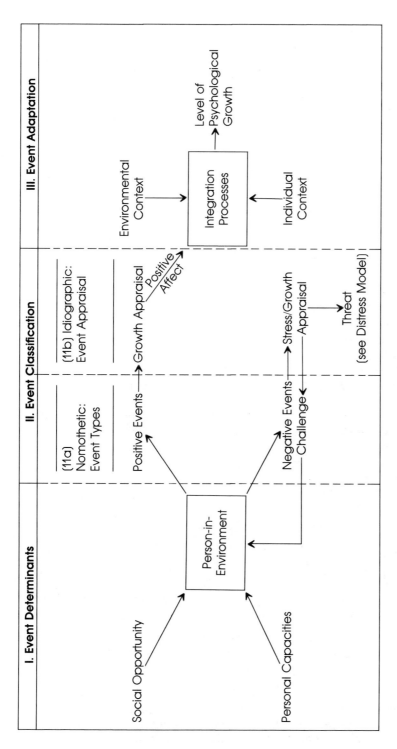

Figure 13–2. Models of distress and growth psychological processes. *(From Zautra, A., & Sandler, I. Life event needs assessments: Two models for measuring preventable mental health problems. Prevention in Human Services, 1983, 2 (4), 38, with permission.)*

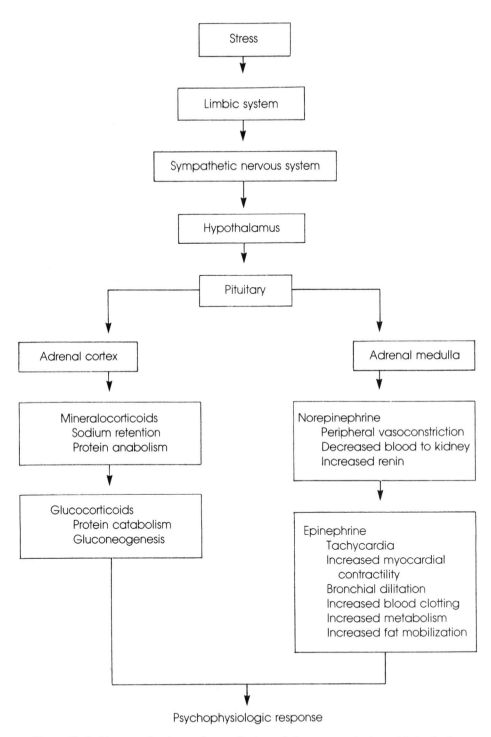

Figure 13–3. Neuroendocrine pathways that mediate response to stress. *(Adapted from Smith, M. J. T., & Selye, H. Reducing the negative effects of stress.* American Journal of Nursing, *79, November 1979, p. 1954.)*

sulting in release of corticoids, norepinephrine, and epinephrine. Thus, limbic signals are converted to autonomical and hormonal processes through the transducing machinery of the hypothalamus and pituitary.[10] Hormones released into systematic circulation appear to be responsible for the myriad effects observed in human beings experiencing stress. Recent work in psychoneuroimmunology presents evidence that the immune system can be markedly weakened by adverse cognitive and behavioral responses to stressors. Borysenko[11] provides an excellent overview of stress, endocrine response and immunity.

APPROACHES TO STRESS MANAGEMENT

At any point in time, an individual or family may be subjected to many sources of potential stress. Multiple stressors can combine synergistically, resulting in cumulative stress. The nurse and client together must assess the level of existing stress and the sources of stress and then determine the appropriate point(s) for intervention to achieve stress reduction.

The primary points for intervention in stress management consist of the following:

- Minimizing the frequency of stress-inducing situations
- Psychological preparation to increase resistance to stress
- Counterconditioning to avoid physiological arousal resulting from stress

Each point of intervention will be discussed in this chapter, and appropriate self-regulatory strategies will be described. Major attention will be given to counterconditioning techniques that can be used by the client to "turn off" physiological responses to stress when tension-producing situations cannot be avoided.[12]

Minimizing the Frequency of Stress-Inducing Situations

In a technological society, the need for adjustment to externally imposed change is continuous. The work of Holmes and Rahe[13] has indicated the importance of "life change" as a risk factor for illness and the impact of change on the level of health. The statistical probability of becoming ill is greater following a period of high life change than after a period of few life changes. Stressful events can include changes in family relationships, work setting, or geographical location. Adaptation reflects the human stabilizing tendency in response to environmental change. In addition, adaptation keeps physiological and psychological parameters within ranges compatible with continuing existence.

How does the client deal with the continuing need to adjust yet avoid the destructive effects of negative tension states? Approaches to assisting clients in preventing stressful situations include (1) habituation, (2) change avoidance, (3) time blocking,[14] (4) time management, and (5) environmental modification.

Habituation. Habit explains much of the behavior about which we have to exercise little conscious thought. Many behaviors are accomplished automatically through routines or stabilized behavior patterns. Routines reduce the need for expenditure of physical and psychological energy, resist change, and thus serve as a stabilizing force. The importance of routines and the threat imposed by their disturbance can be easily seen among hospitalized patients. A major source of stress during hospitalization is the disturbance of usual patterns of living. Every activity takes more energy than is required in the patient's natural setting because it must be done differently. Therefore, during periods of high stress, routines should be supported by health personnel in order to conserve energy that can be reallocated to deal directly with stressful events.

Change Avoidance. During periods of high life change and resulting negative tension states, any unnecessary changes should be avoided. As an example, if a family is experiencing the illness of one of its family members and a subsequent job loss, this may not be the time to consider geographical relocation, pregnancy, or any other change in life style. Negative tension created by multiple changes is synergistic. Each time a distressing change occurs, the potency of previous changes for upsetting stability is increased. Deliberately postponing changes that result in negative tension assists clients in dealing more constructively with unavoidable change and prevents the need for multiple adjustments all at one point in time.

Any changes that are made in life style during periods of high or moderate stress should be self-initiated and provide challenge to the client rather than threat. Increasing positive sources of tension that promote growth and self-actualization can offset the deleterious effects of negative tension. For instance, learning to play tennis, to swim, or to dance may provide an enjoyable challenge to counterbalance stress.

Time Blocking. Girdano and Everly[15] have suggested a time-blocking technique that sets aside specific time for adaptation to various stressors. This block of time may be daily, weekly, or monthly. It offers clients time to focus on a specific change and develop strategies for adjustment. For instance, if a family member has just been diagnosed as diabetic, time must be set aside to meet the new needs of that individual and to learn more about the care and support that family members can provide. Acquisition of new information and thoughtful planning makes a specific change easier to adapt to and allows time for the expression of feelings and emotions that may hinder adjustment. Nurses as health professionals can be a rich resource of information and assistance as clients integrate unavoidable changes into their life style. The major advantage of time blocking is that it ensures that important goals or concerns will be addressed and critical tasks accomplished. This can reduce the sense of time urgency, the level of anxiety, and associated feelings of frustration and failure.

Time Management. This approach to stress management actually refers to managing oneself to accomplish those goals most important in life within the time available. Since lack of time is often given by individuals and families as a reason for not participating in health-promoting activities, assisting clients to manage time better can make a major contribution to their health and fitness. Time-pressured, Type A clients with high risk for cardiovascular disease may be particularly in need of time-management skills.

After clients have used the clarification techniques described in Chapter 7 to identify their values and goals, prioritizing goals can serve as a framework for time management. Identifying time wasted on activities unrelated to personal goals can permit the client to restructure how time is spent. Overcommitment to others or unrealistic expectations of oneself is a frequent source of stress. Time overload can be avoided by learning to say "no" to demands of others that are unrealistic or of low personal or family priority. Overload results in frustration and loss of satisfaction from the work accomplished, since one can seldom expend one's best efforts under strain and pressure.

An important approach to time management is the reduction of a task into smaller parts. A task as a whole may appear as an overload; however, if the task is broken down into smaller segments, accomplishment becomes feasible. An example of this for a client may be learning several effective conditioning exercises before learning a complete conditioning routine, or developing skill with a conditioning routine before beginning a walk–jog activity. To take the whole health-promoting behavior as one task may be overwhelming. Breaking it down into component parts allows mastery and feelings of competence.

Avoiding overload by delegating responsibilities to others and enlisting their assistance is also important. The delegation of responsibilities must be realistic based on the abilities of others so that delegated tasks can be accomplished without excessive supervision. Making use of the skills of others and recognizing their ability to perform assigned tasks provides freedom from the expectation of having to be "all things to all people."

Another important aspect of time management is to reduce the perception of time pressure and urgency. Not all perceptions of time urgency are warranted; some are needlessly self-imposed. The client should differentiate between time urgencies that are valid and others that are needlessly created. Time urgency can also be minimized by avoiding procrastination. Leaving tasks that need to be completed until the last minute can result in needless pressure and stress.[16]

Just as overload can be avoided, periods of low levels of stimulation that produce negative tension can also be anticipated and prevented. Time can be used wisely by planning activities that increase positive tension and promote growth. For example, the salesperson who spends a great deal of time driving between business appointments seldom finds the long trips relaxing. Experiences of boredom are common. This may be the time when audiotapes can be used to present new ideas or assist in the development of new skills. Boredom or sensory monotony can be addressed effectively through adequate planning.

Environmental Modification. Changing the environment is the most extensive approach to minimizing the frequency of stress-inducing situations. Job-related stresses may be avoided by carefully identifying experiences and personalities that are abrasive or stress-producing and minimizing contact to the extent possible. Changing the physical work environment may be difficult unless the client moves to a new position or a new company, but the immediate interpersonal environment can be modified considerably by planning interaction patterns. Committee membership in groups that are stress inducing might be better delegated to someone else who experiences less stress from the activity or who obtains enjoyment from participation.

Stress often results when clients set themselves up for frustration by lack of assertiveness in structuring the immediate work environment. Clients have more control over their work situation than they may realize. Assisting the client in optimally using that control to avoid stress and subsequent physiological arousal is an important role of the professional nurse in comprehensive health counseling. If a job change is required by the client to decrease stress, new employment possibilities should be analyzed to make sure that stress phenomena similar to those already encountered are not an inherent part of the new employment setting.

Psychophysiological Preparation to Increase Stress Resistance

Resistance to stress is achieved through psychological and physical conditioning. Such preparation is an important intervention point in stress management. Psychological conditioning consists of (1) enhancing feelings of self-esteem, (2) increasing assertiveness, (3) developing goal alternatives, and (4) reorienting cognitive appraisal. The major approach to physical conditioning for stress resistance is physical exercise, described in Chapter 11 of this book. Approaches to psychological conditioning will be briefly described.

Enhancing Self-Esteem. While self-esteem as a personality trait is developed over time, studies have shown that the level of self-esteem can be changed. Several methods have been suggested by Girdano and Everly[17] for achieving a positive image of self. One approach is positive verbalization. In using this technique, clients identify positive aspects of self or personal characteristics that they value highly. Each characteristic, one per day, is placed on a 3 × 5 index card, and the cards are placed in a conspicuous place. Each card should be read several times a day. This technique helps clients to become comfortable with positive thoughts about themselves and decreases the amount of time spent in self-devaluation. Identifying positive characteristics of the self can also focus attention on attributes that are admired by others.

Increased self-awareness of positive characteristics and their presence in conscious thought will result in more frequent behavior that reflects these attributes and more positive responses from significant others.

Increasing Assertiveness. Substituting positive, assertive behaviors for negative, passive ones can increase personal capacity for psychological resistance to stress. Assertiveness is the appropriate expression of oneself, one's thoughts, and one's feelings and can result in greater personal satisfaction in living. Assertiveness is more constructive than aggression and deals more effectively than aggression with most problems encountered in the course of living. Many books and articles have been written on assertiveness training. Assertiveness allows individuals to share their perceptions and feelings with others in a way that facilitates rather than inhibits personal or group productivity. Several suggestions for becoming more assertive that clients ought to be encouraged to use include the following:

- Making a deliberate effort to greet others and call them by name
- Maintaining eye contact during conversations
- Commenting on the positive characteristics of others
- Initiating conversation
- Expressing opinions
- Expressing feelings
- Disagreeing with others when holding opposing viewpoints
- Taking initiative to engage in a new behavior or learn a new activity

The webs and constraints that entangle human beings are frequently self-constructed and disappear easily when efforts are made to become more open, assertive, and self-fulfilling. While it is possible for clients through use of simple techniques to become more assertive, very passive and reserved clients might well benefit from more comprehensive assertiveness training by a competent instructor or counselor. The nurse can assist clients in locating such resources for personal development.

Developing Goal Alternatives.[18] Clients must be aware not only of the goals that they have set but of why accomplishment of those goals is rewarding. Similar sources of reward or reinforcement may be possible through accomplishment of alternative goals. For example, a client's wished-for advancement within his or her current work situation may not materialize. If the primary reasons for wanting advancement are recognition and increased income, these rewards may be achieved by accomplishing similar goals. Recognition can come through community or organizational involvement and additional monies may be generated through wise investments. Flexibility on the part of the client permits achievement of desired outcomes through several different approaches. As a result, lack of success in initial attempts to reach goals becomes much less ominous because of the probability of success in similar tasks. The format for assisting clients to develop a goal alternative system is presented in Figure 13–4.

Reorienting Cognitive Appraisal. Personal perception of an event determines whether or not the situation will operate as a stressor for any given individual. Two important aspects of cognitive appraisal are: (1) the internal and external demands perceived in an event and (2) the assessment of personal resources to cope with the envisioned demands.[19] When perceived demands are greater than perceived resources, distress can occur. Cognitive reappraisal can be a powerful tool for lowering stress. For example, criticism from a close family member or friend may be dealt with as if it was a major disaster. However, an individual can reorient cognitive appraisal of the criticism by analyzing the statement perceived to be critical to see if there is any truth in the remark, considering the mood of the critical individual at the time, or placing the critical statement in the context

Step 1: What is the desired goal? _____

Step 2: Is this goal immediately obtainable?
    _____ No
    _____ Yes STOP! Why are you doing this exercise?

Step 3: What is (are) the obstacle(s) that keep(s) you from obtaining this goal?

_____

_____

_____

Step 4: Can this obstacle be removed within a reasonable time period?

    _____ No _____ Yes   If any reasonable methods exist by which you may obtain your goal by removing the obstacle, use them.

Step 5: Consider your desired goal. Take some time and make a list of the specific rewards or desirable characteristics that make that goal desirable to you. Now go back and give each one of those desirable characteristics a score indicative of how important each one is to you. A score of 1 would be the lowest; 10, the highest. Do this very carefully; it is very important.

Figure 13–4. Format for identification of a goal alternative system. (continued on next page). *(From Girdano, D., & Everly, G.,* Controlling Stress and Tension: A holistic approach, *pp. 131–132. Reproduced by permission of Prentice-Hall, Inc. Englewood Cliffs, N.J.)*

	Rewards	Points

Step 6: Are there any other reasonable ways to obtain those *same* rewards listed in Step 5?

_____ Yes
List alternatives, then try them out:

_____
_____
_____
_____

_____ No
If you have arrived at this point, it seems apparent that *all* of those desirable characteristics listed in Step 5 are currently unobtainable. Therefore, instead of feeling sorry for yourself, make a list of alternatives that are *possible* and have at least some of the same desirable characteristics as the original goal. Select the behavior that results in the highest-point score possible. This alternative is your best one because it is most similar to your original behavior, based on the points assigned in Step 5.

	Alternatives	Points

Figure 13–4. (continued)

of all the other interactions with the same individual. As another example, a person who is turned down for a desired job may remark, "This shows how undesirable I am; I'll never amount to anything." The resulting emotions are likely to be worthlessness, hopelessness, and guilt. Others might perceive the rejection differently, as an opportunity to learn why they were not selected for the job, and utilize the feedback obtained from the job interview to seek a position that is better suited to their talents and skills.[20]

Cognitive reappraisal is a structured, short-term intervention intended to help the client identify and change distorted thought patterns that trigger and perpetuate distress. Clients can be taught to recognize cognitive distortions and interrupt self-defeating and stress-producing thoughts. Many potential stressors can be defused if they are examined in an objective manner or within the context of a broad life perspective.

Counterconditioning to Avoid Physiological Arousal

Control of physiological responses to stressful events through counterconditioning techniques is receiving increasing attention within the health community as an approach to stress management. The fact that one can control the autonomical nervous system, which had been thought to be under unconscious control, has been discovered only in recent years through classical conditioning experiments. The goal of counterconditioning is to replace muscle tension and heightened sympathetic nervous system activity produced by stress with muscle relaxation and increased parasympathetic functioning. The three interventions most frequently used to assist the client in accomplishing this are relaxation training, biofeedback, and imagery. Each of these approaches to stress management will be discussed here within the context of the author's private practice.

The clients that the author sees have essential hypertension, are monitored within the hypertension program of the county health department, have a private physician, and are interested in relaxation and biofeedback as an approach to hypertension control. Participation in the program is voluntary. The program is 13 to 16 weeks in length, with 6 months of follow-up.

For the first 4 weeks, clients are seen individually for purposes of assessment. Information is gathered on client history, therapeutic regimen, and life style. In addition, the Modified Health Locus of Control (MHLC) Scale, Health Value Scale, Speilberger State–Trait Anxiety Scale, Twenty Favorite Activities, Signs of Distress, and Stress Charting* are completed by clients. Systolic and diastolic blood pressure (resting) and muscle tension (forearm and forehead) are measured at each visit. Muscle tension is measured by an electromyogram (EMG). In addition, goals of the client for the relaxation program are discussed and clarified. Identifying client expectations and the reality of such expectations is an important activity during initial sessions.

During the second phase of the program, clients attend three group-training sessions in which the physiological effects of stress are discussed and training in progressive relaxation is initiated. The rationale for progressive relaxations and an overview of the approach used by the author in working with clients is presented below.

Progressive Relaxation through Tension–Relaxation Techniques.

Edmund Jacobson, who began his work on relaxation as early as 1908 at Harvard University, proposed that relaxation decreases voluntary muscle activity and activity within the sympathetic nervous system while increasing parasympathetic functioning.[21] There has been an increasing accumulation of evidence in the scientific literature that supports Jacobson's findings that tension levels can be reduced through use of relaxation skills. Relaxation

---

* See Chapter 6 for description of these instruments.

appears to be a way of turning off the body's response to the sympathetic nervous system and of actually decreasing neurohormonal changes that take place in reaction to the experience of negative tension states.[22]

Relaxation is thought to result in the following changes:

- Decrease in the body's oxygen consumption
- Lowered metabolism
- Decreased respiration rate
- Decreased heart rate
- Decreased muscle tension
- Decreased premature ventricular contractions
- Decreased systolic and diastolic blood pressures
- Increased alpha brain waves

The relaxation procedures that the author uses are an adaptation of the basic procedures presented by Bernstein and Borkovec.[23] A very pleasant, quiet, sound-proofed room where lighting can be dimmed to a low level, with reclining lawn or lounge chairs for clients, provides an optimum setting for group relaxation training. External noise is particularly disturbing to clients who are just beginning relaxation training, since the ability to maintain inner awareness or consciousness and to block out external stimuli is a skill developed over time.

Before each session, tight clothing should be loosened, glasses removed, shoes removed, and a comfortable position assumed in the chair. Relaxation should never be taught with clients lying flat. Although this is a common position assumed for rest and sleep, it often results in muscle strain in upper back and neck along with drowsiness, which interferes with training. A reclining position or sitting position is most appropriate. The reclining position recommended by the author for relaxation training of clients is depicted in Figure 13–5.

At the beginning of each session, clients are encouraged to focus on their own breathing as the air moves gently in and out. The purpose of this focusing activity is to increase awareness of self and the often imperceptible functions of the human body. The author guides clients through the relaxation maneuvers one by one. The relaxation sequence is progressively modified throughout the three sessions as indicated below.

Session I. Following the focusing activity, clients are moved slowly through tension and relaxation cycles for each of the major muscle groups listed in Table 13–2, maintaining tension for 8 to 10 seconds and releasing tension instantaneously on cue. The entire tension–relaxation cycle should be repeated twice during the first session to increase clients' awareness of the differences in body sensations during tensed and relaxed periods. The tension–relaxation instructions should be given very slowly, allowing clients to enjoy the feelings of relaxation they are experiencing.

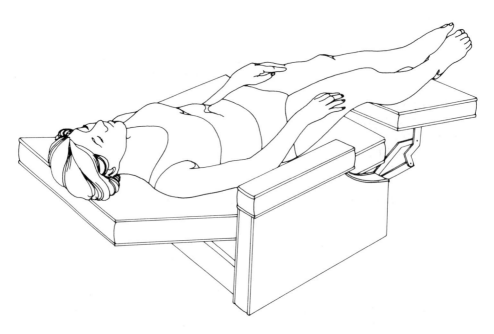

Figure 13–5. Appropriate reclining position for relaxation training.

The guidance provided by the nurse is critical for successful relaxation. A detailed description of the many pertinent considerations is beyond the scope of this book. The reader is referred to other sources for additional information.[24-26]

Session II. After the first group session, training tapes are used by clients at home to facilitate daily practice of relaxation techniques. Clients are also requested to keep a schedule of the frequency and length of time that relaxation is practiced. A self-report sheet is provided. This report is turned in at the beginning of each session. During the first part of the second session, the fifteen-muscle-group tension–relaxation cycle is again reviewed and practiced. In the second half of the session, a relaxation procedure is taught to the group that combines the fifteen muscle groups into seven muscle groups (Table 13–3).

During the seven-muscle-group sequence, clients may report that they did not achieve as deep relaxation as with the 15-muscle-group sequence. This is to be expected. Encourage clients to practice using seven-muscle groups, assuring them that they will develop increasing comfort and skill with the procedure as they engage in home practice. During the second week of practice, clients are encouraged to "think through" the relaxation procedure and do their own coaching. A "prompt sheet" on the sequence of the seven-muscle groups is sent home with them for reference. This is intended

TABLE 13–2. FIFTEEN-MUSCLE GROUP SEQUENCE FOR TENSION–RELAXATION CYCLE

Muscle Group	Abbreviated Instructions
1. Right hand and forearm	Make a fist.
2. Right upper arm	Pull elbow tightly into side.
3. Left hand and forearm	Make a fist.
4. Left upper arm	Pull elbow tightly into side.
5. Forehead	Wrinkle brow.
6. Upper cheeks and nose	Squint eyes and wrinkle nose.
7. Lower cheeks and jaws	Place teeth together and make a "forced" smile.
8. Neck and throat	Pull chin toward chest.
9. Chest, shoulders, and upper back	Take a deep breath. Push shoulder blades toward each other.
10. Upper abdomen	Pull stomach in and hold.
11. Lower abdomen	Bear down against the seat of the chair.
12. Right upper leg	Push down against the foot of the chair.
13. Right lower leg and foot	Point toes toward head and body.
14. Left upper leg	Push down against the foot of the chair.
15. Left lower leg and foot	Point toes toward head and body.

TABLE 13–3. SEVEN MUSCLE GROUPS FOR TENSION–RELAXATION CYCLE

Muscle Group	Abbreviated Instructions
1. Right hand, forearm, and upper arm	Make a fist and pull elbow tightly into side.
2. Left hand, forearm, and upper arm	Make a fist and pull elbow tightly into side.
3. Forehead, upper cheeks and nose, lower cheeks and jaws	Wrinkle brow; squint eyes; wrinkle nose; place teeth together and make a "forced" smile.
4. Neck and throat	Pull chin toward chest.
5. Chest, shoulders, back, upper and lower abdomen	Take a deep breath; push shoulder blades toward each other; pull stomach in and bear down.
6. Right upper leg, lower leg, and foot	Push down against the foot of the chair and point toes toward head and body.
7. Left upper leg, lower leg, and foot	Push down against the foot of the chair and point toes toward head and body.

to move clients toward independent practice of relaxation rather than encouraging reliance on the nurse or the coaching tape as a means of providing relaxation cues.

Session III. During the first part of the third session, self-report sheets on frequency and time of practice are again collected. Clients are encouraged to talk about any difficulties they are having. Some common problems that clients report include:

- Overly rapid self-pacing through the relaxation sequence
- Distraction by environmental noise
- Difficulty keeping attention on own monologue
- Interruption of distracting thoughts during relaxation
- Residual tension in some muscles after tension–relaxation

The problem of overly rapid self-pacing can usually be solved by encouraging clients to slow down internal speech or coaching pace. Phrases like "I feel calm," "I feel very relaxed," and "My arms and legs feel heavy" can be interspersed throughout self-instruction. To avoid distraction by environmental noise, a time of day should be chosen when the client is alone and without interruption. This may be at home in the evening or at the office during the noon hour. Encouraging family members to join in the relaxation practice sessions is another way of minimizing environmental distractions and fostering stress management skills among all members of the family.

Interruption of extraneous thoughts can also be curtailed if clients focus on the physical sensations experienced during relaxation and on the character of their own breathing.

If clients are experiencing any remaining tension after one tension-relaxation cycle in a particular muscle group, the tension-relaxation sequence should be repeated. Generally, after tensing and relaxing a second time, residual tension is considerably diminished.

During the last half of the third session, a relaxation procedure for four muscle groups is taught. While tensing smaller groups of muscles may result in little risk for hypertensive clients, tensing large groups of muscles may significantly increase blood pressure. Therefore, clients with high systolic and diastolic blood pressure should not progress to the four-muscle-group tension-relaxation cycle. Instead, counting down or recall (to be described in the following sections) should be used. For nonhypertensive clients, the seven-muscle groups can be combined into four-muscle groups, as shown in Table 13–4.

Once clients have learned to achieve deep relaxation using the four muscle groups, the entire relaxation procedure, including focusing and tension–relaxation cycles, can be carried out in 10 to 12 minutes. The object of shortening the procedure is not speed per se, but greater flexibility for the client in using relaxation at any time in a variety of settings.

Progressive muscle relaxation lowered blood pressure and decreased

TABLE 13–4. FOUR MUSCLE GROUPS FOR TENSION–RELAXATION CYCLE

Muscle Group	Abbreviated Instructions
1. Entire right and left arms	Make fists with both hands and pull both elbows tightly into sides.
2. Muscles of face, neck, and throat	Wrinkle brow; squint eyes; wrinkle nose; place teeth together; make a "forced" smile; pull chin toward chest.
3. Chest, shoulders, back, upper and lower abdomen	Take a deep breath; push shoulder blades toward each other; pull stomach in and bear down.
4. Entire right and left legs	Push down against the foot of the chair with both feet and point toes toward head and body.

muscle tension in the hypertensive clients with whom this author worked.[27] Following the development of skill with relaxation, hypertensive clients also showed decreased anxiety and increased perception of internal control of health status.[28] Krause and Stryker[29] found that men with internal locus-of-control orientations coped more effectively with stress than those with external locus-of-control beliefs. Thus, if clients can both lower physiological arousal and increase perceptions of control through use of progressive relaxation, this technique can be a useful counterconditioning strategy.

Progressive Relaxation without Tension. While tension–relaxation techniques result in high levels of voluntary muscle relaxation, clients can be taught how to relax without first tensing muscles. Such techniques are taught to clients by the author during individual sessions. They include relaxation through recall, relaxation through counting down, and relaxation through imagery. The major advantage of these techniques is that tension is no longer required. This is particularly important for clients with hypertension, where, as previously indicated, greater elevations in pressure may be caused by prolonged or extensive muscle tensing. Deep relaxation without tension is the goal for the hypertensive client.

Relaxation Through Recall. In this approach, the client is asked to focus on feelings of tension experienced in each of the four-muscle groups used in Session III. With increased sensitivity to muscle sensations, the tension in a particular muscle group should be recognized. The client is asked to recall feelings of relaxation previously experienced in that part of the body and to allow the target muscle group to become similarly relaxed. The sequence of the four muscle groups is the same as the tension–relaxation sequence. The suggestions of relaxation should continue for 30 to 45 seconds for each muscle group. If recall is ineffective at first, the seven- or four-muscle-group tension–relaxation cycle can be repeated, followed immediately by recall to make the sensations of tension and relaxation more vivid. Transition from tension–relaxation techniques to use of recall may be a difficult step for some clients, yet with practice clients can master this self-control technique.

Phrases that can be repeated to facilitate relaxation through recall are listed in Table 13–5. These phrases have been suggested by Elmer and Alyce Green as a result of work in biofeedback at the Menninger Foundation. Such phrases result in physiological imagery that can decrease both sympathetic nervous system activity and tension in voluntary muscles.

Relaxation Through Counting Down. The countdown procedure initially focuses on each of the seven- or four-muscle groups used previously. The

---

TABLE 13–5. RELAXATION-PROMOTING PHRASES

---

1. I feel quiet.
2. I am beginning to feel quite relaxed.
3. My feet feel heavy and relaxed.
4. My ankles, my knees, and my hips feel heavy.
5. My solar plexus and the whole central portion of my body feel relaxed and quiet.
6. My hands, my arms, and my shoulders feel heavy, relaxed, and comfortable.
7. My neck, my jaws, and my forehead feel relaxed. They feel comfortable and smooth.
8. My whole body feels quite heavy, comfortable, and relaxed.
9. I am quite relaxed.
10. My arms and hands are heavy and warm.
11. I feel quite quiet.
12. My whole body is relaxed and my hands are warm—relaxed and warm.
13. My hands are warm.
14. Warmth is flowing into my hands. They are warm, warm.
15. I can feel the warmth flowing down my arms into my hands.
16. My hands are warm, relaxed, and warm.
17. My whole body feels quiet, comfortable, and relaxed.
18. My mind is quiet.
19. I withdraw my thoughts from the surroundings and I feel serene and still.
20. My thoughts are turned inward and I am at ease.
21. Deep within my mind, I can visualize and experience myself as relaxed, comfortable, and still.
22. I am alert, but in an easy, quiet, inward-turned way.
23. My mind is calm and quiet.
24. I feel an inward quietness.

---

client is encouraged to relax each muscle group progressively as the count proceeds from 10 down to 1. When the client has practiced and become skilled with this procedure, total body countdown can be used: relaxing the entire body while silently counting down from 10 to 1. This is a particularly useful procedure for the office or when facing stressful social situations. In 2 to 3 minutes, the skilled client can achieve total body relaxation while in a sitting position with eyes open and focused on a specific object. This is one of the shortest procedures through which relaxation can be accomplished. Mini-relaxation sessions several times throughout the day can promote generalization of relaxation training to everyday life.

Relaxation Through Imagery. The client may find that passively concentrating on pleasant scenes or experiences from the past can greatly facilitate relaxation. Recalling the warmth of the sun, the feeling of warm sand, the sensations of a gentle breeze, the vision of palm trees swaying, or sounds of ocean waves may be comfortable and pleasant for clients. Such recall can promote muscle relaxation.

Each client will vary in those scenes or images that result in actual changes in muscle tension (EMG). For some clients, visualizing specific colors, shapes, or patterns will be as effective as visualizing landscapes or scenes. The important point for the nurse to emphasize to the client concerning use of imagery is that feelings and sensations that accompany specific visualizations should be the primary dimensions for focus, rather than visual detail.

If clients initially have difficulty in using imagery or visualization for relaxation, the nurse may use one of the following techniques:

- Have the client with eyes closed visualize a particular room of his or her house (living room, bedroom, kitchen), focusing on colors, shapes, and specific objects. The client's mind should wander about the room, with the client describing verbally what is seen in as much detail as possible
- Have the client focus on a particular piece of clothing that is a personal favorite. The client should describe the color, texture, design, and trim of the clothing and how it feels when worn (e.g., soft, loose, fitted, light, warm)

As individuals become more vivid in descriptions of concrete objects, their ability to use less concrete imagery for purposes of relaxation increases. Use of imagery can be an important and pleasant adjunct to other relaxation techniques described.

Increasingly, research on relaxation techniques indicates the usefulness of such approaches in the prevention and treatment of a variety of stress-related diseases. Relaxation also has been shown to increase feelings of energy, vitality, and self-control. However, like any other skill, continued use and practice of approaches to relaxation is essential if clients are to experience maximal prevention and health-promotion benefits from their use.[30] The reader is referred to Snyder[31] for further discussion of progressive relaxation as a nursing intervention. Benson[32] and Scandrett and Uecker[33] provide overviews of a variety of other relaxation techniques such as relaxation response, autogenic training, yoga, meditation, and hypnosis.

Biofeedback. During individual sessions following group relaxation training, the author assists clients in acquiring greater skill in relaxation through providing biofeedback regarding level of muscle tension (EMG) and skin temperature. A general discussion regarding use of biofeedback for stress management is presented below; however, a detailed discussion of the many biofeedback modes and how to use them in working with individual clients is beyond the scope of this book.

Biofeedback has in recent years offered the possibility for awareness and control of processes previously thought to be under unconscious rather than conscious control. Biofeedback can be defined as a process in which a person learns reliably to influence physiological responses that are not ordinarily under voluntary control. The four basic operations in biofeedback are as follows.[34]

1. Detection and amplification of bioelectrical potentials
2. Conversion of bioelectrical signals to easy-to-process information
3. Feedback of information to the client
4. Voluntary control of target response through learning based on feedback

The foundations of biofeedback hinge on a very simple idea: Clients need to be provided with information about what is going on inside their bodies, since bodily functions cannot be controlled unless information about them is available to the controller.[35] A wide range of autonomical processes can be controlled through response to feedback. Some of the physiological parameters that have been controlled or modified through feedback include the following:

- *Heart rate*—acceleration and deceleration
- *Heart rhythm*—occurrences of premature ventricular contractions
- *Blood pressure*—systolic and diastolic
- *Peripheral vascular responses*—skin surface temperature
- *Muscle tension*—muscle contractility
- *Alpha wave activity*—brain wave patterns
- *Galvanic skin response*—resistance of skin to passage of electrical current
- *Sexual response*—increased or decreased sexual arousal

Biofeedback is an important modality for facilitating stress management. The ultimate goal is establishing self-regulation that allows the client to control autonomical responses. A permanent change in the target response is desired following training. While biofeedback instrumentation facilitates learning during the training period, the client must learn to read and interpret body signals without the aid of equipment and to function effectively in modifying responses. That is, relaxation rather than tension (fight-or-flight response) should result when stress occurs. It is the belief of the author that relaxation techniques when taught prior to the use of biofeedback provide the client with specific skills for controlling body responses.

The mechanism for biofeedback is illustrated in Figure 13–6. Electrophysiologic studies indicate that every perception of external events (OUTS) has associated electrical activity in both conscious and unconscious central nervous system structures, those involved in both emotional and mental responses. The limbic system is considered primarily unconscious, although neural pathways lead from limbic structures directly to the cortical region,

Normally Conscious Voluntary Domain—Cortical and Craniospinal

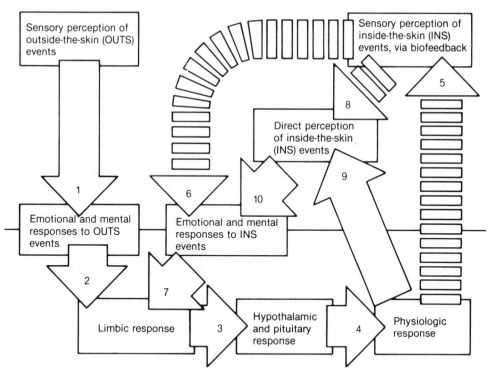

Normally Unconscious Involuntary Domain—Subcortical and Autonomic

Figure 13–6. Simplified operational diagram of "self-regulation" of psychophysiologic events and processes. *(From Green, E., Green, A., & Norris, P. Self-regulation training for control of hypertension.* Primary Cardiology, *March 1980, p. 129. With permission.)*

providing some contact with conscious centers. Emotional states and visceral processes are correlated with electrophysiologic activity in the limbic system. The limbic system is connected to the hypothalamus, where limbic signals are converted to autonomical and hormonal processes through the transducing capacities of the hypothalamus and pituitary. It is a relatively new idea, that one can detect what is going on inside the skin (INS) and change it voluntarily in a direction of choice. However, when an individual is given continuous auditory or visual feedback of physiological information, a new mental–emotional response can be learned. The new response is followed by an appropriate limbic response that combines with, modifies, or replaces the original response. Subsequently, changes occur in the patterns of hypothalamic firing and pituitary response; the physiological state is altered, and this change is fed back via the monitor to the conscious cortex.[36]

Two specific feedback modalities used by the author in her practice will be discussed: electromyograph feedback and skin-temperature feedback. These modalities are frequently used in the clinical setting and appear most relevant for the kinds of clients that nurses would be seeing for stress management; that is, clients learning relaxation as a means of health promotion, prevention, or treatment of stress-related disorders.

Electromyograph (EMG) Feedback. Early experimental work in this area was conducted by Basmajian, using needle electrodes. Subjects learned to control the rate of firing of various motor units within muscles.[37] Electromyograph feedback is now used to train clients to lower tension in whole muscle groups. The most frequent sites of training are the forearm and the forehead (frontalis muscle). The mechanism is that of voluntary muscle control, as opposed to autonomical conditioning as in temperature training. The forearm is easier to train than the frontalis muscle, so it is often recommended for beginning sessions. Once muscle control is achieved in the forearm, training can be moved to the frontalis. It is generally believed that the frontalis muscle is a good indicator of the overall state of body tension.

The EMG measures the amount of electrical discharge in the muscle fibers and quantifies muscle contraction in microvolts, showing this value on a meter as an auditory or visual display. Once clients are aware of what their level of muscle tension is, they can begin to work on bringing about change. Changes in muscle tension levels can be brought about primarily in two ways: by relaxation or by use of imagery.

The EMG feedback technique has been shown to be effective in treating many stress-related disorders, such as chronic back pain, tension headaches, and essential hypertension. It can also be used for muscle reeducation (increasing muscle tension) in clients with cerebrovascular accidents and other central nervous system insults.[38]

The results of EMG training reported by clients in a variety of settings are very impressive. They have reported experiencing decreased muscle strain and discomfort, decreased feelings of mental stress, anxiety, and tension, increased feelings of personal control, increased energy, and enhanced feelings of health and well-being. Positive changes in physiological parameters (e.g., muscle tension, heart rate, and diastolic and systolic blood pressure) are supported in the literature. Further research is needed before the parameters of clinical usefulness are established for this biofeedback modality.

Skin-Temperature Feedback. Historically, the major thrust for use of temperature control as a therapeutic modality came through the work of Elmer and Allyce Green in their laboratory at the Menninger Foundation. They developed the use of temperature training for treatment of migraine headache.[39] More recently, the Greens have used temperature training successfully in the treatment of hypertension, lowering both systolic and diastolic pressures.[40] Temperature training has also been used successfully in treatment of Raynaud's and Buerger's diseases, where spasms of peripheral arteries cause coldness of extremities.

Peripheral skin temperature is regulated by vasomotor control mechanisms. The body responds to external temperature changes through a thermoregulatory response by constriction or dilation of the smooth muscles around the peripheral blood vessels. With decreases in environmental temperature, these vascular changes allow increased blood flow to internal organs and maintenance of constant core temperature. Biochemical factors influencing skin temperature are alcohol, tobacco, histamine, epinephrine, lactic acid, and carbon dioxide. Psychological factors influencing skin temperature include emotional stress, anxiety, and environmental stimuli. Activation of the sympathetic nervous system and subsequent neurohormonal changes result in smooth muscle constriction around the peripheral vessels and decreased skin temperature. Thus, an increase in skin temperature can reflect decreased sympathetic nervous system activity.[41]

Heat flow constitutes an indirect measure of blood flow. In temperature training, a thermistor is attached to the finger, and visual or auditory feedback is used to indicate temperature change. Initial readings, which can range from 75 F to 96 F, can give a clue as to the potential effectiveness of temperature training for any given client. Fuller[42] has indicated that if initial finger temperature readings are above 90 F (32.2 C), the potential for raising temperature is limited compared to when initial readings are between 75 F (23.8 C) and 90 F (32.3 C).

Quiet internal states produced by relaxation or imagery (visualization of warming sensations in the extremities) appear to decrease sympathetic nervous system activity and cause peripheral dilation. This change is reflected in increased finger temperature, which provides helpful feedback to the client.

The effectiveness of temperature training in decreasing physiological responses to stress must be further evaluated through carefully designed clinical research. To date, systematic studies support the potential usefulness of this technique in self-management of hypertension, migraine headache, and other circulation disorders.

Further research is needed concerning the role of biofeedback in health promotion and disease prevention. Schwartz[43] provides an overview of varying theories of biofeedback. The nine theoretical frameworks presented can provide the basis for future psychophysiological research efforts to delineate the usefulness of biofeedback in enhancing well-being.

SUMMARY

A number of different approaches for assisting individuals and families in managing stress have been presented in order to familiarize the reader with the range of strategies available. Some approaches suggested are relatively unstructured, while others are more formally defined and require instrumentation. The decision regarding which strategies to use must be made collaboratively by the client and the nurse. This decision should be based on the characteristics of the client, sources of stress experienced by the client, and general patterns of response to stressful events. The reader is encouraged to consult the references at the end of this chapter for further information on relaxation training and biofeedback.

REFERENCES

1. Selye, H. Introduction. In D. Wheatley (Ed.), *Stress and the heart.* New York: Raven Press, 1977.
2. Hughes, G. H., Pearsons, M. A., & Reinhart, G. R. Stress: Sources, effects and management. *Family and Community Health,* May 1984, 7 (1), 47–58.
3. Selye, op. cit., p. 3.
4. Mueller, D. P., Edwards, D. W., & Yarvis, R. M. Stressful life events and psychiatric symptomatology: Change or undesirability? *Journal of Health and Social Behavior,* 1977, *18,* 307–317.
5. Ross, C. E., & Minowsky, J. A comparison of life event weighting schemes: Change, undesirability, and effect-proportional indices. *Journal of Health and Social Behavior,* 1979, *20,* 166–177.
6. Matheny, K. B., & Cupp, P. Control, desirability, and anticipation as moderating variables between life change and illness. *Journal of Human Stress,* June 1983, 9 (2), 14–23.
7. Zautra, A., & Sandler, I. Life event needs assessments: Two models for measuring preventable mental health problems. *Prevention in Human Services,* 1983, 2 (4), 35–58.
8. Papez, J. W. A proposed mechanism of emotion. *American Medical Association Archives of Neurology and Psychiatry,* 1937, *38,* 725–743.
9. McLean, P. D. Psychosomatic disease and the "visceral brain": Recent developments bearing on the Papez theory of emotion. *Psychosomatic Medicine,* 1949, *11,* 338–353.

10. Greene, E. E., Green, A. M., & Norris, P. A. Self-regulation training for control of hypertension. *Primary Cardiology*, March 1980, *6*, 126–137.
11. Borysenko, J. Stress, coping, and the immune system. In J. D. Matarazzo, S. M. Weiss, J. A. Herd, et al. (Eds.), *Behavioral health: A handbook of health enhancement and disease prevention*. New York: Wiley, 1984, pp. 248–260.
12. Sutterley, D. C. Stress and health: A survey of self-regulation modalities. *Topics in Clinical Nursing*, April 1979, *1*, 1–21.
13. Holmes, T. H., & Rahe, R. H. The social readjustment rating scale. *Journal of Psychosomatic Research*, 1967, *11*, 213–218.
14. Girdano, D., & Everly, G. *Controlling stress and tension*. Englewood Cliffs, N.J.: Prentice-Hall, 1979.
15. Ibid., p. 128.
16. Everly, G. S., Jr. Time management: A behavioral strategy for disease prevention and health enhancement. In J. D. Matarazzo, S. M. Weiss, J. A. Herd, et al. (Eds.), *Behavioral health: A handbook of health enhancement and disease prevention*. New York: Wiley, 1984, pp. 363–370.
17. Girdano & Everly, op. cit., p. 146.
18. Ibid. pp. 129–133.
19. Jaremko, M. E. Stress inoculation training: A generic approach for the prevention of stress-related disorders. *The Personal and Guidance Journal*, May 1984, *62* (9), 544–550.
20. Scandrett, S. Cognitive reappraisal. In G. M. Bulechek & J. C. McCloskey (Eds.), *Nursing interventions: Treatments for nursing diagnoses*. Philadelphia: Saunders, 1985, pp. 49–57.
21. Bernstein, D. A., & Borkovec, T. D. *Progressive relaxation training: A manual for the helping professions*. Champaign, Ill.: Research Press, 1973.
22. Cautela, J. R., & Groden, J. *Relaxation: A comprehensive manual for adults, children, and children with special needs*. Champaign, Ill.: Research Press, 1978.
23. Bernstein & Borkovec, op. cit., pp. 25–32.
24. Cautela & Groden, op. cit., pp. 1–35.
25. Jacobson, E. *Anxiety and tension control*. Philadelphia: Lippincott, 1964.
26. Bernstein & Borkovec, op. cit., 1–56.
27. Pender, N. J. Physiologic responses of clients with essential hypertension to progressive muscle relaxation training. *Research in Nursing and Health*, 1984, *7*, 197–203.
28. Pender, N. J. Effects of progressive muscle relaxation training on anxiety and health locus of control among hypertensive clients. *Research in Nursing and Health*, 1985, *8*, 67–72.
29. Krause, N., & Stryker, S. Stress and well-being: The buffering role of locus of control beliefs. *Social Science and Medicine*, 1984, *18* (9), 783–790.
30. Bernstein & Borkovec, op. cit., pp. 52–70.
31. Snyder, M. Progressive relaxation as a nursing intervention: An analysis. *Advances in Nursing Science*, April 1984, *6* (3), 47–58.
32. Benson, H. The relaxation response and stress. In J. D. Matarazzo, S. M. Weiss, J. A. Herd, et al. (Eds.), *Behavioral health: A handbook of health enhancement and disease prevention*. New York: Wiley, 1984, pp. 326–337.
33. Scandrett, S., & Uecker, S. Relaxation training. In G. M. Bulechek & J. C. McCloskey (Eds.), *Nursing interventions: treatments for nursing diagnoses*. Philadelphia: Saunders, 1985, pp. 22–48.

34. Blanchard, E. B., & Epstein, L. H. *A biofeedback primer.* Reading, Mass.: Addison-Wesley, 1978, pp. 7–9.
35. Gaarder, K. R., & Montgomery, P. S. *Clinical biofeedback: A procedural manual.* Baltimore: Williams & Wilkins, 1977.
36. Green, Green, & Norris, op. cit., p. 128.
37. Basmajian, J. V., Baeza, M., & Fabrigar, C. Conscious control and training of individual spinal motor neurons in normal human subjects. *Journal of New Drugs,* 1965, *5,* 78–85.
38. Fuller, G. D. *Biofeedback: Methods and procedures in clinical practice.* San Francisco: Biofeedback Press, 1977.
39. Sargent, J., Green, E. E., & Walters, E. D. The use of autogenic feedback training in a pilot study of migraine and tension headaches. *Headache,* 1972, *12,* 120–124.
40. Green, Green, & Norris, op. cit., pp. 126–137.
41. Ibid., p. 47.
42. Fuller, op. cit., p. 138.
43. Schwartz, G. E. Biofeedback as a paradigm for health enhancement and disease prevention: A systems perspective. In J. D. Matarazzo, S. M. Weiss, J. A. Herd, et al. (Eds.), *Behavioral health: A handbook of health enhancement and disease prevention.* New York: Wiley, 1984, pp. 308–325.

CHAPTER *14*

Social Support and Health

The nurse responsible for assisting clients of all ages in maintaining and improving health cannot ignore the importance of social networks as the context for personal health behaviors. Social networks such as families, social groups, organizations, and communities can facilitate or thwart efforts directed toward health protection and health promotion. Since social networks appear to influence health status and are amenable to change, the role of the nurse in assisting clients to assess, modify, and develop social support systems will be addressed in this chapter.

SOCIAL NETWORKS

Social networks consist of those persons or groups with whom clients maintain contact and have some form of social bond.[1,2] They exert a powerful influence on how persons think, act, and react. Social networks generally consist of family, neighbors, friends, fellow workers, and other acquaintances with whom the person interacts through work, organizational–political activities, travel, or leisure.[3] Networks can be classified as organized or personal. In an organized network such as a work group or service group, component individuals make up a larger social whole with common aims, interdependent roles, and a distinct subculture. In a personal network, only some, not all component individuals have relationships with one another. The extent to which persons within a social network know one another de-

394

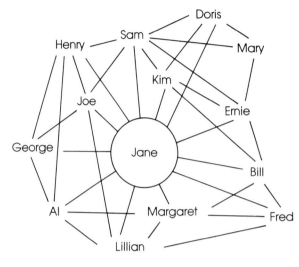

Work Group

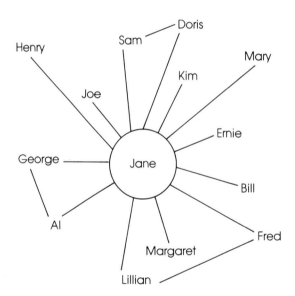

Personal Social Network

―――― = relationship or
acquaintance

Figure 14–1. Comparison of "connectedness" (density) of organized social network versus personal social network. In the work group, it is possible that everyone would know everyone else. In the personal social network, individuals seldom know all other persons in the network.

termines the connectedness of the network.[4] Figure 14–1 contrasts the connectedness of individuals within a hypothetical personal network as opposed to those in a hypothetical work group. The frame of reference for each diagram is a single individual, Jane.

CHARACTERISTICS OF SOCIAL NETWORKS

Social networks have a number of important characteristics of which the nurse should be aware. Key characteristics of social networks include:[5–7]

- Size—the number of people identified as belonging to a specific network. Generally, in order to be included in the network, an ongoing personal relationship must exist that results in some contact at least once a year
- Density—the number of dyadic relationships that exist among members of the network
- Homogeneity—members sharing common demographic, personal, or social characteristics
- Intensity—the amount of time spent in contact, emotional intensity, and intimacy (mutual confiding), and the degree of reciprocity characterizing relationships
- Content—the forms of relationships. The following types of content have been identified:
  Assistance—seeking help or aid from individuals in order to meet own needs
  Value similarity—congruity between desired end states (goals) and means for achieving desired end states
  Concern—extent of altruistic or caring (affective) emotions directed toward individuals
  Trust—using individuals as confidants for sharing information of a private or intimate nature
  Desired interaction—personal affinity or attraction to individuals for interaction–communication and physical proximity
  (Relationships may have one or or more content areas. Generally, the larger the number of content areas, the stronger the dyadic ties.)
- Dispersion—the ease with which network members can make face-to-face contact
- Duration—the length of time relationships within network have been in existence. Mean length of time may be most representative of network history
- Directionality—the extent of movement of component members toward common goal(s)

These characteristics may be applied to any social network in order to describe it in detail. Assessment and diagramming of social networks provide critical information for determining the adequacy of support available to clients.

Functions of Social Networks

Social networks can serve a number of functions for individuals. Social networks may serve any or all of the following three functions[8]

- Support—actions or behavior on the part of individuals within the network that assist the focal person in meeting personal goals or in dealing with the demands of a particular situation. Support can be tangible or intangible
  - Tangible support—money or active assistance
  - Intangible support—encouragement, personal warmth, love and/or emotional support
- Advice—information or guidance on how to achieve a certain goal or complete a certain task
- Feedback—provision of evaluative statements regarding how expectations or requirements for reaching specific goals are being met. Provides information on how well individuals are performing

Individuals within a social network often serve more than one of the above functions. Generally, the more functions each person in a social network serves, the more supportive the network is to the target member.

SOCIAL SUPPORT

Social support can be defined as the subjective feeling of belonging, of being accepted, loved, esteemed, valued, and needed for oneself, not for what one can do for others.[9] Support is provided to any individual by a specific group who constitute that person's social support system. A social support system is the set of personal contacts through which an individual maintains social identity, receives emotional support, material aid, information, and services, and makes new social contacts.[10] The support system represents an enduring pattern of continuous or intermittent ties that play a significant role in maintaining psychological and physical integrity of the individual over time. Social support systems are not static but dynamic, evolving, or changing throughout a person's life span. They provide security for individuals by sustained membership and active involvement in a defined human group.[11]

Five types of social support systems relevant to health have been identified and described in the literature: natural support systems, peer support systems, religious organizations or denominations, organized support systems of care-giving or helping professionals, and organized support groups not directed by health professionals. In most instances, the family (natural support system) constitutes the primary support group. Families, in order to provide appropriate support, must be sensitive to the needs of family members, establish effective communication, respect the unique needs of members, and establish expectations of mutual help and assistance.

Peer support systems consist of people who function informally as generalists or specialists in meeting the needs of others. Generalists are characterized by wisdom in human relations, knowledge about community caregiving systems, and gregariousness. They make contacts easily and enjoy being involved with other people. They maintain a reputation of helpfulness because of support provided to others. Informal care givers who are specialists generally have encountered an experience of major impact in their own life and achieved successful adjustment and growth. Because of extent of insight, their advice is sought primarily in relation to one specific area of concern. Examples include the avid runner, the health-food enthusiast, the widow, or the parents of a retarded child. Successful achievement or coping is the primary credential of the informal care giver who is viewed as a specialist.

Religious organizations or denominations constitute the oldest community support systems evident today. Churches or religious groups represent a congregation of individuals who hold regular meetings, share joint allegiance to theology, a common value system, a body of traditions, and a set of guidelines for living. Even highly mobile individuals may find a ready support system in the local denomination or church.

A third type of support system is composed of care-giving or helping professionals with a specific set of skills and services to offer clients.[12] The professional support system is seldom the first source of help for an individual. Family and close friends or peers are sought out initially for advice and support. It is often only when this source of help is unavailable, interrupted, or exhausted that health professionals enter the support scene.

Organized support systems not directed by health professionals include voluntary service groups and mutual help groups. Voluntary service groups provide assistance to individuals who are in need or for some reason are unable to provide services for themselves. Self-help groups (Alcoholics Anonymous, TOPS, Recovery, Inc.) attempt to effect change in behavior of members or promote adaptation to a life change such as chronic health problem, terminal illness, or disabled family member.[13]

All support systems of a given individual or family are synergistic. In combination, they represent the social resources available to facilitate stability and actualization.

FUNCTIONS OF SOCIAL SUPPORT GROUPS

The functions of social support groups in promoting and protecting health can be conceptualized in four ways, as depicted in Figure 14–2. Social groups

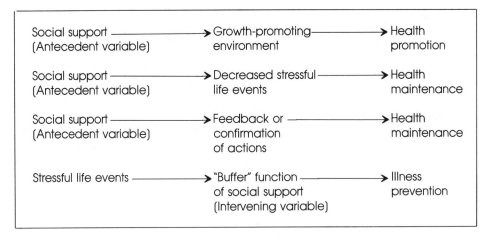

Figure 14–2. Possible impact of social support on health status.

can contribute to health by (1) creating a growth–promoting environment that enhances self-esteem and well-being, (2) decreasing the likelihood of stressful life events, (3) providing feedback or confirmation that actions are leading to anticipated and socially desirable consequences, (4) buffering the negative effects of stressful events by influencing interpretation of events and emotional responses to them, thus decreasing their illness-producing potential.

Personal and contextual factors that mediate the impact of stressful events include: constitutional strengths (e.g., little history of illness in family), extent of social support, health practices, and personal disposition.[14] Kobasa, Maddi, and Kahn describe the personality disposition of hardiness as consisting of commitment and involvement in life, feelings of control or that one is influential rather than helpless, and challenge or the belief that changes rather than stability are normal in life and represent interesting incentives to growth rather than threats to security.[15] Social support appears to be synergistically related to constitutional strengths, health practices, and personality predisposition in promoting and protecting health. Generally, mobilization of personal resources occurs first, followed by mobilization of the social support network. Both types of resources serve a protective or facilitative function.

The extent of integration of individuals within their social support system is a critical factor in mediating the impact of life events.[16] On the whole, poor social integration appears to be a more prevalent condition among individuals and families in the low-income group than at other socioeconomic levels.[17] Stress may also be greater in this group and extent of total supportive resources less. Among low socioeconomic groups, events that result in high levels of life stress, such as job loss, can also disrupt family ties. Thus, a state of high stress and low support may be chronic.[18] Persons with undifferentiated or minimal social support systems exhibit poorer coping behavior and less emotional stability than do those with well-developed, mutually supportive relations. Unfortunately, the fundamental mechanisms underlying the effects of support systems are not well understood.[19]

The relationship between socioeconomic class and pathological stress reactions has two possible explanations. The first is the social selection theory. That is, individuals with coping difficulties suffer from financial exigencies and distresses that result in their attaining and maintaining lower class status. Their lack of coping abilities results in their natural selection into the lower class. Alternative explanations are referred to as social causation theories. The essence of such theories is that the stress from community or neighborhood life is different in intensity and quality from that found in other class environments and the potential for meaningful support is lower, resulting in a high number of pathological reactions to stressful situations.[20]

The primary functions of social support groups are to augment personal strengths of members and promote achievement of life goals.

Within a support aggregate, the persons are dealt with as unique individuals. There is heightened sensitivity to needs that are deemed worthy of respect and satisfaction. The support group also plays an important function in providing accurate feedback. Through collecting and storing cues about the outside world, support groups can be characterized as follows:[21]

- They share common social concerns
- They provide intimacy
- They prevent isolation
- They respect mutual competencies
- They offer dependable assistance in crises
- They serve as referral agents
- They provide mutual challenge

Support During Crises

During a crises period, support groups take on added significance. They often increase in the incidence of supportive behavior for the target individuals or family and relieve the stress and strain of social roles temporarily through role complementarity and role adjustment.[22] Individuals and families are assisted in mobilizing psychological resources as well as attaining material resources to deal with the crisis situation. Increased access to both tangible and intangible resources is usually important during a crises. Unfortunately, low socioeconomic groups may have little access to both. A high level of stress during crises and lack of social support may in combination threaten health and increase the potential for illness.

Family as the Primary Support Group

For most individuals, work and family roles provide the infrastructure of social integration. The family serves an important function during early childhood in orienting individuals to values, beliefs, and behavior styles through social experiences and interaction patterns. These early learning experiences exert continuing influence on behavior throughout life. Resources of the family that can be instrumental in providing support include:

- Family traditions
- Value systems
- Childrearing practices
- Methods of discipline
- Emotional climate
- Curiosity and exploratory behavior
- Patterns of creative behavior
- Recreational pursuits
- Material and economic resources
- Time and money management skills
- Sense of identity and purpose
- Sharing and cooperation
- Coping strategies

Disruption of structural properties of families, such as broken homes because of death, separation, or divorce, have been shown to correlate with increased risk of both physical and emotional disorders.

The emotional support environment within the family of origin has been shown to be curvilinearly related to psychological problems in later adulthood. Too much warmth and overinvolvement on the part of the parents can engulf the child, leaving him or her unable to meet and master life's problems. Too little warmth results in feelings of rejection, powerlessness, lack of worth, and despair. Both support and stress are usually present to some extent in

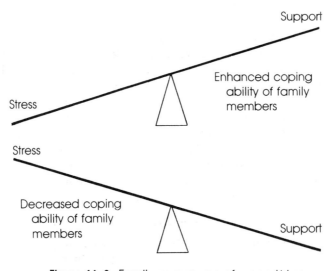

Figure 14–3. Family as a source of support/stress.

all families. The important consideration is the balance achieved.[23] Figure 14–3 depicts two possible combinations of stress and support that may typify any given family. Assessment of support characteristics of families allows the nurse to account more fully for a given client's level of health and adjustment. Lack of support by family members can interact with sources of stress synergistically, creating a high level of individual vulnerability. On the other hand, high-quality emotional support and task-oriented assistance from the family can provide a social context in which the client can grapple successfully with the problems of living.[24] Clark found that the more individuals participated in family activities, the fewer the indicators of ill-health. He hypothesized that family involvement may buffer stress, provide a distancing mechanism through which stressors are put in perspective, or provide security that increases ability to cope.[25]

The Community as a Support Group

The characteristics of a community have a direct bearing on the level of well-being of individuals and families that reside therein. The quality of social interaction and the life experiences of residents can contribute positively to health or negatively to social disorganization and overt illness. Stability within a community tends to promote close-knit ties among residents that mitigate the effects of crises on community members. Stable communities are characterized by value similarity, mutual assistance, mutual trust, and concern for members.

Minority groups frequently lack the backup support of the community since they may be out of phase with the predominant culture, social support systems, and community services. Because of differing values and ethnic background, members of minority groups can become socially isolated within a community, having few, if any, supportive relationships. In interacting with members of minority groups, the professional nurse should be particularly sensitive to the extent of social support available to them. The nurse in her caring role as a health professional may need to personally supplement this support as well as link the minority person with approximate networks within the community.

REVIEWING SOCIAL SUPPORT SYSTEMS

It is important for clients to be aware of sources of social support available to them. Several approaches will be suggested in this chapter for reviewing the social support networks of clients. One or more of the suggested approaches can be useful in giving both client and nurse increased insight into existing support resources.

Support Systems Review

Glaser and Kirschenbaum[26] have suggested a straightforward approach to be used in reviewing sources of social support for clients. In the support systems review the client is asked to list those individuals that provide personal support (financial, emotional, or intellectual). The client is then asked to indicate whether the supportive others are family members, fellow workers, or social acquaintances. By next identifying those individuals that have been sources of support for 5 years or more, the client gains increased awareness of the stability of personal support systems. After examining current sources of support, the client and the nurse can mutually determine the adequacy of support. If inadequate, decisions should be made concerning what can be done to enhance existing social support networks. Figure 14–4 provides a sample support system review for a hypothetical client. Following review of the client's social support systems, the following additional questions can be explored:

- In what areas do you need more support: financial, emotional, intellectual?
- Who within your present support system might provide the support but is not already providing it?
- What other individuals could become a part of your support system?
- What could you do specifically to add the people whom you believe you need in your support system?

Answers to these questions suggest actions that the client could take to expand sources of personal support.

List those individuals below who provide financial, emotional, or intellectual support to you. Indicate the type of support provided by placing the appropriate letter next to each name. F = financial support, E = emotional support, and I = intellectual support. Any individual may provide more than one type of support. Next, indicate whether the supportive other is a family member (FM), fellow worker (FW), or social acquaintance (A). Finally, after each person who has been a source of support for 5 years or more, place the number 5.

John	F, E, I, FM (husband), 5	Nancy	E, A
Peter	E, FM (son), 5	Larry	E, I, A
Carmen	E, FM (daughter), 5	Arlene	E, I, A
Helen	E, FM (mother), 5	Duane	I, A, 5
Ted	E, FM (father), 5	Elaine	I, A, 5
Audrey	E, FM (cousin), 5	Margaret	E, I, FW
Andrew	E, I, FM (cousin), 5	Marlene	E, I, FW
Jane	E, I, A	Frances	I, FW
David	E, I, A	Rose	I, FW
Tom	I, A, 5	Karen	I, FW
Elsa	E, I, A, 5	Theresa	I, FW
Jack	E, A	Diane	I, FW

Figure 14–4. Support systems review.

The individuals identified on the previous page should be grouped in the following way:

Sources of Emotional Support

FAMILY	WORK	SOCIAL GROUP
John	Margaret	Jane
Peter	Marlene	David
Carmen		Elsa
Helen		Jack
Ted		Nancy
Audrey		Larry
Andrew		Arlene

Sources of Intellectual Support

FAMILY	WORK	SOCIAL GROUP
John	Margaret	Jane
Audrey	Marlene	David
Andrew	Frances	Tom
	Rose	Elsa
	Karen	Larry
	Theresa	Arlene
	Diane	Duane
		Elaine

Sources of Financial Support

FAMILY	WORK	SOCIAL GROUP
John		

Sources of Support for More than 5 Years

FAMILY	WORK	SOCIAL GROUP
John		Tom
Peter		Elsa
Carmen		Duane
Helen		Elaine
Ted		
Audrey		
Andrew		

Figure 14–4. (continued)

List below in the left-hand column those individuals who have visited your home during the past 3 months. In the right-hand column, list those individuals whose home you have visited during the past 3 months. Then code each individual in the following way:

FM = Family Member
FW = Fellow Worker
 A = Social Acquaintance

SR = Similar Religion
DR = Different Religion
SE = Similar Ethnic Background
DE = Different Ethnic Background
SV = Similar Values
DV = Different values

 H = Individuals that I was happy to see when they came or that I believe were happy to see me
 X = Individuals that I was not particularly happy to see or that were not particularly happy to see me

Persons Who Have Visited My Home	Persons Whose Homes I Have Visited

Identify below those persons with whom you have one or more similarities and whom you were happy to see. These individuals are likely to provide the core of your extended family or social support system. Consider what you can do specifically to further strengthen these relationships to enhance the social support available to you.

Figure 14–5. Mutual support patterns. *(Reprinted by permission of A & W Publishers, Inc. from* Values Clarification: A handbook of practical strategies for teachers and students, *revised edition by Sidney B. Simon, Leland W. Howe, and Howard Kirschenbaum. Copyright © 1972, 1978. Hart Publishing Co., Inc.).*

Mutual Support Patterns

A second approach to reviewing social support networks has been described by Simon et al.[27] The format for this approach to assessing mutual support patterns is presented in Figure 14–5. Clients are asked to identify those individuals who have been to their home for a meal or visit within the past 3 months. Clients are also asked to list those individuals who have invited them to their house within the same time period. With the client as the point of reference, persons within the support network are coded in the following way: similar religion (SR) or different religion (DR), similar age (SA) or different age (DA), similar ethnic background (SE) or different ethnic background (DE), and similar values (SV) or different values (DV). Clients are to place an H by those individuals that they were happy to see when they came and an X by those individuals whom the clients do not look forward to seeing again.

Through this review, clients can identify individuals within their support networks with whom they have mutual interests and backgrounds as well as mutually supportive relationships. The nurse can provide appropriate follow-up for this exercise by discussing with the client ways in which mutuality of caring relationships can be strengthened.

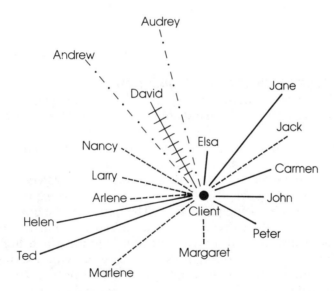

Legend: ————— Strong emotional support

— · — · – Moderate emotional support

- - - - - - Weak emotional support

+++++ Relationship in which conflict currently exists

Figure 14–6. Emotional-support diagram.

Emotional-Support Diagram

Sources of emotional support can also be diagrammed in such a way that strength of support is readily apparent. Figure 14–6 presents a sample emotional-support diagram that is coded to indicate strong, moderate, and weak sources of support, as well as current conflicts with supportive individuals. The length of each line can be used to indicate geographical proximity to the client. This approach is particularly appropriate for clients who need a more visual presentation of their emotional support system in order to take action effectively to sustain or enhance emotionally satisfying relationships.

Accepting and Giving Emotional Support

Caplan et al.[28] have presented an approach for determining the extent to which clients can both give and receive emotional support. This questionnaire is presented in Figure 14–7, with only minor modifications. The questionnaire was initially developed in order to evaluate social support and its impact on adherence to medical regimens. However, the tool can also be used for the general purpose of determining the extent of mutual emotional support within a given client's social network. The following areas are addressed: number of friends and social visits, emotional support from significant others, and ability to give emotional support. The questionnaire is interesting and easy to fill out, yet it provides a great deal of helpful information for the client and the nurse to use as a basis for actions to enhance sources of personal support at home, at work, or in the community.

Dyadic Support or Marital Adjustment

An important part of emotional support is that provided in the husband–wife relationship. The degree of marital adjustment can set the tone for the support climate that the entire family experiences. While many tools are available to measure both marital and sexual adjustment, the short questionnaire presented in Figure 14–8 provides a general indication of marital adaptation. The questions included are taken from *The Adaptation Potential for Pregnancy Scale* developed by Nuckolls[29,30] for assessing the extent of social support available to women during pregnancy. The nature of the questions included in the scale permit their use as a general measure of marital adjustment or satisfaction. Since marital adjustment and happiness is a highly personal topic for clients, this questionnaire should be used with discrimination and the client assured of the confidentiality of the information. The nurse should be ready to listen to the client and provide support if use of the questionnaire is emotionally distressing.

Review of social support systems can be an integral part of the action phase of health behavior. Through review, the client is assisted in recognizing current sources of support and in identifying barriers in social relationships that may thwart desirable health actions. The nurse must always be alert to client situations where social support is minimal or nonexistent. Extensive review of support systems may cause anxiety and depression for the client. In this case, a more informal, nonthreatening approach should be used.

For each of the questions below, fill in or circle the appropriate response.

A. *Number of Friends and Social Visits*

　1. How many close friends do you have who live within 45 minutes travel?

　　_____ FRIENDS

　2. How many times have you visited with any of these close friends in the past 4 weeks? _____ TIMES

B. *Social Support*

Please read what Mike and Jim are like. Then indicate the extent to which the following people are like Mike and Jim.

Mike　　　*Jim*

Mike is a warm, friendly person. When something concerns a person, Mike listens sympathetically and attentively. Mike gives people encouragement and praises people's efforts, no matter how small those efforts may be. Most of all, Mike is very understanding and accepting of others' feelings.

Jim is a cold, businesslike person. People rarely talk to Jim about their concerns, and when they do, he appears unsympathetic and inattentive. Jim shows his disappointment in people and their concerns. He rarely praises others' efforts. People often feel that Jim is not very understanding or accepting of their feelings.

How much does each of the following persons resemble Mike or Jim?
CIRCLE ONE NUMBER FOR EACH ITEM.

1. Your immediate supervisor at work? If you have no boss or don't work check here ☐.

Exactly or a lot like Mike	Somewhat like Mike	Halfway between	Somewhat like Jim	Exactly or a lot like Jim
1	2	3	4	5

Figure 14-7. Receiving and giving emotional support (continued on next page). *(From Caplan, R. D., Robinson, E. A., & French, J. R., Adhering to medical regimens: pilot experiments in patient education. 1976. © Institute for Social Research, University of Michigan, Ann Arbor, Mich.).*

2. *Your spouse* (if you are not married, rate your closest relative).

Exactly or a lot like Mike	Somewhat like Mike	Halfway between	Somewhat like Jim	Exactly or a lot like Jim
1	2	3	4	5

3. *Your best friend or acquaintance within 45 minutes of where you live.*

Exactly or a lot like Mike	Somewhat like Mike	Halfway between	Somewhat like Jim	Exactly or a lot like Jim
1	2	3	4	5

C. Supportive Behavior

How often did someone do each of the following for you *during the past week?*
CIRCLE ONE NUMBER FOR EACH ITEM.

	Not at all	Once	Twice	Three times	Four or more times
1. Showed warmth or friendliness toward you when you were troubled about something.	0	1	2	3	4
2. Listened attentively to you when you needed to talk about something.	0	1	2	3	4
3. Encouraged you or showed approval for something you did.	0	1	2	3	4
4. Showed understanding when you felt upset or irritable.	0	1	2	3	4

D. *Concern of Others*

How much real concern about you and your well being has been shown within the past week by each of the following people?
CIRCLE ONE NUMBER PER ITEM.

Figure 14–7. (continued)

	Almost none	A little	Some	A lot
1. Your immediate supervisor?	1	2	3	4
2. Your closest friend?	1	2	3	4
3. Your spouse (if no spouse, a close relative or friend)?	1	2	3	4
4. Your closest neighbor?	1	2	3	4

E. *Giving Social Support*

How often did you *do* each of these activities during the past week?
CIRCLE ONE NUMBER PER ITEM.

	Not at all	Once	Twice	Three times	Four or more times
1. Showed warmth or friendliness toward someone when he or she was troubled by something.	0	1	2	3	4
2. Listened attentively to someone who needed to talk about something that was bothering him or her.	0	1	2	3	4
3. Encouraged or showed approval to someone who needed encouragement.	0	1	2	3	4
4. Showed understanding with someone who felt upset or irritable.	0	1	2	3	4

F. *Ability to Accept Social Support*

How *comfortable* do you usually feel about friends doing each of the following *for you*?
CIRCLE ONE NUMBER PER ITEM.

1. Showing warmth or friendliness toward you when you are troubled about something.

Very Comfortable	Somewhat Comfortable	Somewhat Uncomfortable	Very Uncomfortable
1	2	3	4

Figure 14–7. (continued)

2. Listening attentively to you when you need to talk about something.

Very Comfortable	Somewhat Comfortable	Somewhat Uncomfortable	Very Uncomfortable
1	2	3	4

3. Encouraging you or showing approval for something you do.

Very Comfortable	Somewhat Comfortable	Somewhat Uncomfortable	Very Uncomfortable
1	2	3	4

4. Showing understanding when you fell upset or irritable.

Very Comfortable	Somewhat Comfortable	Somewhat Uncomfortable	Very Uncomfortable
1	2	3	4

G. *Trust in Others*

Generally speaking, would you say that
☐ most people can be trusted.
OR
☐ you can't be too careful in dealing with people.
Would you say that most of the time
☐ people try to be helpful.
OR
☐ they are mostly just looking out for themselves.
Do you think that most people
☐ would try to take advantage of you if they got the chance.
OR
☐ would try to be fair.

Figure 14–7. (continued)

SOCIAL SUPPORT AND HEALTH

The intent of this section is to provide the reader with an overview of completed research that has explored the relationship between social support and health or illness. Several key questions will be addressed in this section:

- What is the role of social support in promoting health?
- What role does lack of support play in increased susceptibility to illness or as a direct causative factor?
- What are the mechanisms by which social support exerts its impact on human health and well-being?

Please indicate for each of the following scaled items, the response that best fits your current feelings about your marital relationship.

1. Has marriage been for you:

| Very happy | Quite happy | About average | Somewhat unhappy | Extremely unhappy |

2. Do you consider your marriage a success in accomplishing the goals you want your marriage to achieve?

| Very definitely | Mostly | Somewhat | In many ways, no | Quite unsuccessful |

3. Has your marriage brought you many disappointments?

| None at all | Almost none | Only a few | Some | Quite a few |

4. What kind of an adjustment do you feel that you and your husband or wife have made to each other in marriage?

| Extremely good | Very good | Satisfactory | Somewhat unsatisfactory | Poor |

5. Has your marriage brought you satisfactions that you could not have achieved otherwise?

| Very many | Many | Some | Few | None |

6. Has marriage given you the personal satisfactions which you believe marriage should bring?

| To the fullest extent | Very much so | Somewhat | Very little | Not at all |

Figure 14–8. Review of marital relationship (continued on next page). *(Adapted from The Potential for Pregnancy Scale in Nuckolis, K. B., Psychosocial assets, life crisis and the prognosis of pregnancy.* Doctoral dissertation, University of North Carolina at Chapel Hill, 1970. With permission.)

7. Are you satisfied with the extent of emotional support provided to you by your husband or wife?

| Perfectly satisfied | Very well satisfied | Well satisfied | Satisfied | A little bit Dissatisfied | Very disatisfied |

8. Is sexual intercourse between you and your husband or wife a satisfying expression of love and affection?

| Always | Usually | Sometimes | Hardly ever | Never |

9. How would you describe your husband or wife for each of the following characteristics?

(A)

| Very easy-going | Fairly easy-going | Somewhat irritable | Very irritable |

(B)

| Placid and calm | Fairly placid | Sort of nervous | Very nervous |

(C)

| Very even temper | Fairly even temper | Quick temper | Uncontrollable temper |

(D)

| Very permissive | Sort of permissive | Sort of strict | Very strict |

10. To what extent would you be inclined to marry the same person again if you were unmarried?

| Very much | Quite a bit | Somewhat | A little bit | Not at all |

Figure 14–8. (continued)

Role of Social Support in Health Promotion

The relationship between social support and health is a relatively new field for exploration within the social sciences. While the amount of information available is limited, several studies that address the relationship between social support and positive health states will be cited.

In a study of 153 women Brim[31] explored the relationships between reported happiness or life satisfaction (a dimension of health) and five dimensions of social networks: concern, trust, value similarity, assistance, and desire for interaction. The pattern of correlations between these dimensions differed for married and unmarried women, as illustrated in Figure 14–9.

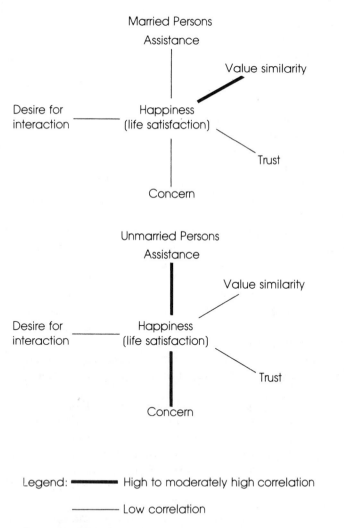

Figure 14–9. Strength of relationship to expressed happiness and life satisfaction for five dimensions of social support networks.

Married women considered value similarity as the most important dimension of support relationships; unmarried women gave less importance to value similarity. Assistance available from the relationship and concern evidenced on the part of the other were significantly correlated with happiness or life satisfaction for unmarried women. It is possible that the tangible assistance and continuing concern generally experienced by married women from their husbands made this dimension of social support less important to them. On the other hand, single women who had no one readily available to rely on were more aware of the need for assistance with life tasks and for show of concern on the part of individuals close to them.

While this study does not directly address health per se, happiness and life satisfaction are important dimensions of health that need to be considered in any holistic approach to health assessment. The study results provide information helpful to the professional nurse in understanding the dimensions of human support relationships generally important to married and single women. Additional data are needed on married and single men.

In a study of 678 elderly residents aged 60 or above, Minkler, Satariano, and Langhuaser[32] found that in persons below 75 years of age, there was a significant relationship between extent of social ties and self-rated health. Persons who rated their social ties as high also had higher rating on personal health. It is interesting to note that this relationship was not significant in the "old-old," or persons over 75 years of age. This suggests that with advanced age, social ties may not be as strongly associated with health status as they are for younger persons. A significant relationship was also found between the seeking of advice through support networks and self-reported health status. Advice provided by significant others may be an important contributor to health status among the elderly.

Baldassare, Rosenfeld, and Rook[33] studied a sample of 1050 elderly individuals living in 50 communities in northern California. Social relations were found to be a significant predictor of psychological well-being. Perceived lack of companionship was consistently related to decreased levels of well-being. The findings illustrate the need to distinguish among the various types or dimensions of social support in order better to understand the mechanisms through which social support contributes to the health and well-being of older adults.

In studying the experience of widowhood, Walker et al.[34] found that during the initial stage of bereavement, needs of the new widow were met by strong ties within a small but dense social support network that provided high levels of empathy. However, it was interesting to note that in the stage of psychosocial readjustment following the initial bereavement period, the needs of widows changed, making the support system that had fulfilled needs at the onset inappropriate or maladaptive. The small, dense network with strong ties maintained the identity of the widow during the initial loss crisis but entrapped the widow when she sought to change her identity and adjust to a new life style. The small group seemed to offer a limited set of normative expectations, restricted information, and few new social contacts. Transition to new social roles was better served by interacting with individuals who had bridging relationships to other groups in addition to the target group. If there were individuals who were part of other social groups, the likelihood was increased that widows would meet compatible people with potential for strong tie relationships.

From these findings, it appears evident that every individual needs both intimate ties within a primary group and less intimate ties with individuals in other groups that can expand horizons and offer new social possibilities.

Role of Support in Prevention

The role of social support in prevention has been demonstrated by the findings of a number of studies. The "buffer" effect of social support appears to be instrumental in the prevention of both physical and psychological disorders.

Nuckolls[35] explored the relationship between social support, life change, and complications of pregnancy. A large number of variables were measured in order to determine the extent of social support available to more than 150 pregnant women. Measures of social support included the quality of marital relationships, extent of interaction with extended family, and level of adjustment within the community. The extent of life change experience was determined from responses to the social readjustment rating scale.

While neither extent of life change nor support resources alone predicted ease of pregnancy, those women with high life change and also high support scores had only one-third the complications of women with many life changes and low support scores. The study provides evidence for the "buffer" effects of strong social relationships. In spite of life change, support appeared to prevent complications during pregnancy.

In a study that explored the relationship between social support and illness symptoms, Gore[36] studied 100 rural and urban, married, blue-collar workers who had suffered job loss. The mean age of the men was 49 years, with average employment seniority of 20 years. These men were compared to a control group of 74 men employed in comparable jobs in four other companies. The focus of the study was on the effect of social support in moderating the health consequences of unemployment. Social support was measured by 13 items covering the individual's perception of wife, relatives, and friends as supportive; frequency of activities outside the home with the above individuals; and perceived opportunities to engage in social activities that were satisfying and allowed him to talk about his problems. The health outcomes measured were level of serum cholesterol, illness symptoms, depression, and self-blame.

The rural men were more supported than were urban men, possibly because of the ethnic cohesion of the rural area and the economic threat posed to the entire community by the massive layoffs. The mean cholesterol level dropped over time following the layoff except for men who were unemployed and unsupported at the time of the last interview. The number of reported illness symptoms was higher initially after job loss than at later interviews, but social support did not have a significant effect on this variable.

Perceived economic deprivation was significantly associated with depression *only* for those men who were unsupported. In addition, the majority of men who exhibited self-blame were among the unsupported. It appeared from this study that social support buffered the severity of physiological and psychological responses to unemployment. While unemployment resulted in loss of instrumental accomplishments important to self-worth, self-esteem appeared to be maintained through supportive relationships with significant others.[37] Social support also appeared to play a key role in sustaining mental health despite job loss.

Life change does appear to result in stress that can be the initiating or exacerbating factor in mental illness. Dohrenwend and Dohrenwend[38] found a significant correlation between life change and ratings of psychological impairment in urban adults. Schwab and Schwab[39] found that frequency of contact with friends correlated significantly with rated psychological impairment. That is, the fewer the social contacts with significant others, the higher the probability of mental impairment or difficulties. This suggests that social support can be instrumental in maintaining mental health and in preventing the catastrophic effects of life stress.

The findings of Tolsdorf[40] support those of Schwab and Schwab in that he found in comparing medical and psychiatric patients that medical patients had a higher number of mutually reciprocal relationships than did psychiatric patients. Psychiatric patients engaged in more unilateral relationships where they received more from others than they gave and received support from fewer persons than did the medical patients studied. The medical patients appeared to share more of themselves with others so that people could be genuinely helpful. They also used the advice of others and used the support provided by others more effectively than did psychiatric patients.

Lin et al.[41] in studying the Chinese-American population within the United States found that social support correlated -0.36 with psychiatric symptoms, while stressful life events correlated at 0.21. Social support rather than life change was a stronger predictor of extent of psychiatric symptoms. This gives credence to the idea that social support rather than life change may be the key variable in the prevention of mental illness or in the amelioration of distressing psychological symptoms.

Social Support and Health Behavior

The question must be raised concerning the extent to which support networks affect observed health behavior. It is well known that significant others function as an important lay referral system for individuals making decisions to seek professional care for health promotion, illness prevention, or care in illness. The priority given to health-related needs often depends on the previous experience of significant others with the same problem or dilemma. The individual passes through the lay referral system not only during the decision phase, concerning whether to seek care, but also during the action phase. Physician and nurse behavior, diagnosis, prescriptions for medication, and life changes recommended by the professional care system are discussed with others. Concurrence by the lay referral system often determines the extent to which advice or counseling by health professionals will affect self-care.

When a client is a member of a subculture that differs markedly from that of the health professionals available, an extended lay-referral and consultant structure may be available that actually retards seeking professional care. Folk practices, religious incantations, or other rituals that do not have therapeutic value may be applied before health professionals are consulted.

In subcultures that approximate that of health professionals available, the lay system is usually truncated or does not exist at all. Contact with health personnel is generally made early in the course of a problem or concern.

The importance of social support, particularly from spouse, was apparent in a study by Heinzelmann and Bagley[42] of 239 men participating in a physical exercise program. Although few men reported joining the program because of pressure from their wives, 80 percent of the men with wives exhibiting positive, supportive attitudes toward the program had good adherence. Only 40 percent of the men with wives exhibiting neutral or negative attitudes established a good record for participation in the program.

The importance of social support in facilitating health protection is also evident from the work of Pratt.[43] In studying a large group of married couples, he found that couples with traditional conjugal relationships (unequal power in decision making, strong sex-role differentiation, and low companionship) had poorer preventive health behaviors when socioeconomic status was controlled than did couples with more egalitarian conjugal relations.

A final study to be cited in this section is that of Langlie,[44] who studied the relationship between social group characteristics and direct and indirect risk behavior of individuals. Her primary concern was whether variations in preventive health behavior were a result of differences in personal health beliefs or characteristics of social groups with which the individual was affiliated. The direct risk behaviors studied were driving behavior, pedestrian behavior, smoking, and personal hygiene. The indirect risk behaviors studied were seat-belt use, medical checkups, dental care, immunization, diagnostic screening, exercise, and nutrition. The health belief variables employed in the study were perceived vulnerability, perceived benefits, perceived barriers or costs, salience of health, and attitudes toward providers. Social network variables studied were neighborhood socioeconomic status, family socioeconomic status, conjugal structure (single, egalitarian wife works, traditional wife does not work), kin interaction, nonkin interactions, and religious affiliation.

The Health Belief Model variables of perceived susceptibility and salience of health had little predictive power in this study. Social network variables were related to the extent of indirect risk behavior but not to direct risk behavior. Persons who were Protestant, above the mean in neighborhood and family socioeconomic status, and had frequent interaction with nonkin were more likely to have higher than average preventive health behavior related to indirect risk factors. Individuals who consistently participated in preventive behaviors related to direct and indirect risk behavior had higher socioeconomic status, interacted more frequently with nonkin, had more positive attitudes toward providers, were older, and were more likely to be female than were nonparticipants. It also appeared that individuals with social groups exhibiting norms close to that of health professionals were more likely to receive information on how to prevent disease and where to go for various health services.

While many retrospective studies have been done to determine the impact of social support on health behavior, prospective studies are needed in which networks of social support are identified and differences between health-promotion and illness-prevention behaviors are observed. The results from early studies appear promising, but additional research is needed to delineate more clearly the impact of social support on health and the salient dimensions of support that exert the greatest impact on well-being.

Help-Seeking Behavior

In studying help-seeking behavior among adults, Brown[45] observed that help seeking in coping with life stresses was the rule rather than the exception. Of the individuals in his study who sought help, 48 percent sought help from their social network, thus substantiating the importance of the lay referral system; 12 percent reported using formal systems of professional assistance; and 40 percent reported using both. Those people most likely to seek help were individuals with resources already available to them, rather than individuals with sparse resources. Those individuals who did not report seeking help with life change or crisis fell into two separate and distinct groups representing opposite ends of a continuum: (1) those who possessed the most social and psychological resources and felt that they could handle the problem themselves and (2) those individuals with poor personal and social resources who felt that no one was available, that seeking help required too much effort, or that seeking help would draw attention to their problems and result in personal embarrassment.

It appeared that the social group was the first point of contact for help. Following contact with the social group, if further help was needed, it was sought from self-help groups or professional care providers. Social networks of family and friends influenced the nature of help-seeking in the following ways.

- They buffered the impact of stress, which obviated the need for additional help
- They precluded the need for professional assistance through provision of instrumental and affective support

- They acted as screening and referral agents to professional services
- They transmitted attitudes, values, and norms about help seeking[46]

The degree to which a target life event is perceived as stressful or threatening influences the extent of help-seeking behavior. Interestingly, help-seeking behavior decreases with age, is more prevalent among whites than among blacks, and is generally sought from family and friends, depending on the nature of the problem, before professionals are consulted. Young, well-educated, white, middle-class females are the individuals most likely to seek professional assistance when faced with a life crisis.

Self-Help Groups

This chapter would not be complete in exploring social support networks if self-help groups were not included in the discussion. While family and friends generally serve as primary sources of support, self-help groups are an important source of assistance within most communities. Examples of self-help groups include Mended Hearts, Compassionate Friends, Weight Watchers, and physical fitness clubs. Characteristics of self-help groups include a critical mass sufficient to form a group, a form of publicity or recruitment to attract appropriate members, and a central goal or activity that gives the group purpose and sustains the psychological investment of its members. The question has been raised as to why individuals use self-help groups rather than other resources such as professional services. Two hypotheses have been offered: (1) self-help groups arise in society to fulfill a need for services not being offered, or (2) self-help groups arise because of disappointment with the inadequate assistance or lack of meaningful resources within the community.

Self-help groups have been found to share the following common characteristics:

- Membership consists of those who share a common condition, situation, heritage, symptom, or life experience
- The group is self-regulating and self-governing, emphasizing peer solidarity rather than hierarchical governance
- Members advocate self-reliance and require intensive commitment and responsibility
- The group has a code of precepts, beliefs, and practices
- Members maintain a face-to-face or phone-to-phone support network
- The more experienced members provide anticipatory guidance
- Members provide empathy for one another
- The group provides specific guidance in dealing with a dilemma or life problem
- Members can suggest practical ways for handling day-to-day problems[47]

In studying 20 self-help groups, Levy[48] identified the following four types of self-help groups by purpose: behavioral control or conduct reorganization, stress coping and support, survival orientation, and personal growth or self-actualization. The process operating within the groups appeared to be behaviorally and cognitively oriented.

Behaviorally oriented processes included:

- Direct and vicarious social reinforcement for the development of desirable behaviors and the elimination of troublesome behaviors
- Training, indoctrination, and support in the use of various kinds of self-control behaviors
- Modeling of methods of coping with stresses and changing behaviors
- Providing members with agenda of actions they can engage in to change the social environment

Cognitively oriented processes were the following:

- Removal of members' mystification over their experience
- Provision of normative and instrumental information and advice
- Expansion of the range of alternative perceptions of members' problems and circumstances and of the actions they might take to cope with their problems
- Support for change in attitudes toward self, one's own behavior, and society
- Social comparison and consensual validation leading to reduction or elimination of members' uncertainty and sense of isolation or uniqueness regarding their problems and experiences
- The emergence of an alternative or substitute culture within which members can develop new definitions of their personal identity and new norms upon which they can base their self-esteem

In all, 28 different support or help-giving activities that the group used for mutual assistance of members were identified. The nine help-giving activities that were most frequently used included positive reinforcement, self-disclosure, sharing, mutual affirmation, empathy, morale building, personal goal setting, explanation, and catharsis.[49]

Self-help groups are a valuable source of support within many communities. Their records of success in assisting millions of individuals in coping with a variety of different life experiences attest to their continuing viability as an integral part of community health resources.

Enhancing Social Support Systems

The importance of social support in relation to health has been discussed in this chapter. In addition, approaches for evaluating social support systems of clients have been presented. At this point, strategies for assisting clients to enhance or strengthen their social support systems will be discussed. Support-enhancing strategies have three goals: assisting individuals and families to strengthen existing supportive relationships, helping individuals and families to establish satisfying interpersonal ties, and preventing disruption of ties from evolving into or contributing to mental or physical illness.

Approaches to enhancing social support or alleviating loneliness have been categorized as follows:[50]

- Facilitating social bonding
     Changing characteristics of the lonely client
     Providing new opportunities for social contacts
- Enhancing coping with lack of support or loneliness
     Offering social loss transition programs
     Assisting in development of solitary skills
- Prevention of loss of support or loneliness
     Identification of high-risk groups
     Educational approaches

Facilitating Social Bonding. Social skills training represents one approach to changing the characteristics of clients to enable them to develop supportive interpersonal relationships with others. Training can be carried out with individual clients or with groups of people who have similar skills deficits, such as dysfunctional families.[51] Social skills training is based on the belief that socially competent responses can be learned just like other behaviors. Initially, training is directed toward assessing and modifying perceptions of appropriate behavior in social situations. In addition, persons are taught to re-evaluate their thoughts about themselves in a more positive manner. Attempts are made to improve social interaction patterns through modeling, role playing, performance feedback (e.g. videotapes), coaching, and homework assignments. Skills to be taught can include initiating conversations, speaking fluently on the telephone, giving and receiving compliments, handling periods of silence, enhancing physical attractiveness, nonverbal methods of communication, approaches to physical intimacy, and dealing with criticism and conflict. Training sessions may last 10 to 12 weeks.[52] Within the school setting, training in social skills and problem solving can be provided in the classroom as an approach to preventing the acquisition of socially alienating behaviors. To complement such work, the broader aspects of the school environment should be assessed to determine the extent to which they facilitate or inhibit students' opportunities for and skills in developing social ties.[53]

Providing opportunities for new social contacts is important in order to enlarge the potential pool of supportive others available to any given individual or family. Frequently, persons with poor interpersonal skills have not cultivated friendship circles. Also, lack of time or money to participate in social activities and distance from others represent very basic constraints. The degree of match between a person and their social environment may also present problems. Widows' social lives are frequently determined by the number of widows that live in the same neighborhood.[54] Integration of individuals into existing hobby, recreational, or other special-interest groups is one approach to providing new opportunities for social contacts. Church groups also provide an existing mechanism for reaching out to people who feel alone or alienated.

Enhancing Coping. Preventing the lack of social ties from resulting in serious psychological and physical problems is particularly important during developmental or situational transition periods. Seminars or groups for widows, children of separated or divorce parents, parents who have lost a child, or relatives of persons imprisoned can assist such persons in coping with life stress. Benefits from such programs include: help in understanding puzzling and disturbing emotional reactions, reducing feelings of alienation, and assisting people to cope with the crisis and move ahead into the future. It is important that programs be tailored to the unique needs of the populations served in terms of content and composition.[55]

Persons who have experienced recent loss may or may not have the skills necessary to spend time alone in productive and satisfying activities. Thus, assisting such persons to develop hobbies or skills that can be carried out alone may increase feelings of self-sufficiency and self-confidence. Such activities may be particularly useful to persons who are geographically isolated or who are disabled and cannot participate in formal or informal group activities.

Preventing Loss of Support and Loneliness. Preventing loneliness is a more desirable approach than treatment of loneliness and isolation after it has occurred. Two approaches to prevention include the identification of high-risk groups and educational interventions for persons of all ages focused on developing social support ties.[56] Young, unmarried, unemployed, and low-income persons appear particularly vulnerable to lack of support and loneliness. Obstacles to social participation such as lack of transportation for the elderly or constant caretaking responsibilities for middle-aged women with elderly parents can create high-risk populations. When such groups are identified, programs can be planned to decrease aloneness and isolation. Possible programs include transportation vehicles manned by volunteers for those in need, respite programs to provide relief for caretakers and support groups for families with disabled or impaired members (e.g., Alzheimer's disease, multiple schlerosis).

Educational approaches to prevention include classroom experiences for schoolchildren that help them gain experience in making friends, working cooperatively with others, and resolving differences or conflict. Over the past 30 years there is a growing body of evidence that poor social functioning of children often leads to serious personal adjustment problems in later life. Most experts would agree that children require the security of positive reciprocal relationships with their peers, parents, and teachers for maximum growth and development.[57]

For older adults, public service announcements concerning the importance of building sound relationships with relatives and friends may be the cues needed to initiate support-enhancing behavior. In addition, pamphlets, community programs, and neighborhood activities can be geared to helping persons build their own relationships or to reaching out to others in need of friendship and companionship.

Other general suggestions for enhancing social support include:

- Mutual goal setting with significant others to achieve common directions in actions and efforts
- Providing additional encouragement, personal warmth, and love to significant others
- Dealing constructively with conflict between oneself and support group members
- Offering assistance more frequently to individuals within personal social network to show concern and promote trust
- Seeking counseling, if needed, to enhance marital adjustment
- Making use of the nurse and other health professionals as community support resources
- Capitalizing on ties to a number of social groups in order to expand horizons for new growth opportunities

Many references are available in the areas of parenting, marital relationships, social assertiveness, interpersonal relationships, and self-help groups that the reader should consult for additional information on building strong bonds within social networks. A number of references appear at the end of this chapter. In attempting to enhance personal support networks, clients should be encouraged to identify specific goals to be achieved. By focusing on one or two changes at a time relevant to goals of highest priority, clients can often markedly alter the breadth and depth of social support available to them.

SUMMARY

With the important role that social support appears to play in the health and well-being of clients, the nurse cannot provide comprehensive health-protective and health-promotive care without considering the social context of the client, be it individual or family. Social support groups appear to be instrumental in assisting clients to cope with everyday hassles and major stressful life experiences. The extent to which stressful events threaten well-being and health may well depend on the support available from core (family) or extended (community and professional) social networks.

Additional research is needed in order to understand the fundamental mechanisms underlying the effects of social support on human health more fully. Longitudinal studies are needed to identify the health benefits derived over time and at various developmental stages from social support.[58] Also, the types of social support most helpful in given situations or life circumstances need to be ascertained. Various approaches to developing and strengthening social support systems also need to be empirically tested. Wallston and her colleagues describe in detail needed areas of research.[59] The area of social support and its impact on health status is a fertile area for nurse-researchers interested in developing the knowledge base for prevention and health promotion.

REFERENCES

1. Brim, J. Social correlates of avowed happiness. *Journal of Nervous and Mental Disease*, 1974, *158*, 432–439.
2. Tolsdorf, C. Social networks, support and coping: An exploratory study. *Family Process*, 1976, *15* 407–417.
3. Liem, R. & Liem, J. Social class and mental illness reconsidered: The role of economic stress and social support. *Journal of Health and Social Behavior*, June 1978, *19*, 139–156.
4. Bott, E. *Family and social networks*. London: Tavistock, 1971.
5. Brim, op. cit., p. 434.
6. Walker, K. N., MacBride, A., & Vachon, M. L. S. Social support networks and bereavement, *Social Science and Medicine*, 1977, *11*, 35–41.
7. Tolsdorf, op. cit., p. 408.
8. Ibid.
9. Moss, G. E. *Immunity and social interaction*. New York: Wiley, 1973.
10. Walker, MacBride, & Vachon, op. cit., pp. 35–37.
11. Cobb, S. Social support as a moderator of life stress. *Psychosomatic Medicine*, 1976, *38*, 300–314.
12. Liem & Liem, op. cit., pp. 139–156.
13. Lieberman, M. A., & Borman, L. D. *Self help groups for coping with crisis*. San Francisco: Jossey-Bass, 1979.
14. Hammer, M. "Core" and "extended" social networks in relation to health and illness. *Social Science and Medicine*, 1983, *17*, (7), 405–411.
15. Kobasa, S. C., Maddi, S. R., & Kahn, S. Hardiness and health: A prospective study. *Journal of Personality and Social Psychology*, 1982, *42*, (1), 168–177.
16. Lin, N., Ensel, W. M., Simeone, R. S., & Wen, K. Social support, stressful life events and illness: A model and an empirical test, *Journal of Health and Social Behavior*, June 1979, *20*, 108–119.
17. Hammer, op. cit., p. 409.
18. Brown, G. Meaning, measurement and stress of life events. In B. S. Dohrenwend & B. P. Dohrenwend (Eds.), *Stressful life events: Their nature and effects*. New York: Wiley, 1974, pp. 217–243.
19. Jung, J. Social support and its relation to health: A critical evaluation. *Basic and Applied Social Psychology*, 1984, *5* (2), 143–169.
20. Dohrenwend, B. S. Social status and stressful life events. *Journal of Personality and Social Psychology*, 1973, *28*, 222–235.
21. McKinley, J. B. Social networks, lay consultation and help-seeking behavior. *Social Forces*, March 1973, *51*, 275–292.

22. Baker, G. W., & Chapman, D. W., *Man and social disaster.* New York: Basic Books, 1962, p. 212.
23. Petroni, F. Significant others and sick role behavior: A much neglected sick role contingency, *Sociological Quarterly,* Winter 1969, *10,* 32–41.
24. Liem & Liem, op. cit., p. 151.
25. Clark, A. W. The relationship between family participation and health. *Journal of Occupational Behaviour,* 1983, *4,* 237–239.
26. Glaser, B., & Kirschenbaum, H. Using values clarification in a counseling setting. *Personnel and Guidance Journal,* May 1980, *59,* 569–575.
27. Simon, S. B., Howe, L. W., & Kirschenbaum, H. *Values clarification: A handbook of practical strategies for teachers and students.* New York: Hart, 1972.
28. Caplan, R. D., Robinson, E. A., & French, J. R. *Adhering to medical regimens: Pilot experiments in patient education and support.* Ann Arbor: Research Center for Group Dynamics, Institute for Social Research, University of Michigan, 1976.
29. Nuckolls, K. B. *Psychosocial assets, life crisis and the prognosis of pregnancy.* Doctoral dissertation, University of North Carolina at Chapel Hill, 1970. *Dissertation Abstracts International,* 1970, *31,* 2796B. (University Microfilms No. 70–21, 219).
30. Nuckolls, K. B. Psychosocial assets, life crisis and the prognosis of pregnancy, *American Journal of Epidemiology,* 1972, *95,* 431–441.
31. Brim, op. cit., pp. 432–439.
32. Minkler, M. A., Satariano, W. A., & Langhauser, C. Supportive exchange: an exploration of the relationship between social contacts and perceived health status in the elderly. *Archives of Gerontology and Geriatrics,* 1983, *2,* 211–220.
33. Baldassare, M., Rosenfeld, S., & Rook, K. The types of social relations predicting elderly well-being. *Research on Aging,* December 1984, *6* (4), 549–559.
34. Walker, MacBride, & Vachon, op. cit., pp. 35–41.
35. Nuckolls, 1970, op. cit.
36. Gore, S. The effect of social support in moderating the health consequences of unemployment. *Journal of Health and Social Behavior,* 1978, *19,* 157–165.
37. Moss, G. E. *Immunity and social interaction.* New York: Wiley, 1973.
38. Dohrenwend, B. S., & Dohrenwend, B. P. (Eds.), *Stressful life events: Their nature and effects.* New York: Wiley, 1974.
39. Schwab, J., & Schwab, R. The epidemiology of mental illness. Paper presented at the American College of Psychiatrists, Sixth Annual Seminar for Continuing Education of Psychiatrists, New Orleans, 1973.
40. Tolsdorf, op. cit., pp. 412–417.
41. Lin et al., op. cit., pp. 111–119.
42. Heinzelmann, F., & Bagley, R. W. Response to physical activity programs and their effects on health behavior. *Public Health Reports,* 1970, *85,* 905–911.
43. Pratt, L. Conjugal organization and health. *Journal of Marriage and the Family,* 1972, *2,* 85–95.
44. Langlie, J. K. Social networks, health beliefs and preventive health behavior. *Journal of Health and Social Behavior,* September 1977, *18,* 244–260.
45. Brown, B. Predicting patterns of help-seeking in coping with stress in adulthood. Doctoral dissertation, University of Chicago, 1979. (Unpublished.)
46. Lieberman & Borman, op. cit., p. 121.
47. Ibid., p. 14.

48. Levy, L. Processes and activities in groups. In Lieberman, M. A., & Borman, L. D. (Eds.), *Self help group for coping with crisis.* San Francisco: Jossey-Bass, 1979.
49. Ibid., pp. 260–263.
50. Rook, K. S. Promoting social bonding: Strategies for helping the lonely and isolated. *American Psychologist,* December 1984, *39* (12), 1389–1407.
51. Eisler, R. M. Promoting health through interpersonal skills. In J. D. Matarazzo, S. M. Weiss, J. A. Herd, et al. (Eds.), *Behavioral health: A handbook of health enhancement and disease prevention,* New York: Wiley, 1984, pp. 351–362.
52. Rook, K. S., op. cit., p. 1393.
53. Mitchell, R. E., Billings, A. G., & Moos, R. H. Social support and well-being: Implications for prevention programs. *Journal of Primary Prevention,* Winter 1982, *3* (2), 77–98.
54. Rook, K. S., op. cit., p. 1304.
55. Ibid., p. 1396.
56. Ibid., p. 1397.
57. Eisler, op. cit., p. 359.
58. Dreessen Kinney, C. K., Mannetter, R., & Carpenter, M. Support groups. In G. M. Bulechek & J. C. McCloskey (Eds.), *Nursing interventions: Treatments for nursing diagnoses,* Philadelphia: Saunders, 1985, pp. 185–197.
59. Wallston, B. S., Alagna, S. W., DeVellis, B. M., & DeVellis, R. F. Social support and health. *Health Psychology,* 1983, *2* (4), 367–391.

PART V

Sociopolitical Strategies and Future Directions for Prevention and Health Promotion

Changes in individual and family behavior must be complemented by changes in social policy, changes in group health practices, and changes in the environment if the health of the public is to be maximized. The importance of altering society and the environment to support preventive and health-promoting behavior will be discussed in Chapter 15. Social change can expand the range of health-protecting and health-promoting options available and decrease opportunities for health-damaging behavior. The extent to which social change can be imposed is an important ethical question. However, failure to work for a better society and environment in which to live results in "victim blaming" and frustration for individuals and families attempting to improve their life styles.

In Chapter 16, economic incentives for illness prevention and health promotion will be discussed. Information pertaining to the potential cost-effectiveness of prevention and health-promotion efforts will be presented.

Finally, in Chapter 17, future directions for research, education, and practice in the area of health promotion will be charted.

CHAPTER 15

Protecting and Promoting Health Through Social and Environmental Change

Health is both an individual and a social responsibility. Since personal health practices are only one of the determinants of health, a comprehensive approach to health promotion requires that attention be given to the environmental, cultural, and social constraints imposed on individuals and families in their quest for health. It is now accepted that behavioral, social, and environmental factors play a significant role in the etiology of major chronic health problems. In the United States, 20 percent of mortality is attributed to environmental factors. Needless pollution of the environment continues and harmful social conditions such as poverty, hunger, and ignorance persist. A new environmental and social ethic is needed.[1] This can best be achieved through influencing policy and program decisions at the local, state, and national levels. Through changes at the policy level, the public can create better health care systems and positively influence the health of present and future generations.

The possible choices that individuals and families can make and the range of health behaviors available are highly dependent on the values of the society in which they live. Therefore, any strategy for health promotion that focuses only on behavior change is doomed to failure without simultaneous efforts to alter the environment and collective behavior. In the Health Promotion Model proposed in Chapter 3, interpersonal influences (social environment), situational factors (health-promoting options available), and behavioral factors (past experience with health-promoting actions) are proposed as affecting decisions to engage in health-promoting behaviors. Vuori[2] has commented on the importance of developing a "value atmosphere" within society that allows the use of societal means such as legislation, production policies, and price control to improve the health behavior of populations. In order to accomplish this, it is his belief that health education must be a visible and integral part of the educational system of the nation as well as a service offered within health care delivery settings. Internalization of positive health values occurs most effectively during early childhood. Therefore, parents, early socialization groups, and the educational system bear the major responsibility for teaching children to be activated health care consumers.

The intricate interplay between freedom of the individual and societal responsibility was well stated in a paper presented by Gustave Weigel at the Center for the Study of Democratic Institutions in 1958:

> Man is not for society but society for man. This does not mean that society exists to grant man the objects of his caprice and uncriticized impulses. The individual has rights which society cannot nullify, and the commonwealth has rights which it cannot abdicate. All historical malaise comes from the failure of either the individual to respect the rights of the collectivity, or the collectivity's tyrannical suppression of the rights of the individual.[3]

The mutuality that exists between the goals and efforts of individuals, groups, and society mandates a multidimensional approach to improving the health status of the population. This chapter focuses on communities, society, and the environment as the milieu for health behavior.

COMMUNITY APPROACHES TO CHANGING BEHAVIOR

The realities of the home, work, and community environments must be dealt with in developing prevention and health-promotion programs directed at life-style change. Given the high potential of the social collective for impact on individual and family behavior, a number of arguments can be made for community-based programs. The strengths of such programs over individual approaches to the delivery of care include the following:[4]

1. The power of intervention is greater due to the opportunity for diffusion and change of social norms
2. Public awareness of health-promoting behaviors and barriers to such behaviors is increased, providing a basis for informed social action
3. Programs are geared to the "real world" in which people live
4. Programs can be delivered to larger groups than services targeted to individuals in circumscribed clinical settings
5. Costs are generally lower for community programs than for one-on-one clinical services
6. Cues can be provided in the community environment to "trigger" health actions

7. An environment of social support can be developed for risk-lowering and health-enhancing behaviors
8. Conclusions can be drawn through program evaluation that are applicable to populations with a wide range of demographic characteristics

The theoretical S-curve of diffusion of a new health practice resulting from community-level intervention is compared with the usual individual adoption curve in Figure 15–1. The benefits of altering collective behavior can be seen in examining the effectiveness of the Three Community Study, a community-based, risk-reduction program described in Chapter 4. An experimental mass media program to change life styles was conducted in one of the three participating communities along with individual counseling for high-risk individuals. Decrease in the level of dietary fat intake and smoking cessation appeared to be the primary factors responsible for lowered risk of

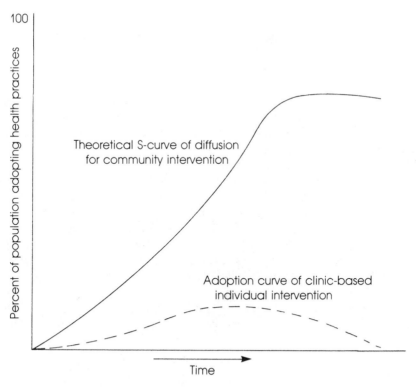

Figure 15–1. Comparison of the theoretical S-curve of diffusion through community-directed intervention with the usual adoption curve of clinic-based individual intervention. *(From Farquhar, J. W., The community-based model of life style intervention trials.* American Journal of Epidemiology, *August 1978, 108, 103–111.)*

cardiovascular disease following the extended community education effort.[5] The social dynamics that played a part in the success of the program need to be analyzed in order to provide greater insight into the diffusion and support mechanisms underlying successful community-based programs.

Miller and Cantor[6] examined the effectiveness of differing forms of mass media in disseminating health information on cancer, substance abuse, and sickle cell anemia to a target community in South Carolina. In the community survey, which followed repeated presentation of educational material via radio, television, and newspaper, residents were queried concerning receipt of the health education information. Findings indicated that overall the newspaper was the most effective means of disseminating information about all three major health problems. In exploring patterns of dissemination of information, differences were noted. In small towns, as opposed to urban areas, television was more effective than either radio or newspaper in disseminating information about cancer prevention. In providing information about substance abuse, newspaper and television were superior to radio throughout the county. However, information about sickle cell anemia was more frequently acquired from the newspaper or radio than from television. Interesting differences also emerged based on race. Black participants received information on all three health problems more frequently on radio than did white participants, indicating differential patterns of exposure to mass media.

The results of this study emphasize the importance of population characteristics in determining the most effective program of information dissemination within a given community. The optimum approach, of course, is to use all three mass media if monies permit. However, if this is not possible, careful attention to life style patterns and use of mass media by the target population is critical in order to maximize the effectiveness of health education efforts. Timpke[7] discussed television as a valuable resource for nurses to use in teaching communities about illness prevention and health promotion.

Other major studies currently in progress in the United States to determine the impact of community-level programming for prevention include the Stanford Five City Project,[8] the Pawtucket Heart Health Project,[9] and the Minnesota Heart Health Program.[10]

In many communities, population based programs for primary and secondary prevention currently exist in a variety of areas. These include:[11]

• Accident prevention
• Early detection of disabilities among children
• Immunization
• Case finding and contact investigation (communicable diseases)
• Substance abuse control
• Suicide prevention

- Family planning
- Industrial hygiene and occupational health
- Environmental sanitation and pollution control

Ubel[12] has stressed the ultimate impact of even a 3- to 5-percent population change per year in any specific health practice. This rate of change is sufficient to create a social milieu supportive of the "target practice" within only a few years, since there is accelerating collective pressure for the desired behaviors to become the social norm.

The following guidelines for community health programming have been identified from analysis of the experimental risk-reduction programs conducted to date:

1. Use a population-based approach involving as many small groups, organizations, interorganizational networks, and community-wide structures as possible
2. Obtain official endorsement of program from governmental agencies (mayor's office, city council, governor's office, local and state health departments)
3. Base program on an aggregate–population theoretical framework
4. Focus on intensive community action with a trained and well-organized health service structure as backup
5. Ensure that the program has legitimacy by involving respected community leaders and reputable health professionals
6. Plan the time sequence of program components so that adequate time is allowed for each program phase and the overall time frame is manageable
7. Throughout the program, develop a sense of community ownership and control of the program
8. Enlist community volunteers as change agents to promote participant modeling
9. Incorporate strategies to promote both acquisition and maintenance of healthful life styles
10. Attend to ethnic and sociocultural aspects of the community in designing the program and in tailoring health-promotion strategies to subpopulations
11. Develop means for monitoring and evaluating the success of the program and for providing feedback to participating populations concerning progress in reaching program goals

Communities frequently need help in organizing to deal with their health needs, just as individuals require help in coping with their individual problems.[13] Nurses conversant with national, state, and local health issues and skilled in population-based health promotion strategies can provide valuable assistance to communities in planning and implementing health-promotion efforts.[14]

EXPANDING CHOICES AND BEHAVIORAL OPTIONS IN SOCIETY

Milio[15] has presented six propositions that place personal choice making in the context of societal option setting. These propositions emphasize the importance of the social context in achieving major changes in health status for a significant proportion of any target population. The propositions are as follows:

1. The health status of populations is the result of deprivation and excess of critical health-sustaining resources
2. Behavioral patterns of populations are a result of habitual selection from limited choices, and these habits of choice are related to (a) actual and perceived options available and (b) beliefs and expectations developed and refined over time by socialization, formal learning, and immediate experience
3. Organizational behavior (decisions or policy choices made by governmental–nongovernmental, national–nonnational; nonprofit–for profit, formal–nonformal organizations) sets the range of options available to individuals for personal choice making
4. The choice making of individuals at a given point in time concerning potentially health-promoting or health-damaging selections is affected by their efforts to maximize valued resources
5. Social change may be thought of as changes in patterns of behavior resulting from shifts in the choice making of significant numbers of people within a population
6. Health education, as the process of teaching and learning health-supporting information, can have little significantly extensive impact on behavior patterns, that is, on personal choice-making of groups of people, without the easy availability of new, or newly perceived, alternative health-promoting options for investing personal resources

The American population experiences many chronic illnesses that are partially caused by excesses or deprivation. Many of these illnesses are unrelated to socioeconomic status, while others are clearly more prevalent in low-income groups. Malnutrition is a good example. It is prevalent at all socioeconomic levels, but for different reasons. Malnutrition among the affluent results from consumption of calorie-rich, nutrient-poor foods that have popular appeal or are convenient to eat or prepare. Individuals and families that can afford to eat frequently in restaurants where food costs are high often consume nutrient-poor meals that are cost-effective for restaurants to offer. Food eaten outside the home is likely to be high in fat and simple carbohydrates but low in protein, complex carbohydrates, vitamins, and minerals. Lower socioeconomic groups are often malnourished because of deprivation due to inability to purchase nutritious foods with limited resources. In addition, low-income families may not fully understand how to invest their food dollars for maximum nutritional quality. If individuals feel powerless in controlling their environment and lives, they may continue to limit personal choices even when a broader range of health-promoting options becomes available.

Milio[16] contends that health-damaging options are more accessible in relation to health-promoting options among low-income groups than among groups with higher levels of income:

> Low-income Americans are not only more vulnerable to acute disease relative to their affluent counterparts, but also sustain more of the chronic degenerative illnesses and accidents which are integral to the affluence of the wider society. The cigarettes, sucrose, cars, pollutants and tensions are readily available to the poor, while at the same time they are deprived of the level of protection afforded by the quality of food, shelter and environment which sustain the more affluent.

Compounding the problem of choices for all socioeconomic groups, health-damaging options are not only more readily accessible but often are more attractively packaged and less costly than health-promoting options. While individual and family behavior can be changed, often such changes must be made in the face of counterforces consisting of advertising, reference group norms, and the prevalent American life style.

Organizational control of advertising, production, and pricing policies sets the parameters of choice for many Americans. Advertising appeals to the emotions, priorities, preferences, and even self-concept of many Americans. Influential, attractive, and successful people are used to promote products that are actually health-damaging or that divert resources away from more desirable purchases that are health-promoting. Control of production dictates the products and related services that will be available for purchase and the extent of safety of those products. The current campaign to promote the safety of toys manufactured for children is evidence of the need for continuing efforts to ensure that the products offered to the public are safe and not detrimental to health. Another vivid example of the impact of production on individual behavior is in auto safety. Even with reduced speed limits of 55 miles per hour, cars made to go 120 miles per hour will be driven at that speed by irresponsible individuals. With lowered speed limits and interest in fuel conservation, cars of lower horsepower are beginning to appear on the market.

In discussing the impact of organizational policies on the nation's employees, Navarro[17] has pointed out the limited control available to many workers over their occupational environment and thus over their own personal health. Eighty percent of Americans have little control over the setting in which they work, since actual control of work environments is in the hands of 5 percent of the population, which own 75 percent of organized industry and business. This 5 percent exert an overwhelming amount of influence over economic and political institutions because of the capital that they control. An example of the negative impact of organizations on health is the resistance of many industries to government regulations controlling exposure of workers to toxic substances. Many lawsuits have been filed by industries against the Environmental Protection Agency (EPA) to show technical defects in the laws and thus negate the need to comply with federal regulations. In addition, concern about carcinogens has been trivialized with a new rhetoric that "life is inescapably risky." The case is made that the increase in risk of cancer from certain types of work must be "put in perspective" against the advantages of employment and the resultant products useful to society. This attitude persists despite the fact that one in four Americans is exposed to health hazards on the job, 4 million workers contract occupational diseases annually, and at least 100,000 die from them each year.[18]

Milio[19] has proposed that choice-making behavior at any point in time reflects individual and organizational efforts to maximize valued resources. The value atmosphere or hierarchy characteristic of a particular society will determine those resources that are valued and consequently maximized. In Western culture, many individuals and groups make choices based on cost versus actual or perceived gain. As an example, for some individuals the cessation of smoking may be perceived as too great a sacrifice for the benefit of healthy lungs 15 to 25 years hence. For industry, the profit available from the manufacture of tobacco products appears to offset any concerns about the potentially lethal effects of smoking. Thus, profit from the manufacture and sales of products that put the health of individuals and society at risk is a powerful financial incentive for industries, organizations, and the government itself.

Because health promotion represents a new direction in health policy, the profit-generating potential of health-protecting and health-promoting products and services is virtually untapped. The public's interest in preventing illness and experiencing high-level wellness will hopefully create a greater demand for health-enhancing products and less of a demand for those that are health-damaging.

Murrell and Norris[20] have proposed that quality of life (QOL), rather than strictly a profit motive, be used for making political and business decision. They define QOL as a measure of global or holistic well-being within a given population. The higher a population's resources relative to its stressors, the higher its QOL. Murrell and Norris suggest that analysis of resource-stressor discrepancies can indicate those life domains where monies ought to be spent to increase QOL. This in turn can give direction to production and programming initiatives.

The major approach for expanding choices and behavioral options within society is through influencing health policy. Since the nation's politicians are the individuals who ultimately make health care policy decisions, nurses and consumers alike should become involved in political activities directed toward enacting health-protecting and health-promoting legislation. Storfjell and Cruise identified the following strategies for affecting health policy:

1. Testify regarding identified community health needs before policy- and law-making bodies
2. Lobby decision makers regarding health issues
3. Attend city or county board meetings and other legislative sessions to voice your perspectives and opinions
4. Use the media to educate community residents regarding health concerns
5. Participate in interorganizational networks to achieve mutual policy goals that promote the public good

Additional strategies include:

1. Run for local, state, or federal public office
2. Develop positive working relationships with legislators, public health administrators, and leaders within the executive branch of government
3. Seek appointment to health and health-related boards and commissions that will influence current and future health policy
4. Join or organize consumer groups to increase the public's impact on policy issues
5. Use public television as a medium for expressing personal opinions regarding health issues

Interested consumers, concerned health professionals, and informed health policymakers are essential for constructive social change supportive of health and well-being. The bureaucracy inherent in organizational structures, resistance from vested interest groups, and monetary expenditures required for change all retard progress. Sustained efforts, often over a long period of time, are required of groups attempting to make changes in health policy.

PROMOTION OF HEALTH THROUGH ENVIRONMENTAL CONTROL

The chemical environment in which Americans live can be hazardous to health. Higginson[22] has addressed the importance of environmental factors in the etiology of human cancer. Currently, exogenous and environmental stimuli are considered to play a role in at least 30 to 40 percent of human cancers within the United States. In industrialized societies it is unknown to what extent material gain has been associated with unforeseen environmental hazards.

Current cancer patterns represent reactions to substances present in the environment 20 to 50 years ago, often making the exact substance(s) responsible for the development of cancer hard to identify. Reactions of human populations to newly manufactured chemicals will only be evident after years of continuing exposure. While animal studies provide some useful information about toxicity, reactions of human populations may differ from laboratory findings. Examples of cancers thought to be partially caused by the cultural, occupational, or physical environment include the following:

- *Lung cancer*—smoking (cultural environment), asbestos (occupational contaminant), side stream smoke, and air pollution (physical environment)
- *Esophageal and liver cancer*—excessive drinking (cultural environment) exaggerated by exposure to specific chemicals associated with liver pathology (occupational environment)
- *Skin cancer*—excessive exposure to sun without adequate protection (cultural environment, e.g., looking tan, and occupational environment, e.g., farming)
- *Colon cancer*—exposure to high fat content in diet, low fiber, and charcoal-broiled meats (cultural environment)[23]

Cancers clearly of occupational origin appear to represent at least 5 to 7 percent of all tumors in industrialized states. Not only do workers suffer exposure in the immediate environment, but industrial chemicals have become widespread in the general environment, resulting in higher than anticipated exposures on the part of large populations. It is unknown to what extent the presence of a wide variety of chemicals of industrial origin in the general environment is responsible for nonoccupationally related cancers. Information on human health effects of long-term exposure to low levels of air pollution is crucial for the establishment of rational standards for air pollutants. The effects of interaction of pollutants must also be considered.[24]

In looking at environmental control from an even broader perspective, the EPA estimates that fully one-third of the 1500 active ingredients in pesticides are toxic, although only a few are restricted. In the matter of toxic substances alone, every week new threats or side effects of toxic substances are discovered that were not previously suspected. Adequate testing procedures are not currently available for determining the full extent of toxic effects of many substances, nor are adequate laws available that require the testing of products and technologies that go on the market to make sure that they are safe before there is wide distribution and use.[25]

It has been estimated by the EPA that 20 percent of the 70,000 chemicals in commercial use are carcinogens. For example, cadmium, which is not yet regulated, has been linked to birth defects, cancer, and damage to kidneys and liver. Cadmium is discharged into sewage systems from electroplating and rubber tire industries (from deteriorating tires) and poses a threat to water supplies.

With an incidence of cancer at 300 per 100,000 per year, or one in four Americans during their lifetime, control of environmental carcinogens is critical. It is interesting to note that in migrants, the cancer pattern of the adopted country becomes apparent during the individual's lifetime or at the latest in the second generation. While individual susceptibility of racial or genetic origin to specific cancers cannot be ruled out, it appears highly likely that environmental factors play a strong role in causation. With deaths from malignant neoplasms much lower in other countries than in the United States, attention must be given to the potential health-damaging effects that accompany industrialization.

Control of environmental hazards demands not only the actions of legislative bodies, organized industry, and health professionals but also the efforts and collaboration of an informed public. Therefore, accurate information about risks should be made available to the public as soon as possible and expressed in a clear and concise way. For a long time, Americans seemed willing to pay any price for progress. Now, people refuse to accept an environment that menaces their health and lowers their enjoyment of life. An increasing number of persons are embracing a new public expectation that includes environmental consciousness and a profound sense of their place in nature.[26]

Organizing community groups is an important strategy for addressing health concerns relative to the environment. Freudenberg[27] has described the formation process for environmental monitoring and action groups from a survey of 110 such groups in 31 states. The first stage of organization is information gathering. Survey respondents reported that the following activities were critical to their group becoming informed to deal knowledgeably with environmental issues: attending conferences or meetings dealing with environmental quality or specific toxic products, reading relevant government reports, meeting with activists from local or national environmental groups, consulting experts on specific topics, and following press coverage of environmental issues.

In the survey conducted by Freudenberg, 88 percent of the groups reported that they had difficulty getting information about the particular environmental issues of concern. Almost half, 45 percent, reported that they perceived governmental agencies as obstructive rather than facilitative in their attempts to learn more about environmental health issues. All groups indicated that they eventually did obtain enough relevant information to monitor their own immediate environment and take organized action.

Lee[28] described the formation of environmental interest groups in the work setting. He stressed the importance of educating employees regarding aspects of the work environment that pose immediate or future threats to health or that can enhance well-being. Important strategies for environmental change include:

1. Worker training programs that enable knowledgeable employees to spot potential hazards and monitor safety of work procedures
2. Worker training programs that focus on augmenting the aesthetic and health strengthening aspects of the environment

3. Organized programs for employee monitoring of work performance areas
4. Inspection committees and environmental improvement committees with employee members
5. Employee consultants to management on environment issues

The quality of the psychosocial environment should also be monitored. For instance, the stress level of the work environment should be carefully evaluated. An environment in which workers are harrassed, verbally abused, and unrecognized as contributors is a major threat to health and well-being. While persons are surprisingly resilient and can adapt to short periods of stress, repeated stressful experiences and conditions that create chronic stress are detrimental to physical and mental health.

In addition to prevention, which has monopolized the attention of many citizen action groups during past years, health promotion through improvement of the aesthetic, social, and economic dimensions of the environment is beginning to receive more attention. Health-promotion concerns go beyond toxic waste, air pollution, and water pollution to considerations of the aesthetics or attractiveness of the environment, mental health or social wellness of the population, and the quality of school and work environments.[29]

Taylor[30] views the environment as a health-strengthening field. He describes health promotion in the environment as designing surroundings to influence populations positively so that individuals and groups can maximize their potential.

VOLUNTARY CHANGE VERSUS LEGISLATIVE POLICY

It has been stated that matters that benefit survival and security are predominantly subject to regulatory decisions, while matters where risks are not clearly vital to general health and welfare are issues for personal decision and action. In our society, even vital risks may be left to individual decision, providing that they do not infringe on the rights of others. The question can be posed as to what government's role is in legislating environmental and behavioral changes that promote good health and increased longevity. If the government uses the means at its disposal for regulating changes in behavior, it may be faced with problems of an ethical nature. On the other hand, education and individualized approaches may fall short in widely inducing changes in self-damaging behaviors.

Government involvement in life style reform is to some extent supported by the long-standing role of the federal government as a health care provider. Faced with the costs of almost insatiable demands for health care, it could be cost effective for the government to consider legislation that required individuals to assume more self-care responsibility. While such federal regulations might be cost effective if health-promotion interventions are shown to reduce health care costs substantially, many individuals would resist legislation of preventive and health-promotion measures as unethical or undue intrusion upon individual freedom. Ethical issues, including individual autonomy, must be thoughtfully considered in matters of health.

Pellegrino[31] has suggested certain guidelines in considering trade-offs between individual freedom and social responsibility.

1. Certain life styles result in disease, disability, and death, with economic consequences damaging to the whole society. Thus, there is a social mandate to encourage healthier life styles in all citizens
2. In a civilized and democratic society, individual freedom must be protected and is to be limited only when it violates the freedom of others. In an interdependent society, free acts are subject to justifiable restriction
3. Coercive measures should be considered only when their effectiveness is unequivocal for large numbers of people and when control extends over a limited sector of life
4. Even if a societal control measure meets all of the above criteria, it must accommodate as closely as possible the democratic principle of self-determination. Voluntary measures must be clearly inadequate at the outset or must have failed before coercive measures are contemplated

These principles can provide basic ethical premises for social policy formulation.

While government regulation is sometimes deemed necessary for the public good, self-direction is valued by Americans because most individuals believe that they themselves are the best judge of what is good for them, and the process of choosing is considered a good in itself even when the outcomes are health-damaging. Some persons may voluntarily opt for a brief life span full of unhealthy practices. It can be argued that if the practices are non-detrimental to others and carried out in full awareness of the consequences, these people should be allowed to pursue the course they want. However, the role of society is to make sure that individuals have as much information as possible on which to base informed decisions concerning life style and health-related behavior. Approaches to maintaining social conditions that support informed and voluntary choice include the following:[32]

- Make sure that individuals and groups are well aware of the consequences of their acts and the extent to which given behaviors are health promoting or health damaging
- Create conditions in which health-related decisions can be made free from social or commercial manipulation
- Structure situations for choice making in which individuals are not under severe mental stress or compulsion
- Prevent undue external constraints on individual choice making

Deciding whether social changes to enhance health should be voluntary or mandatory presents society with a complex dilemma for which there is no easy answer. Should coercion be used, and if so, how and to what extent? Is it coercive to increase cigarette tax in order to help defray the cost of smoking-induced disease? Would such a move also imply that highly refined sugar products and high-cholesterol foods should also be taxed more heavily to pay for the cost of obesity—and atherosclerosis-induced health problems? Should tax on large, high-speed automobiles be proportionately higher than taxes on smaller cars with limited speed and greater fuel economy? Should overweight individuals pay higher taxes than individuals of normal weight, with the excess taxes and interest to be paid back at the time individuals lose weight and arrive at the norm for their height-weight category? Which life-style, organizational, and social changes should be voluntary and which should be mandatory through enactment of legislation? Some blend of voluntary and mandatory action is needed. However, the ethical dimensions of such health-related decisions should be given careful consideration.

SUMMARY

The focus of this chapter has been on society as a collective, and the impact of the cultural, occupational, and physical environments on the health status of individuals and families. Prevention and health promotion are both individual and social problems and consequently must be dealt with at both levels. Individual changes in behavior without a supportive environment to make continuing enactment of change possible will result in frustration and failure of health-promotion efforts.

A balanced approach to prevention and health promotion within the United States requires avoidance of a "blame-the-victim" ideology to the exclusion of concerns for the quality of the environment. On the other hand, environmental and occupational control measures should not be funded to the exclusion of funds for personal health services and community-based programs that facilitate health-promoting changes in individual life styles. It is the responsibility of professional nurses to become well informed on prevention–promotion issues so that they can play a significant role in supporting appropriate voluntary and legislative initiatives.

REFERENCES

1. Michael, J. M. The second revolution in health: health promotion and its environmental base. *American Psychologist*, August 1982, *37* (8), 936–941.
2. Vuori, H. The medical model and the objectives of health education. *International Journal of Health Education*, 1980, *23*, 12–19.
3. Weigel, G. Paper presented at the Center for the Study of Democratic Institutions. Chicago, Ill., 1958.
4. Farquhar, J. W. The community-based model of life style intervention trials. *American Journal of Epidemiology*, August 1978, *108*, 103–111.

5. Ibid., p. 107.
6. Miller, M. C., & Cantor, A. B. A comparison of mass media effectiveness in health education. *International Journal of Health Education*, 1980, *23*, 49–54.
7. Timpke, J. Television—A resource for nurse educators to teach the community about health maintenance and disease prevention. *Journal of Nursing Education*, May 1984, *23* (5), 217–218.
8. Farquhar, J. W., Fortmann, S. P., Maccoby, N., et al. The Stanford Five City Project: An Overview. In J. D. Matarazzo, S. M. Weiss, J. A. Herd, et al, (Eds.), *Behavioral Health: A Handbook of Health Enhancement and Disease Prevention.* New York: Wiley, 1984, pp. 1137–1139.
9. Lasater, T., Abrams, D., Artz, L., et al. Lay volunteer delivery of a community-based cardiovascular risk factor change program: The Pawtucket experiment. In J. D. Matarazzo, S. M. Weiss, J. A. Herd, et al. (Eds.), *Behavioral health: A handbook of health enhancement and disease prevention.* New York: Wiley, 1984, pp. 1166–1170.
10. Blackburn, H., Luepker, R., Kline, F. G., et al. The Minnesota Heart Health Program: A research and demonstration project in cardiovascular disease prevention. In J. D. Matarazzo, S. M. Weiss, J. A. Herd, et al. (Eds.), *Behavioral Health: A handbook of health enhancement and disease prevention.* New York: Wiley, 1984, pp. 1171–1178.
11. Jonas, S. Hospitals adopt new role. *Hospitals,* October 1979, *53*, 84–86.
12. Ubel, E. Health behavior change: A political model. *Preventive Medicine*, 1972, *1*, 209–221.
13. Washington, W. M. An interactive model for wellness: A systems approach. *Family and Community Health*, 1985, *7* (4), 44–52.
14. Pender, N. J. Health promotion: Implementing strategies. In Logan, B., & Dawkins, C. (Eds.), *Family-centered nursing in the community.* Menlo Park, Calif.: Addison-Wesley, 1986, pp. 295–334.
15. Milio, N. A framework for prevention: Changing health-damaging to health-generating patterns. *American Journal of Public Health*, May 1976, *66*, 435–439.
16. Ibid., p. 436.
17. Navarro, V. Justice, social policy and the public's health. *Medical Care*, May 1977, *15*, 363–370.
18. Taylor, R. C. R. The politics of prevention. *Social Policy*, Summer 1982, *13* (1), 32–41.
19. Milio, op. cit., p. 437.
20. Murrell, S. A., & Norris, F. H. Quality of life as the criterion for need assessment and community psychology. *Journal of Community Psychology*, April 1983, *11*, 88–97.
21. Storfjell, J. L., and Cruise, P. A. A model of community focused nursing. *Public Health Nursing*, 1984, *1* (2), 85–96.
22. Higginson, J. A. A hazardous society? Individual versus community responsibility in cancer prevention. *American Journal of Public Health*, April 1976, *66*, 359–366.
23. Brammer, S. H., & DeFelice, R. L. Dietary advice in regard to risk for colon and breast cancer. *Preventive Medicine*, 1980, *9*, 544–549.
24. Aubry, F., Gibbs, G. W., & Becklake, M. R. Air pollution and health in three urban communities. *Archives of Environmental Health*, September–October 1979, *34*, 360–368.
25. Cahn, R. The case for an environmental ethic. *The Center Magazine*, March 1980, *13*, 5–13.
26. Michael, op. cit., p. 939.

27. Freudenberg, N. Citizen action for environmental health: Report on a survey of community organizations. *American Journal of Public Health*, May 1984, *74* (5), 444–448.
28. Lee. J. S. Cadmium, mercury and lead—the heavy metal gang. *Family and Community Health*, 1984, 7 (3), 8–14.
29. Pender, N. J., op. cit.
30. Taylor, C. W. Promoting health strengthening and wellness through environmental variables. In J. D. Matarazzo, S. M. Weiss, J. A. Herd, N. E. Miller, and S. M. Weiss (Eds.), *Behavioral health: a handbook of health enhancement and disease prevention*. New York: Wiley, 1984, pp. 130–149.
31. Pellegrino, E. D. Health promotion as public policy: the need for moral groundings. *Preventive Medicine*, May 1981, *10*, 371–378.
32. Wikler, D. I. Persuasion and coercion for health: Ethical issues in government efforts to change lifestyle. *Milbank Memorial Fund Quarterly*, Summer 1978, *56*, 303–338.

CHAPTER *16*

Economic Incentives for Prevention and Health Promotion

Albert R. Pender

Within the past decade, prevention and health promotion have emerged as dominant themes in national health policy within the United States. Still, national health care resources are largely devoted to curative, hospital-based services. Major obstacles that exist to integrating prevention and promotion services into the health care system include:

1. Professional preference for acute illness problems
2. National preoccupation with financial and defense issues as opposed to health considerations
3. Reluctance on the part of consumers to admit they share responsibility for their health
4. Strong financial and political resistance to any change in medical benefits
5. Stereotype of the increasing number of aged adults as too old or disabled for effective prevention and health promotion[1]

Our dependence on diagnosis and treatment of disease as an avenue to improved health and increased longevity is not only economically anchored but also socially rooted in our culture. As a society, Americans have been willing to spend escalating proportions of both personal and public dollars on more medical care services. Health care costs have increased at an average of 15 percent each year over the past decade, with only limited public concern about the burgeoning costs of health care and the decreasing benefits from traditional medical care.[2]

Since economic resources in any country are limited, citizens must make decisions concerning how discretionary dollars will be spent. The pattern of health care expenditures depends on the structure of the health care reimbursement system, the various services available, and the number and types of providers from which consumers can make selections. Fueled by economic concerns, major shifts in national health policy have occurred within recent years. While policy should direct the health care delivery system, large-scale programmatic shifts in health care have not followed policy changes. Thus, it appears that the time is right to consider restructuring the health care system to achieve a better balance among prevention, promotion, and treatment services consistent with current policy.

Changing megasystems within society such as health care requires that both human value issues and economic concerns be addressed. Thus, if prevention and health-promotion services are to be made widely available to consumers in the twenty-first century, the public must be convinced of the value of staying well, the effectiveness of prevention and promotion programs, and the economic and human advantage of shifting a portion of health care dollars from the treatment of illness to keeping people healthy. Since value issues have been addressed in Chapter 15, the economics of prevention and health promotion will be the primary focus in this chapter.

THE COST OF ILLNESS

In 1982, health care expenditures in the United States totaled $322.4 billion, an average of $1365 per person. These expenditures represented 10.5 percent of the 1982 Gross National Product (GNP). In 1983, health care expenditures had increased to $355.4 billion.[3] These figures represent the direct costs of health care and do not include other associated indirect costs. Calculation of indirect costs is generally based on the economic value of the individual in terms of losses in productivity or wages due to morbidity and mortality. When both the direct and indirect costs of illness are considered together, total monetary expenditures for health care during 1985 totaled 22 to 25 percent of the GNP. Continued rise at the current inflation rate will result in direct costs for health care of $416.4 billion by the year 2000.[4] It has been estimated that currently for every $1500 spent on illness care only $50 is spent on prevention and health promotion. Is it possible that this disparity is responsible for the rapidly escalating health care budget?

Figure 16–1 presents an interesting picture of national expenditures for illness care and preventive care and associated changes in life expectancy. While expenditures for prevention are barely perceptible at the bottom of the graph, illness expenditures have been rising consistently. The increased cost of care without proportional health benefits leads one to ponder the wisdom of continuing current patterns for health care expenditures.

An analysis of mortality in the United States in 1976 attributed more

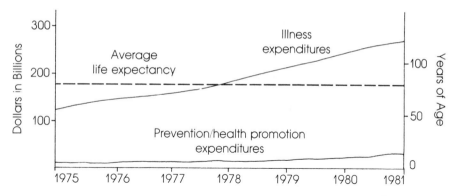

Figure 16–1. Life expectancy trend versus national expenditures for illness care, 1975–1981.

than 50 percent of premature deaths to unhealthy behavior or life style, 20 percent to environmental factors, 20 percent to human biological factors, and 10 percent to inadequacies in health care.[5] Thus, it appears that increased resources must be focused on assisting individuals, families, and communities to modify personal health habits and the environment if noticeable improvements are to be achieved in the life span and health status of the population and in the quality of life experienced.[6]

By looking at expenditures related to specific illnesses induced or aggravated by life style or the environment, health care costs can be examined from a different angle. For example, smokers are reported to experience a 45-percent greater rate of absenteeism than nonsmokers. Kristein[7] has estimated that a smoker costs a company $350 per year in absenteeism, loss of productivity, and insurance costs. Other researchers have estimated excess annual company costs for smokers over nonsmokers at $600 to $1500 per employee. In an average work span of 20 years, a company loses a minimum of $7000 per smoking employee.[8] In 1982, in Wisconsin alone, 1600 deaths were attributed to lung cancer resulting directly from cigarette smoking. The treatment of smoking-related cancers in Wisconsin is estimated to total $70 million per year. The state's estimated cost for treating all smoking-related disorders, including cancer, heart and blood vessel disease, chronic bronchitis, and emphysema, approaches $200 million per year.[9]

Alcohol abuse is another expensive health problem of increasing frequency among adults and adolescents within the United States. It is estimated that alcoholism costs industry more than $40 billion a year. Total health care costs resulting from alcoholism include direct costs of treating the problem and relating disorders as well as indirect costs resulting from lost earnings. Additional costs are also incurred from alcohol-related motor vehicle accidents, crimes, and fire losses. Fortunately, alcoholism is receiving increasing attention as a risk factor for a number of illnesses and as a significant health problem in its own right. This brief discussion of the costs of preventable illnesses will provide a foundation for examining the potential cost-effectiveness of prevention and health promotion programs and services.

APPROACHES TO COST ANALYSIS OF PREVENTION AND HEALTH-PROMOTION PROGRAMS

Because of marked inflation in health care costs, new health programs are being critically scrutinized as never before. The economic impact of prevention and health-promotion programs must be assessed if they are to compete successfully with treatment-oriented programs for health care dollars. The question has been raised as to whether preventive–promotive care will decrease health care costs or only add to current health expenditures.

Two approaches have been proposed for studying health care costs: cost-effectiveness analysis (CEA) and cost-benefit analysis (CBA). The nurse should be aware of the basic principles and concepts underlying each of these cost study methods and the differences between the methods. Both CEA and CBA require that significant costs and desired results be identified, measured and compared. However, CEA answers the question: What results are obtained for the money spent? In contrast, CBA answers the question: What financial returns are received from the money spent?[10] In CEA, benefits or outcomes do not have to be expressed in dollars and cents. Outcomes measured might be days of illness prevented or number of well years. However, programs to be compared by CEA must use the same criteria for success in order to determine whether one program is more effective than the other for the same monetary outlay. For example, CEA can be used to compare the effectiveness of health programs that have the same goals but employ different methods. Consider comparison of two weight-loss programs, one using behavior-modification techniques and the other using stimulus-control methods. The cost of each program per pound lost by participants could be calculated and compared.

In CBA, both costs and outcomes in monetary terms are measured. Then a ratio between monetary benefit and cost is constructed. Benefit-cost ratios standardize cost data so that comparisons can be made among widely differing programs regardless of program focus or desired results.[11] To illustrate the use of such a ratio, consider the impact of an aerobic exercise program on level of absenteeism among female clerical employees. The levels of absenteeism before and after entry into the program are compared. If absenteeism decreases, the dollars saved can be compared to the cost of offering the program. A benefit-to-cost ratio of 1:1 indicates that the program broke even; a ratio of 2:1 indicates that the benefits exceeded the costs; and a ratio of 1:2 indicates that the program was more costly than economically beneficial.[12]

Issues to be addressed in setting up cost-analysis studies are: standardization of methods to permit accurate comparisons, quality and availability of the data required for sound analyses, and the time frame needed to measure program results appropriately.[13] Factors that must be considered in the cost analysis of various prevention and health-promotion interventions are: (1) the magnitude of the problem, (2) the number of cases preventable or the health gains to be realized with current intervention methods, (3) the cost of prevention and health promotion versus the cost of cure or care in illness, (4) the likely rate of adoption of preventive–promotive practices, (5) the time frame in which cost savings can be realized, and (6) the appropriate target populations for intervention.[14]

For many prevention and health-promotion programs, costs are incurred now and benefits derived later. While an extended time period between costs and benefits can be reconciled mathematically with cost-analysis procedures, it is important to consider how much consumers are willing to spend to improve their health status when they feel well or to protect themselves from a health problem with 20 years' latency. Emphasizing short-term as well as long-term benefits may enhance consumer acceptance of prevention–promotion services. The extent of acceptance of any given health service or health practice markedly affects its actual versus its potential impact on the health of a given group or population. The difference between potential and actual effectiveness is indicated in the following equations:

Potential Effectiveness = Identification and intervention with all eligible individuals × maximal participation and optimal health benefits from intervention

Actual Effectiveness = Identification and intervention with a finite number of eligible individuals × limited rate of participation and partial health benefits from intervention

For example, evaluation of past antismoking efforts indicate a 25-percent (actual effectiveness) rather than 100-percent (potential effectiveness) success rate for those persons participating in smoking cessation programs. As another example, screening for hypertension is relatively inexpensive, yet many individuals do not successfully control their hypertension after detection. As many as 55 to 85 percent of individuals with hypertension fail to adhere to prescribed medical regimens. Thus, the cost-effectiveness of screening is greatly compromised by noncompliance.[15] The actual, rather than the potential effectiveness of prevention and health-promotion interventions determines the extent to which public and private resources should be invested in facilities, programs, and personnel for implementation.

Still another important consideration related to the economic impact of preventive–promotive care is the dose–response relationship. Not only must differing approaches to intervention such as mass screening, mass education, screening at-risk populations, personal health services, and environmental measures be considered as possible modes of intervention, but the extent of each intervention necessary to produce desired effects must be determined. Questions to be asked include:

1. Should intervention be short-term, long-term, continuous, or intermittent to maximize effectiveness and control cost?
2. At what point does the dose result in diminishing returns or negative effects?
3. What factors alter the dose–response relationship, that is, decrease or increase the extent of dose necessary?
4. After reviewing dose–response relationship of various interventions, which offers the higher human and/or cost advantage?

Shepard and Thompson have identified six important steps in evaluating prevention and health-promotion services for cost-effectiveness:

1. Identify the epidemiological or causal link between illness or health and the target intervention
2. Define precisely the program to be analyzed, its focus, processes and limits
3. Compute the net monetary cost for prevention or health-promotion activities within the proposed program
4. Identify possible negative effects of the program and compute related costs
5. Compute the positive health effects or benefits
6. Establish policy or make program decisions based on net costs and net health effects or monetary benefits[16]

The bottom line in considering the effectiveness of any prevention and health promotion effort is what the public is willing to pay directly or indirectly for access to such services.[17] While alternative modes of care and new preventive–promotive services can be made available, they must enter the health marketplace and compete for dollars now spent by government, third-party payers, and consumers on treatment services.[18]

Can money spent on curative or supportive care be diverted to prevention and promotion? Knobel[19] questions the extent to which this is possible in government given the current economic climate. He views the chances as slim that individual states will provide significant support for health promotion, considering the established health programs that will be competing for the limited block-grant funds available. He sees industry, insurance carriers, hospitals, and voluntary agencies, rather than government, as playing a major role in shifting more resources to prevention and health promotion. Willingness of third-party payers to offer new benefits for prevention and health promotion to enrollees will undoubtedly increase as cost-effectiveness data become available concerning specific interventions. It is only as the public learns to value preventive–promotive services and is willing to pay directly or demand insurance coverage for them that such services will have an impact on personal and family health.

EFFECTIVENESS OF PREVENTION

The early detection of diseases for which primary prevention is not yet available has been the major approach to decreasing morbidity and mortality from chronic illness. In screening for early signs of chronic disease, the following cost factors must be considered:[20]

1. Cost of persuading people to be screened
2. Cost of transportation and time devoted to screening visits
3. Cost of the professionals, facilities, and equipment used in screening
4. Cost of follow-up and treatment of people who are found to be abnormal on the screen
5. Cost of any deleterious (iatrogenic) effects of the screen, follow-up, and treatment

Numerous screening efforts for major chronic illnesses have been initiated in recent years. Several of these programs will be reviewed in terms of their cost and effects on health status.

Shapiro[21] reported the results of a randomized clinical trial in the Health Insurance Plan of Greater New York to determine whether periodic screening with mammography in addition to palpation would result in reduced mortality from cancer. The picture that emerged from the long-term study was a 10-percent reduction in mortality from breast cancer when mammography was used in addition to palpation. Interestingly, all the gains from use of mammography in screening were at age 50 or above. The decrease in mortality reported in this study represented a considerable savings in terms of earnings that would have been cut short by death or disability. In addition, the cost of more complex medical services necessary to treat advanced disease were also decreased.

Alderman and Kristein[22] reported on the cost effectiveness of a work-based hypertension detection program. The total cost of the hypertension screening and follow-up program was $94,187 for 1 year. This represented a cost of $250 per capita for all individuals treated and a cost of $363 per capita for all individuals who were controlled (blood pressure decreased to below 148/90 on follow-up) or improved (10-percent decrease in diastolic). At the 1-year follow-up, 60 percent were controlled and 74 percent were improved. It is estimated that hypertensive individuals spend approximately $250 on medical care annually and may experience an average loss in wages of $794 a year because of illness or premature death. This total amount of $1044 a year is obviously greater than the cost of intervention, even when intervention costs are calculated conservatively on the basis of controlled or improved hypertensive individuals rather than total persons screened.

Early detection of disease or risk factors and appropriate treatment can be effective in lowering health care costs. Continuing evaluation of new screening methods as they become available is necessary to optimize the cost-effectiveness of secondary prevention. Meanwhile, the search for primary prevention measures for chronic diseases must continue, with secondary prevention serving as a stopgap measure until proven primary prevention measures are available.

EFFECTIVENESS OF HEALTH PROMOTION

The cost-effectiveness of health promotion has received much less attention in the literature than the cost-effectiveness of prevention. There are several reasons for this disparity. First of all, interventions to improve general health status are less well defined than interventions for avoidance of specific diseases; thus, expected outcomes of health-promotion activities are difficult to specify. Secondly, many preventive strategies for specific diseases have been in use for decades, while strategies for health promotion are in their developmental stages. Third, most health-promotion programs are so new that the period of time that has elapsed since their start-up is too short to allow evaluation of important long-term effects. Fourth, most existing programs combine emphases on health promotion and prevention.

In this section, data published by various companies regarding the economic impact of health promotion activities at their worksites will be reported. In most instances, little information is available concerning the approaches to program evaluation used by the various companies. Thus, the methodological adequacy of the studies from which the data were obtained cannot be evaluated. However, the data suggest the potential for substantial economic impact if health-promotion programming is widely adopted at worksites.

Kimberly-Clark found that when 90 percent of the company employees were screened to determine cardiovascular status, 25 percent began using company-furnished exercise facilities. Retesting of employees at a later date indicated significant reductions in blood pressure and triglyceride levels and increased treadmill capacity. Concurrently, the number of sick days—and thus lost production time—was reduced among employees using exercise facilities.[23]

For the past 8 years, New York Telephone Company has sponsored a balanced health care management program for its 80,000 employees. The components of the comprehensive health program include: smoking cessation, cholesterol reduction, hypertension control, fitness training, stress management, alcohol abuse control, colon and breast cancer screening, and a low-back-disability program. The nine programs cost New York Telephone approximately $2.8 million in 1980. The savings reportedly accrued from reduced absenteeism and lowered treatment costs in the same year were estimated to be $5.5 million, which provided the company with net savings of $2.7 million.[24]

Johnson and Johnson reported considerable impact on employee health status with their program, "Live for Life." Participants averaged a weight loss of 13 pounds, smoking cessation close to 100 percent, and success in development of relaxation skills. These program results were credited with lower absenteeism, less employee turnover, and lower insurance costs for the company.[25]

Since 1979, Mesa Petroleum Company has provided an on-site fitness center at no cost to its 350 employees and their families. Employees must exercise on their own time, but a flexible work schedule allows employees to include fitness as part of their work day. In 1982, Mesa employees who participated in the fitness program averaged only $173 per person in medical care expenses paid by the company, while employees not participating in the fitness program averaged $434 in medical care costs. The differences in medical costs between the two groups amounted to nearly $200,000 per year. Nonparticipating employees averaged 44 hours of sick time, while participating employees averaged only 27 hours of sick time.[26]

At Purdue University, a physical fitness program designed for 100 men 35 to 55 years old showed that men who jogged or engaged in vigorous recreational sports for 1 1/2 hours, three times per week, had medical care claims totaling $3965. Claims for those who dropped out of the program were $7698.[27]

The New York State Education Department's exercise training class has been in existence for 5 years. When 847 men and women participating in exercise were evaluated, 55 percent charged less sick leave time during their first year in the program than for the prior year—36.1 hours versus 66.5 hours. Metropolitan Life Insurance Company studied two groups of employees at its Canadian main office and found that employees involved in the fitness program averaged 4.8 sick days, while members in a nonexercising control group averaged 6.2 sick days.[28]

The author of this book and her colleagues conducted a study of the impact of participation in a corporate fitness program on absenteeism, productivity, anxiety, and job-related strain among clerical employees in Signature Corporation, a subsidiary of Montgomery Ward. Over a 10-month period, findings revealed that persons participating in the fitness program had significantly lower absenteeism rates and significantly higher productivity levels than nonparticipants. There was no statistically significant difference between participants and nonparticipants on anxiety and reports of job-related strain.

Control Data Corporation is an example of one company that has committed resources to a long-term evaluation of the impact of their comprehensive "Stay Well Program" on employee health. Over 18,000 employees participate in the program. The 5-year research effort begun in 1982 will collect data on program costs, changes in employee health status, productivity, and absenteeism.[29]

Large-scale, long-term studies are critical for appropriate evaluation of the impact of health-promotion programs. Future transfers of economic resources from diagnosis and treatment to wellness and prevention programs will depend on a continued accumulation of favorable cost-effectiveness and cost-benefit data as well as societal pressure for changing the current health care system.[30]

FINANCIAL INCENTIVES FOR PREVENTION

Current insurance coverage offers little in the way of incentives to increase motivation for engaging in health-protecting and health-promoting activities. As Figure 16–1 illustrates, rapidly increasing illness care expenditures have not markedly altered the life expectancy of Americans for a number of years. Additional expenditures for care in illness are not likely to result in significant changes in the quality of life for individuals and families or in major changes in morbidity and mortality. How can increasing amounts of money be spent annually to pay for a health care system that does not commensurately improve health? For example, 90 percent of the population has insurance coverage for hospital care, yet few have coverage for health promotion services because such services cannot be related to a specific diagnosis or medical complaint.

While the federal government itself extols the virtues of prevention and health promotion, it prohibits reimbursement by Medicare for many preventive services despite the fact that Medicare expenditures are approaching 2 percent of the Gross National Product.[31] In the federal government, prevention suffers from a double standard with respect to cost-benefit considerations. Although Medicare prohibits the consideration of cost with respect to new diagnostic or therapeutic procedures, cost considerations are routinely used to forestall the coverage of preventive services.[32] In exploring health maintenance for the elderly, the Technical Committee on Health Maintenance and Health Promotion of the 1981 White House Conference on Aging recommended that "future service delivery should be developed within the framework of health promotion, prevention, and health maintenance rather than take the more narrow approach of treatment and long-term care."[33] In recent years, an increasing number of health-promotion programs have been conducted specifically for older populations. However, most of these programs have not been evaluated systematically in terms of resultant changes in health status of the population served and subsequent impact on health care utilization and health care costs. Virtually none of the programs have been supported by organized insurance plans.

Prepaid health care plans such as Health Maintenance Organizations (HMOs) have particular potential for incorporating health-promotion activities into the services provided. However, at present, health-promotion activities in HMOs are limited. Deeds[34] concludes that even though many HMOs sponsor educational programs, they are more often geared to helping sick people get well than to preventing well people from getting sick. Emphasis by HMOs on illness in educational programming undoubtedly reflects the dominance of a medical orientation. Thus, the nature of services offered in many HMOs must be carefully examined in light of their supposed mission of keeping people healthy.

In 1980, the Health Care Finance Administration (HCFA) within the federal government took a step toward a preventive orientation by funding five demonstration projects in which Medicare beneficiaries were allowed to join existing HMOs. The participating organizations were reimbursed prospectively on a capitation basis. These projects demonstrated that:

1. Care of the elderly within an HMO costs Medicare less than other services purchased in the community
2. Savings generated could be returned to beneficiaries in the form of more comprehensive benefits than previously covered under Medicare
3. Older adults are willing to join HMOs[35]

Although the demonstration projects covered preventive services such as immunizations, physical examinations, and screening tests that had not been formerly covered by Medicare, the programs, for the most part, did not emphasize health-promotion activities. A noted exception was MedCenter Health Plan in Minneapolis, Minnesota, which developed wellness programs.[36] Staffed primarily by nurse-practitioners and a social worker, special services included telephone information, home visits, and health education programs. Education programs included a support group, course on aging, and a community-based exercise program.

The success of the Medicare HMO prospective payment demonstrations led to the program's full-scale adoption in the Tax Equity and Financial Responsibility Act (TEFRA) of 1984. Now, all Medicare enrollees covered by Parts A and B have the option of joining an HMO or another prepaid health plan. The Social/Health Maintenance Organization (S/HMO), an experimental program, is currently being tested in four national sites. These S/HMOs are based on a commitment to the integration of health care with psychosocial, environmental, and informal supports to reduce dependency in the elderly. The S/HMO is geared to coordination of services rather than fragmentation and to maximizing functional capacity of older adults in the least restrictive environment.[37]

Both HMOs and other alternative health care systems represent an important strategy for decreasing health care costs and for providing a broader array of preventive and promotive services, not only to older adults but to other populations. The HMO model, if implemented properly, could provide many incentives for prevention and health promotion.

Present reimbursement patterns for health care limit consumer choice among alternative systems and alternative providers and present barriers to the delivery of prevention and health-promotion services. Rather than discouraging prevention and health promotion, as our present reimbursement system does, economic advantages for use of such services should be brought directly to consumers. The following suggestions for financial incentives are offered:

1. Expand insurance coverage to ambulatory care services for prevention and health promotion as warranted by demonstrated impact on quality of life and results of cost-analysis studies
2. Offer partial insurance premium refunds for maintaining good health or for improving health status
3. Offer health-promotion and prevention services or facilities as part of employee fringe benefits
4. Develop a sliding scale for insurance premiums based on documented attendance at health-education programs or involvement in health promotion activities in the community or at the worksite
5. Provide prevention and health-promotion literature free of charge to insurance subscribers

MANPOWER FOR PREVENTION AND HEALTH PROMOTION

Provision of appropriate prevention and health-promotion services to the public on a nationwide basis will require the use of a variety of health care personnel. While physicians have been concerned traditionally with diagnosis and cure, the emphasis in professional nursing has been on care in illness, prevention, and health promotion. Nurses are concerned with assisting clients in regaining and maintaining a high level of health even in the presence of a physical disease or disability. Professional nurses by virtue of their education are in a key position to synthesize knowledge from the physical and behavioral sciences as a basis for providing quality prevention and health-promotion services to clients. Thus, nurses can provide leadership to a cadre of other health professionals such as nutritionists, physical fitness specialists, psychologists, and health educators in developing comprehensive health-promotion programs in a variety of settings.

To maximize the cost-effectiveness of health-promotion programs, physician services should be minimally utilized. Physicians can serve as program consultants as the need arises for medical expertise. The competencies and skills of various nonphysician providers should be well utilized and appropriately coordinated to provide comprehensive health-promotion services to individuals, groups, and communities. Flexibility to hire those health professionals needed to meet the prevention and health-promotion needs in any given setting or geographic location is essential in order to tailor services to various populations of clients.

SUMMARY

This chapter has provided information relevant to the potential economic impact of prevention and health-promotion services. It has also described some of the possible economic incentives to encourage consumer participation in prevention and health promotion. With inflation in health care costs, it is imperative that better use of professional and client self-care resources be achieved. Health professionals and consumers must be clear on the appropriate health personnel to deliver a variety of prevention and health-promotion services in the most effective and cost-efficient way. Attention must be given to the continuity of care provided throughout the life span.

Increased federal and private expenditures on prevention and health-promotion programs are needed in order to allow for adequate evaluation of the costs and benefits of various interventions directed toward health enhancement. Improved measures of health status must also be developed as a basis for determining the extent to which prevention and health-promotion services improve the quality of life and extend life expectancy. The results of the cost-analysis studies to date look promising in regard to the potential of prevention and health promotion for improving the health status of the American people.

REFERENCES

1. Somers, A. R. Why not try preventing illness as a way of controlling Medicare costs? *New England Journal of Medicine*, 1984, *311* (13), 853–856.
2. Rentmeester, K. L. The economics of wellness promotion: values versus economics. *Health Values: Achieving High Level Wellness*, 1984, *8*, 6–9.
3. Caserta, J. E., & Addiss, S. The economics of community health: Dealing with realities. In *The economics of health care and nursing*, Presidential Address and Papers, 1984 Annual Meeting and Scientific Session of the American Academy of Nursing, pp. 43–63.
4. Scheffler, R. M. The economic evidence on prevention. In *Health people: The Surgeon General's report on health promotion and disease prevention.* (U. S. Public Health Service Publ. No. 79-55071) Washington, D.C.: Government Printing Office, 1979.
5. *The Surgeon General's report on health promotion and disease prevention.* (U. S. Public Health Service Publ. No. 79-55071) Washington, D.C.: Government Printing Office, 1979.
6. McNerney, W. J. Control of health-care costs in the 1980s. *The New England Journal of Medicine*, November 6, 1980, *303* (19), 1088–1095.
7. Kristein, M. The economics of health promotion at the worksite. *Health Education Quarterly*, 1982, *9*, 27–35.
8. Rentmeester, op. cit., p. 7.
9. Wisconsin Department of Health & Social Services, Division of Health. *It's Time.* Madison, Wis., October 1982.

10. LaRosa, J. H., & Kiefhaber, A. Cost analysis and workplace health promotion programs. *Occupational Health Nursing*, 1985, *33*, 234–236, 262.
11. Rogers, P. J., Eaton, E. K., & Bruhn, J. G. Is health promotion cost effective? *Preventive Medicine*, 1981, *10*, 324–339.
12. LaRosa & Kiefhaber, op. cit., p. 235.
13. Ibid., p. 236.
14. Peddecord, K. M. Competing for acute care dollars: The economics of risk reduction. *Family and Community Health*, May 1980, *3*, 25–40.
15. Stason, W. B., & Weinstein, M. C. Public health rounds at the Harvard School of Public Health: Allocation of resources to manage hypertension. *New England Journal of Medicine*, 1977, *296*, 732–739.
16. Shepard, D. S., & Thompson, M. S. First principles of cost-effectiveness analysis in health. *Public Health Reports*, November–December 1979, *94*, 535–543.
17. Breslow, L. Risk factor intervention for health maintenance. *Science*, May 1978, *200*, 908–912.
18. Peddecord, op. cit.
19. Knobel, R. J. Health promotion and disease prevention: Improving health while conserving resources. *Family and Community Health*, February 1983, *5*, 16–27.
20. Lave, J. R., & Lave, L. B. Cost-benefit concepts in health: Examination of some prevention efforts. *Preventive Medicine*, 1978, *7*, 414–423.
21. Shapiro, S. Measuring the effectiveness of prevention, Part II. *Milbank Memorial Fund Quarterly*, 1977, *55*, 291–305.
22. Alderman, M. H., & Kristein, M. M. *Costs of a worksite hypertension program.* Unpublished paper, 1978.
23. Knobel, op. cit., p. 19.
24. LeRoux, M. Cashing in on wellness. *Business Insurance*, September 21, 1981, 1–36.
25. Knobel, op. cit., p. 19.
26. Reduced costs, increased worker production are rationale for tax-favored corporate fitness plans. *Employee Benefit Plan Review*, November 1983, 21–23.
27. Ibid.
28. Ibid.
29. Knobel, op. cit., p. 24.
30. Rentmeester, op. cit., p. 9.
31. Gibson, R. M., Waldo, D. R., & Levit, K. R. National health expenditures, 1982. *Health Care Finance Review*, 1983, *5* (1), 1–31.
32. Somers, A. R. Sounding Board—Why not try preventing illness as a way of controlling Medicare costs? *The New England Journal of Medicine*, September 27, 1984, *311* (13), 853–856.
33. Report of the Technical Committee on Health Maintenance and Health Promotion. Washington, D.C.: White House Conference on Aging, 1981, p. 33.
34. Deeds, S. G. Overview: The HMO environment in the eighties and related issues in health education. *Health Education Quarterly*, 1981, *8*, (4), 281–291.
35. Galblum, T., & Trieger, S. Demonstrations of alternative delivery systems under Medicare and Medicaid. *Health Care Finance Review*, 1982, *3* (3), 1–11.
36. Interstudy: Final report: A Medicare multiple choice program for Minneapolis. HCFA Contract 500-78-0081, April 2, 1984.
37. Glazer, E., Snyder, C. A., & Kodner, D. L. Aging populations and the emergence of prepaid health plans: a health-promotion opportunity. *Family and Community Health*, May 1985, *7*, 59–71.

CHAPTER 17

Health Promotion: Directions for the Future

The challenge of bringing to fruition a health care system with major emphasis on health promotion and prevention lies ahead. Changes in national health policy and the increasing interest of the public in health-promoting activities and life-style change are precursors of such a system. Despite some progress, the tide of change has been slowed by vested interests in the economic gains inherent in "illness-oriented" care and by political concerns about the national debt and the high cost of health services. However, as John Naisbitt has so poignantly stated in *Megatrends*, the shift from institutional care to self-care is a reality. Interest in health promotion is a growing trend, not a passing fad.[1]

More individuals than ever before have the potential of living well into their eighth and ninth decades. It is estimated that more than 35,000 people in the United States are over 100 years of age. This number will continue to increase in the coming years. The quality and productivity of added years will become critical as an increasing proportion of the American population moves toward "maximum lifespan."[2]

Individuals, families, organizations, communities, and the public and private sectors of society will all play a vital role in the "health-promotion" evolution in health care. Yet it is the efforts of consumers, facilitating change from the bottom up, that will continue to "unfreeze" the current system of health care delivery and third-party reimbursement.

Nurses and other health care professionals with a vision for the future can provide leadership in developing new initiatives in research, education, and practice focused on health promotion. However, these initiatives must be supported by redirection of a significant portion of public and private monies into health- rather than illness-oriented activities. Currently, the federal government pays 40 percent of the national health care bill. Less than 5 percent of the federal health budget is spent on prevention and health promotion. The question of whether changes in life style and the environment can significantly improve the quality of life for individuals and families throughout the life span and decrease morbidity and mortality will only be answered through funding and evaluation of large-scale health-promotion programs in many communities over an extended period of time.

Within this chapter, future directions for nursing research, education, and practice within the area of health promotion are charted. The ideas presented here should provide "food for thought" for students and encourage nurse-researchers, nurse-educators, and nurses in practice to launch out boldly into the uncharted but promising "waters" of health promotion.

DEVELOPING A SCIENTIFIC BASIS FOR HEALTH PROMOTION

There is a dearth of research that focuses on understanding healthy human functioning and the underlying fundamental mechanisms. While as early as 1859, Florence Nightingale viewed the laws of nursing as synonymous with the laws of health, the primary focus of nursing research has been on the care of people in illness. Thus, nurse-scientists need to conduct basic research that explores the physiological, cognitive, and behavioral processes that characterize human wellness. Examples of questions to be addressed in basic research include: What cellular-level changes occur as a result of regular exercise? What physiological mechanisms underlie the positive effects of social support? What alterations in nutrition can optimize cellular functioning and increase longevity? What behavioral mechanisms account for acquisition and maintenance of exercise behavior? Collaboration on the part of basic scientists in nursing and other disciplines around these and similar research questions could contribute a great deal to our understanding of health as an evolutionary process of human patterning.

Another question with which nurse-scientists and theorists must deal is: "What is health?" Health as a concept needs to be operationalized so that salient dimensions of health can be measured in individuals, families, communities, and society as a whole. What are the characteristics of high-level community wellness? What are the dimensions on which the level of health of a society can be assessed? While, in name, many health indices exist, these are really illness indices. That is, they measure health by its absence—morbidity and mortality—rather than as a positive human experience. Nurse-scholars need to focus on identifying the patterns characteristic of healthy functioning of individuals, families, and larger social groups so that varying levels of health can be identified at all system levels.

Throughout nursing literature, scholars exhibit concern for (1) the principles and laws governing life processes; (2) patterns of behavior as humans interact with the environment during critical life situations such as birth, loss, illness, hospitalization, and death; and (3) the processes that bring about positive changes in a person's health status.[3] Based on predictions concerning consumers of nursing services, health care systems, and nursing in the twenty-first century, the American Nurses' Association Cabinet on Research has identified the following two research priorities with particular relevance to health promotion for scientists within the discipline of nursing:

Develop knowledge that will enable nurses to:

- Promote health, well-being, and ability to care for oneself among all age, social, and cultural groups
- Develop integrative methodologies for the holistic study of human beings as they relate to their families and life-styles[4]

Goals and strategies for goal attainment necessary to achieve these priorities are also described. Thus, the statement of the Cabinet provides direction for the efforts of nurse-theorists and nurse-researchers in health promotion as the profession moves into the twenty-first century.

Pender[5] has identified the need for an integrative theoretical framework for studying specific health-promoting behaviors and the more global phenomenon of health-promoting life style. The Health Promotion Model presented in Chapter 3 offers an organizing schema for variables thought to affect the occurrence of positive health practices. The model is derived from social learning and is currently being tested to determine its validity in explaining health-enhancing behavior. Kenneth[6] has identified social learning theory as a "powerful framework" for guiding investigation of health-promoting behaviors.

Bender[7] has suggested a phenomenological approach for studying human health phenomena. She identifies the need for in-depth case studies of individuals who exhibit high levels of health behaviors over a sustained time period. These data could provide valuable insights into human patterning in health and enrich theoretical endeavors. Nurse-scientists are becoming increasingly eclectic in their approaches to research. Use of multiple methods, both qualitative and quantitative, and integrative analytical approaches can provide new information about human beings as complex wholes and their health generating interactions with the environment.

Development of instruments and technology to measure health phenomena is critical. Since health promotion is a relatively new area of investigation, measurement tools are sparse. Reliable and valid tools for measuring health perceptions, health beliefs, health attitudes, and health behavior patterns need to be developed. New technological instrumentation will also be crucial for measurement of variables such as human energy fields and man–environment energy exchange as health states fluctuate or ebb and flow throughout life. Nurse-scientists should take the initiative to contact research and development departments within appropriate corporations to determine their interest in university–industry partnerships for the development of technology to be used for health assessment and health promotion. Premature use of inadequately developed instrumentation can lead to erroneous conclusions from the research conducted. Careful psychometrical and technological evaluation of the tools developed and controlled distribution of instruments prior to full-scale evaluation is critical.

Developmental studies with a longitudinal perspective could assist nurse-researchers in understanding the emergence of health behaviors in children. Factors facilitating or inhibiting development of health-protecting, health-promoting, and health-damaging behaviors need to be identified. The adolescent period may be of particular importance in stabilizing health behaviors acquired in childhood. During adolescence, individuals may be highly vulnerable to changes in long-standing positive health habits. The roles of modeling, peer pressure, and social support in encouraging or discouraging health behaviors in adolescents need to be investigated further.

Cross-cultural studies of health beliefs and health behavior patterns would provide valuable information about cultural differences that may lead to diverse definitions of health, differences in beliefs concerning control of health, and variations in beliefs concerning the benefits of health-promoting behaviors. Nurses provide health care services to people with differing ethnical and cultural heritages. Theories that address similarity and diversity in health beliefs, attitudes, and behaviors across cultures could assist nurses in providing more culturally appropriate, health-promotive care.

As basic and applied research as well as theoretical efforts contribute to our understanding of human health and health behavior, nursing interventions based on empirical data need to be developed, evaluated, and refined. Since nursing is a discipline that offers a service to society, the development of prescriptive theory can provide direction for nursing interventions. Failure to base practice on current knowledge derived from research can greatly compromise the quality of health-promotion services provided by nurses.

EDUCATION FOR HEALTH PROMOTION

With the escalating changes in health care that are occurring and will continue to occur into the twenty-first century, nursing curricula need to be evaluated for relevancy to the current health care needs of society. Since health promotion is a major emphasis in health care policy, nursing faculty who have not already done so should consider what health-promotion concepts they believe are important to present in the curricula. The philosophy and objectives of both undergraduate and graduate programs should be reviewed to determine to what extent a commitment to health promotion and wellness is evident.

In the opinion of this author, nursing students should be introduced early in their professional education to the concepts of health, health-protecting behaviors, health-promoting behaviors, and health-damaging behaviors. At present, many undergraduate nursing students are oriented to the concepts of illness behavior and sick-role behavior, with little emphasis placed on behaviors directed toward maximizing health. The idea of health should be presented to students as a positive state, an ongoing experience of human beings throughout the life span. Normal growth and development can provide a basis for understanding the impact of developmental transitions on wellness.

An excellent approach for teaching health concepts to undergraduate students is by concrete experience. Thus, faculty in baccalaureate programs should consider working with their university health centers, nurse-managed centers, or other appropriate student service units to develop a student wellness program. Through such a program, students can assess their own personal health as well as develop a Health Protection–Promotion Plan and follow through with implementation. Students of college age can develop positive health practices with greater ease than older adults. The college years offer access to on-campus recreational facilities and health programming that may be less accessible when students become working adults.

Once nursing students have developed and implemented their own health-enhancement plans, opportunities can be provided for them to serve as peer counselors for other students attempting to make life style changes. This can be carried out on a volunteer basis or as a clinical experience within the nursing education program. Active involvement in health-promotion experiences can make the concept of health "alive and meaningful" to undergraduate students. Without the opportunity to experience the health-promotion process, health and health behavior concepts may seem irrelevant and vague. A schema that can serve as an organizing framework for orienting undergraduate students to prevention and health-promotion concepts appears in Figure 17–1.

Specialists in health promotion should be prepared at the graduate level. However, given the current emphasis on health promotion within our society, no graduate nursing student, regardless of major, should receive an advanced degree without an understanding of major health-promotion concepts. In addition, all graduate students should be introduced to theoretical models that are currently being offered as explanations of health-protecting and health-promoting behavior. Integrated discussion of health concepts, theoretical models, and empirical findings from health promotion research can assist graduate students in understanding the interrelationship of theory, research, and practice.

For graduate students seeking specialization in health promotion, this area of emphasis, if offered, frequently is a part of the graduate community health nursing program. However, faculty in a program may decide to distribute responsibility for teaching health-promotion concepts across several

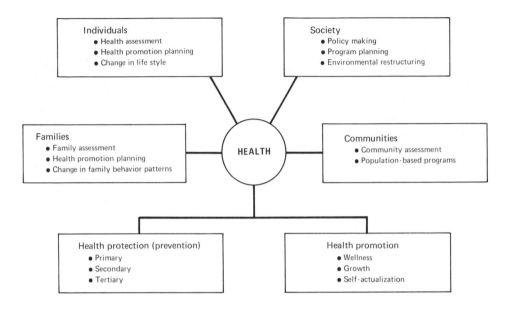

Figure 17–1. Organizing framework for presentation of health-promotion concepts in the undergraduate nursing curriculum.

departments according to the system level being addressed: individual, families, communities, or society as a whole.

The nursing interventions and strategies in which graduate students specializing in health promotion should become skilled will vary with the systems level at which they will be functioning upon completion of graduate studies. Some of the strategies useful in working with individuals are: comprehensive health assessment; health education and counseling; development of individualized health-promotion plans; life style modification techniques; progressive relaxation, including biofeedback; exercise prescription; nutrition counseling; and social-skills training. Strategies appropriate for work with families include: family assessment, developing a family Health Protection–Promotion Plan, group approaches to life style modification, family education and counseling, and intergroup support building. For nurses working with communities in the area of health promotion, useful strategies include: community assessment, community-based program planning, program evaluation, policy formulation, policy analysis, interorganizational networking, use of mass media, political process, and marketing.

Clinical experiences must be provided for graduate students to enable them to develop skill in the application of health-promotion strategies. It is highly desirable that students gain experience in health-promotion programs where a variety of health professionals are employed. Experience in health-promotion settings with other health professionals assists graduate students in understanding the valuable contributions of exercise physiologists, nutritionists, psychologists, and health educators to the health-promotion team. The best comprehensive health-promotion programs offer individuals and families the services of a variety of health care professionals.

Doctoral education in health promotion should prepare nurse-scholars who are competent in theory development, instrumentation, and research. Currently, several existing doctoral programs in nursing offer advanced preparation in the area of health promotion. The number of programs offering such preparation should be increased in the future. Graduates of these programs will have major responsibility for developing and testing explanatory, predictive, and prescriptive theories useful in understanding client health and health behaviors and in providing health promotion services to individuals, families, and communities.

A word is needed concerning the preparation of nursing faculty to teach health-promotion concepts and skills. Deans and directors of undergraduate and graduate programs should provide opportunities for interested faculty to acquire knowledge and skills in the area of health promotion to enhance their competence in planning and providing appropriate learning experiences for students. Schools, worksites, nursing centers and various community agencies offer excellent opportunities for faculty learning and practice in the area of health promotion.

DESIGNING DEMONSTRATION PROJECTS FOR THE DELIVERY OF HEALTH-PROMOTION SERVICES

Nurse-administrators and nurse-researchers should provide leadership to other health professionals in preparing and submitting proposals for community-based health-promotion demonstration projects. Well designed, population-based intervention projects involving several communities would be well received by public and private funding sources. Testing the impact of nurse-managed and nurse-administered health-promotion programs in multiple sites can provide valuable information concerning the impact of community-based programs on the health of specific populations.

A major criticism of health-promotion efforts to date is the restricted population that they serve. Health promotion has been primarily a middle-class phenomenon. Nurses could gain considerable national visibility in the area of health promotion by designing demonstration projects to be offered to low socioeconomic groups or to blue-collar workers in heavy industry. While the health of these workers is likely to be in greater jeopardy than that of white-collar, middle-class employees, few published studies can be found that describe comprehensive health promotion programs for industrial laborers.

Many questions can be raised concerning the response of industrial laborers to health-promotion efforts. What health-promotion programs are industrial workers likely to attend? What intervention strategies are most successful in altering life style? What reinforcements or rewards motivate involvement in health-promoting behaviors? What is the perception of control of health among industrial workers? What are the major occupational stressors that low-income workers in industries face? Demonstration projects applying innovative change strategies to low-income groups could provide valuable information concerning aproaches to health promotion most effective with this population.

Developing sound evaluation plans for demonstration projects mandates that economic variables be included in the analyses. However, many nurses are unprepared to apply analytical techniques such as cost-effectiveness analysis and cost-benefit analysis to program evaluation. Thus, consultation should be sought in this area from health economists or health administrators skilled in such techniques. With the current emphasis on cost of health programs, no demonstration project should be undertaken without a highly sophisticated plan for economic analysis.

Nurses have had only limited involvement in planning large community-based health demonstration projects in the past. It appears timely for nurses to become more involved in developing proposals for such projects and publishing the results in nursing and other health care journals. Wide dissemination of results through articles, newspapers, radio, and television would increase public awareness of the important role of nurses in health-promotion.

SUMMARY

In this chapter, future directions for the nursing profession in the area of health promotion have been proposed. While the changing health care scene is a major challenge to nurses, it also represents a significant opportunity for growth as a health profession. The "mainstreaming" of nursing research in the federal government through creation of The National Center for Nursing Research within the National Institutes of Health should greatly augment the capacity of nurses to meet the challenge of generating knowledge about human health processes. Progressive nursing-education programs can provide competent and qualified practitioners to assume health-promotion responsibilities. Well-planned demonstration projects can permit nurses in practice to evaluate the effectiveness of community-based health promotion endeavors. Through research, education, and practice, nurses can make valuable contributions to the national health-promotion effort.

REFERENCES

1. Naisbitt, John. *Megatrends: Ten new directions transforming our lives.* New York: Warner Books, 1982.
2. Walford, R. *Maximum lifespan.* New York: Norton, 1983.
3. American Nurses' Association, Cabinet on Nursing Research, *Directions for nursing research: Toward the twenty-first century.* Kansas City, Mo.: American Nurses' Association, 1985.
4. Ibid.
5. Pender, N. J. Health promotion and illness prevention. In H. H. Werley & J. J. Fitzpatrick (eds.), *Annual Review of Nursing Research, Volume 2,* New York: Springer, 1984, pp. 83–105.
6. Kenneth, H. Y. *The benefits, costs, and sources of social support associated with establishing and maintaining physical activity among employed adults.* Unpublished doctoral dissertation, University of California-San Francisco, 1984.
7. Bender, R. C. *Health definition and health behavior of well adults.* Unpublished master's thesis, Texas Women's University, Denton, Texas, 1985.

APPENDIX

Summary Chart of Selected Nutrients

Nutrients	Importance	Sources	Deficiency Symptoms	Toxicity Level
Choline	Important in normal nerve transmission Aids metabolism and transport of fats Helps regulate liver and gallbladder	Egg yolks Organ meats Brewer's yeast Wheat germ Soybeans Fish Legumes Lecithin	Fatty liver Hemorrhaging kidneys High blood pressure	No known oral toxicity, even with intake as high as 50,000 mg daily for 1 week
Folic acid (folacin)	Important in red blood cell formation Aids metabolism of proteins Necessary for growth and division of body cells	Dark-green leafy vegetables Organ meats Brewer's yeast Root vegetables Whole grains Oysters Salmon Milk	Poor growth Gastrointestinal disorders Anemia B_{12} deficiency	No toxic effects. Single doses up to 400 μg are available without prescription
Inositol	Necessary for formation of lecithin May be indirectly connected with metabolism of fats, including cholesterol Vital for hair growth	Whole grains Citrus fruits Brewer's yeast Molasses Meat Milk Nuts Vegetables Lecithin	Constipation Eczema Hair loss High blood cholesterol	No known toxicity. Single doses up to 500 mg are available without prescription

Nutrient	Function	Food Sources	Deficiency Symptoms	Dosage/Notes
Niacin (nicotinic acid, niacinamide)	Necessary for carbohydrate, fat, and protein metabolism. Helps maintain health of skin, tongue, and digestive system	Lean meats, Poultry and fish, Brewer's yeast, Peanuts, Milk and milk products, Rice bran, Desiccated liver	Dermatitis, Nervous disorders	100–200 mg nicotinic acid orally or 30 mg intravenously may produce side effects for some individuals. No effects with niacinamide
PABA	Aids bacteria in producing folic acid. Acts as a coenzyme in the breakdown and use of proteins. Aids in formation of red blood cells. Acts as a sunscreen	Organ meats, Wheat germ, Yogurt, Molasses, Green leafy vegetables	Fatigue, Irritability, Depression, Nervousness, Constipation, Headache, Digestive disorders, Graying hair	Single doses of 100 mg are available without prescription. Continued high ingestion may be toxic.
Pangamic acid	Helps eliminate hypoxia. Helps promote protein metabolism. Stimulates nervous and glandular system	Brewer's yeast, Rare steaks, Brown rice, Sunflower, pumpkin, and sesame seeds	Diminished oxygenation of cells	500 mg tolerated daily with no toxic effect
Carbohydrate	Provides energy for body functions and muscular exertions. Assists in digestion and assimilation of foods	Whole grains, Sugar, syrup, and honey, Fruits, Vegetables	Loss of energy, Fatigue, Excessive protein breakdown, Disturbed balance of water, sodium, potassium, and chloride	Intake should not exceed what is needed to maintain desirable weight.

Nutrients	Importance	Sources	Deficiency Symptoms	Toxicity Level
Fat	Provides energy Acts as a carrier for fat-soluble vitamins A, D, E and K Supplies essential fatty acids needed for growth, health, and smooth skin	Butter and margarine Vegetable oils Fats in meats Whole milk and milk products Nuts and seeds	Eczema or skin disorders Retarded growth	Intake should not exceed what is needed to maintain desirable weight.
Protein	Necessary for growth and development Acts in formation of hormones, enzymes, and antibodies Maintains acid–alkali balance Source of heat and energy	Meats, fish, and poultry Soybean products Eggs Milk and milk products Whole grains	Fatigue Loss of appetite Diarrhea and vomiting Stunted growth Edema	Intake should not exceed what is needed to maintain desirable weight
Vitamins Vitamin A (carotene)	Necessary for growth and repair of body tissues Important to health of the eyes Fights bacteria and infection Maintains healthy epithelial tissue Aids in bone and teeth formation	Liver Eggs Yellow fruits and vegetables Dark-green fruits and vegetables Whole milk and milk products Fish–liver oil	Night blindness Rough, dry, scaly skin Increased susceptibility to infections Frequent fatigue Loss of smell and appetite	50,000 or more IU may be toxic if there is no deficiency. 10,000 IU is the maximum single dose that can be bought without a prescription.

Vitamin	Functions	Sources	Deficiency Symptoms	Toxicity
Vitamin B complex	Necessary for carbohydrate, fat, and protein metabolism; Helps functioning of the nervous system; Helps maintain muscle tone in the gastrointestinal tract; Maintains health of skin, hair, eyes, mouth, and liver	See individual B vitamins	Dry, rough, cracked skin; Acne; Dull, dry, or gray hair; Fatigue; Poor appetite; Gastrointestinal tract disorders	See individual B vitamins; relatively nontoxic
Vitamin B₁ (thiamine)	Necessary for carbohydrate metabolism; Helps maintain healthy nervous system; Stabilizes the appetite; Stimulates growth and good muscle tone	Brewer's yeast; Whole grains; Blackstrap molasses; Brown rice; Organ meats; Meats, fish, and poultry; Egg yolks; Legumes; Nuts	Gastrointestinal problems; Fatigue; Loss of appetite; Nerve disorders; Heart disorders	No known oral toxicity. Single doses of up to 500 mg are available without prescription.
Vitamin B₂ (riboflavin)	Necessary for carbohydrate, fat, and protein metabolism; Aids in formation of antibodies and red blood cells; Maintains cell respiration	Brewer's yeast; Whole grains; Blackstrap molasses; Organ meats; Egg yolks; Legumes; Nuts	Eye problems; Cracks and sores in mouth; Dermatitis; Retarded growth; Digestive disturbances	No known oral toxicity. Single doses of 100 mg are available without prescription.

Nutrients	Importance	Sources	Deficiency Symptoms	Toxicity Level
Vitamin B$_6$ (pyridoxine)	Necessary for carbohydrate, fat, and protein metabolism Aids in formation of antibodies Helps maintain balance of sodium and phosphorus	Meats Whole grains Brewer's yeast Blackstrap molasses Wheat germ Legumes Green leafy vegetables Desiccated liver	Anemia Mouth disorders Nervousness Muscular weakness Dermatitis Sensitivity to insulin	No known oral toxicity. Single doses up to 100 mg are available without prescription.
Vitamin B$_{12}$ (cyanocobalamin)	Essential for normal formation of blood cells Necessary for carbohydrate, fat, and protein metabolism Maintains healthy nervous system	Organ meats Fish and pork Eggs Cheese Milk and milk products	Pernicious anemia Brain damage Nervousness Neuritis	No known oral toxicity even with intake as high as 600–1200 µg
Vitamin B$_{13}$ (orotic acid)	Needed for metabolism of some B vitamins	Root vegetables Liquid whey	Degenerative disorders	No known toxicity
Biotin	Necessary for carbohydrate, fat, and protein metabolism Aids in use of other B vitamins	Egg yolks Liver Unpolished rice Brewer's yeast Whole grains Sardines Legumes	Dermatitis Grayish skin color Depression Muscle pain Impairment of fat metabolism Poor appetite	No known oral toxicity. Single doses up to 50 µg are available without prescription.

Nutrient	Functions	Food Sources	Deficiency Symptoms	Comments
Pantothenic acid	Aids in formation of some fats; Participates in the release of energy from carbohydrates, fats, and protein; Aids in the use of some vitamins; Improves body's resistance to stress	Organ meats; Brewer's yeast; Egg yolks; Legumes; Whole grains; Wheat germ; Salmon	Vomiting; Restlessness; Stomach stress; Increased susceptibility to infection; Sensitivity to insulin	10,000–20,000 mg as a calcium salt may have side effects in some people
Vitamin C	Maintains collagen; Helps heal wounds, scar tissue, and fractures; Gives strength to blood vessels; May provide resistance to infections; Aids in absorption of iron	Citrus fruits; Rose hips; Acerola; Cherries; Alfalfa seeds, sprouted; Cantaloupe; Strawberries; Broccoli; Tomatoes; Green peppers	Bleeding gums; Swollen or painful joints; Slow-healing wounds and fractures; Bruising; Nosebleeds; Impaired digestion	Essentially nontoxic. 5000–15,000 mg daily over a prolonged period may have side effects in some people.
Vitamin D	Improves absorption and use of calcium and phosphorus required for bone formation; Maintains stable nervous system and normal heart action	Salmon; Sardines; Herring; Vitamin-D fortified milk and milk products; Egg yolks; Organ meats; Fish liver oils; Bone meal	Poor bone and tooth formation; Softening of bones and teeth; Inadequate absorption of calcium; Retention of phosphorus in kidney	25,000 IU may be toxic in some individuals over extended period of time. 400 IU is the maximum single dose that can be purchased without a prescription.

Nutrients	Importance	Sources	Deficiency Symptoms	Toxicity Level
Vitamin E	Protects fat-soluble vitamins Protects red blood cells Essential in cellular respiration Inhibits coagulation of blood by preventing blood clots	Cold-pressed oils Eggs Wheat germ Organ meats Molasses Sweet potatoes Leafy vegetables Desiccated liver	Rupture of red blood cells Muscular wasting Abnormal fat deposits in muscles	Essentially nontoxic. 4–12 g (4000–30,000 IU) of tocopherol for prolonged periods produces side effects in some persons.
Vitamin K	Necessary for formation of prothrombin Needed for blood coagulation	Green leafy vegetables Egg yolks Safflower oil Blackstrap molasses Cauliflower Soybeans	Lack of prothrombin, increasing the tendency to hemorrhage	Synthetic vitamin K may have side effects in newborn infants. Available in alfalfa tablet form.
Bioflavonoids	Help increase strength of capillaries	Citrus fruits Fruits Black currants Buckwheat	Tendency to bleed and bruise easily	No known toxicity
Minerals Calcium	Sustains development and maintenance of strong bones and teeth	Milk and milk products Green leafy vegetables	Tetany Softening bones Back and leg pains Brittle bones	Excessive intakes of calcium may have side effects in certain persons.

Mineral	Functions	Sources	Deficiency symptoms	Toxicity
	Assists normal blood clotting, muscle action, nerve function, and heart function	Shellfish Molasses Bone meal		No known oral toxicity
Chlorine	Regulates acid–base balance Maintains osmotic pressure Stimulates production of hydrochloric acid Helps maintain joints and tendons	Table salt Seafood Meats Ripe olives Rye flour	Loss of hair and teeth Poor muscular contractibility Impaired digestion	Daily intake of 14–28 g of salt (sodium chloride) is considered excessive. Excess intake of chlorine may have adverse effects.
Chromium	Stimulates enzymes in metabolism of energy and synthesis of fatty acids, cholesterol, and protein Increases effectiveness of insulin	Corn oil Clams Whole-grain cereals Brewer's yeast	Depressed growth rate Glucose intolerance in diabetics Atherosclerosis	No known toxicity
Cobalt	Functions as part of vitamin B_{12} Maintains red blood cells Activates a number of enzymes in the body	Organ meats Oysters Clams Poultry Milk Green leafy vegetables Fruits	Pernicious anemia Slow rate of growth	Excessive intake of cobalt may have side effects in certain people. Available by prescription only.

Nutrients	Importance	Sources	Deficiency Symptoms	Toxicity Level
Copper	Aids in formation of red blood cells Part of many enzymes Works with vitamin C to form elastin	Organ meats Seafood Nuts Legumes Molasses Raisins Bone meal	General weakness Impaired respiration Skin sores	20 times RDA over prolonged period may cause toxicity.
Fluorine	May reduce tooth decay by discouraging the growth of acid-forming bacteria	Tea Seafood Fluoridated water Bone meal	Tooth decay	Excessive intake of fluorine may have side effects in some persons
Iodine	Essential part of the hormone thyroxine Necessary for the prevention of goiter Regulates production of energy and rate of metabolism Promotes growth	Iodized salt	Enlarged thyroid gland Dry skin and hair Loss of physical and mental vigor Cretinism in children born to iodine-deficient mothers	Up to 1000 μg daily produced no toxic effects in persons with a normal thyroid.
Iron	Necessary for hemoglobin and myoglobin formation Helps in protein metabolism Promotes growth	Organ meats and meats Eggs Fish and poultry Blackstrap molasses Cherry juice Green leafy vegetables	Weakness Paleness of skin Constipation Anemia	100 mg daily over prolonged period of time may be toxic in some individuals

Mineral	Important functions	Sources	Deficiency symptoms	Toxicity
Magnesium	Acts as a catalyst in the use of carbohydrates, fats, protein, calcium, phosphorus, and possibly potassium	Dried fruits Desiccated liver Seafood Whole grains Dark-green vegetables Molasses Nuts Bone meal	Nervousness Muscular excitability Tremors	30,000 mg daily may be toxic in certain individuals with kidney malfunctions.
Manganese	Enzyme activator Plays a part in carbohydrate and fat production Necessary for normal skeletal development Maintains sex-hormone production	Whole grains Green leafy vegetables Legumes Nuts Pineapples Egg yolks	Paralysis Convulsions Dizziness Ataxia Blindness and deafness in infants	Excessive intake may have side effects in certain people. Single doses of up to 60 mg are available without prescription.
Molybdenum	Acts in oxidation of fats and aldehydes Aids in mobilization of iron from liver reserves	Legumes Whole-grain cereals Milk Liver Dark-green vegetables	Premature aging	5–10 ppm is considered toxic.
Phosphorus	Works with calcium to build bones and teeth Uses carbohydrates, fats, and proteins	Fish, meats, and poultry Eggs Legumes Milk	Loss of weight and appetite Irregular breathing Pyorrhea	No known toxicity

Nutrients	Importance	Sources	Deficiency Symptoms	Toxicity Level
	Stimulates muscular contractions	Milk products Nuts Whole-grain cereals Bone meal		
Potassium	Works to control activity of heart muscles, nervous system, and kidneys	Lean meats Whole grains Vegetables Dried fruits Legumes Sunflower seeds	Poor reflexes Respiratory failure Cardiac arrest	No known toxicity
Selenium	Works with vitamin E Preserves tissue elasticity	Tuna Herring Brewer's yeast Wheat germ and bran Broccoli Whole grains	Premature aging	5–10 ppm is considered toxic.
Sodium	Maintains normal fluid levels in cells Maintains health of the nervous, muscular, blood, and lymph systems	Seafood Table salt Baking powder and baking soda Celery Processed foods Milk products Kelp	Muscle weakness Muscle shrinkage Nausea Loss of appetite Intestinal gas	Excessive sodium intake may have adverse effects Intake of 14–28 g of sodium chloride (salt) is considered excessive.

Nutrient	Function	Sources	Deficiency	Comments
Sulfur	Part of amino acids Essential for formation of body tissues Part of the B vitamins Plays a part in tissue respiration Necessary for collagen synthesis	Fish Eggs Meats Cabbage Brussel sprouts		Not available for over-the-counter sales
Vanadium	Inhibits cholesterol formation	Fish		No known toxicity
Zinc	Component of insulin and male reproductive fluid Aids in digestion and metabolism of phosphorus Aids in healing process	Sunflower seeds Seafood Organ meats Mushrooms Brewer's yeast Soybeans	Retarded growth Delayed sexual maturity Prolonged healing of wounds	Relatively nontoxic. 50 mg available without prescription
Water	Part of blood, lymph, and body secretions Aids in digestion Regulates body temperature Transports nutrients and body wastes	Fruit juices Fruits Vegetables	Dehydration	

Index

UNIVERSITY BOOK STORE
RETAIN RECEIPT 92-3

2600277   36.95
SUB TTL   36.95
8.2% SALES TAX 3.03
4464505762003761/03381600
/24/92   6 BANK CARD   TTL   39.98

CUSTOMER COPY
PLEASE RETAIN THIS COPY FOR
YOUR RECORDS